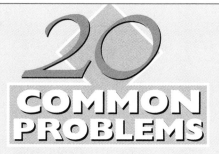

Ethics in Primary Care

Notice

Medicine is an ever-changing science. As new research and clinical experience broaden our knowledge, changes in treatment and drug therapy are required. The editor and publisher of this work have checked with sources believed to be reliable in their efforts to provide information that is complete and generally in accord with the standards accepted at the time of publication. However, in view of the possibility of human error or changes in medical sciences, neither the editor nor the publisher nor any other party who has been involved in the preparation or publication of this work warrants that the information contained herein is in every respect accurate or complete, and they are not responsible for any errors or omissions or for the results obtained from use of such information. Readers are encouraged to confirm the information contained herein with other sources. For example and in particular, readers are advised to check the product information sheet included in the package of each drug they plan to administer to be certain that the information contained in this book is accurate and that changes have not been made in the recommended dose or in the contraindications for administration. This recommendation is of particular importance in connection with new or infrequently used drugs.

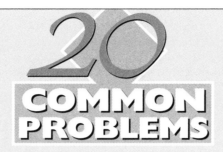

Ethics in Primary Care

JEREMY SUGARMAN, M.D., M.P.H., M.A.

Director, Center for the Study of Medical Ethics and Humanities
Associate Professor of Medicine and Philosophy Duke University
Durham, North Carolina

Series Editor
BARRY D. WEISS, M.D.
Professor of Clinical Family and Community Medicine
University of Arizona College of Medicine
Tucson, Arizona

McGraw-Hill
Health Professions Division

New York   St. Louis   San Francisco   Auckland   Bogotá   Caracas   Lisbon   London   Madrid
Mexico City   Milan   Montreal   New Delhi   San Juan   Singapore   Sydney   Tokyo   Toronto

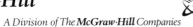

McGraw-Hill

A Division of The McGraw·Hill Companies

20 COMMON PROBLEMS—ETHICS IN PRIMARY CARE

1234567890 DOCDOC 01234567890

ISBN 0-07-063369-X

This book was set in Garamond by Better Graphics.
The editors were Susan Noujaim and Barbara Holton.
The production supervisor was Rick Ruzycka.
The index was prepared by Jerry Ralya.
Cover photos by John Moses.
R.R. Donnelley and Sons, Inc., was the printer and binder.

This book was printed on acid-free paper.

Library of Congress Cataloging-in-Publication Data is on file for this title at the Library of Congress.

I dedicate this book to my parents, Barbara
and Daniel Sugarman, who have in many ways made it
possible for me to pursue interesting projects.

Contributors

Robert M. Arnold, M.D.
Associate Professor of Medicine
Director, Section of Palliative Care and Medical Ethics
Montefiore University Hospital
Pittsburgh, PA

Paul Bascom, M.D.
Assistant Professor of Medicine
Director, Comfort Care Team
Division of General Internal Medicine
Oregon Health Sciences University
Portland, WA

Clarence H. Braddock III, M.D., M.P.H.
Assistant Professor, Medicine and Medical History
   and Ethics
University of Washington
Center for Education and Development
VA Puget Sound Health Care System
Seattle, WA

Allan S. Brett, M.D.
Professor of Medicine
Center for Bioethics and Department of Medicine
University of South Carolina School of Medicine
Columbia, SC

Howard Brody, M.D., Ph.D.
Professor of Family Practice
Director, Center for Ethics and Humanities
   in the Life Science
Michigan State University
East Lansing, MI

Jeffrey H. Burack, M.D., M.P.P., B.Phil.
Assistant Adjunct Professor of Bioethics
   and Medical Humanities
University of California, Berkeley
Assistant Clinical Professor of Medicine
University of California, San Francisco
East Bay AIDS Center
Berkeley, CA

David Casarett, M.D., M.A.
Instructor of Medicine
Division of Geriatric Medicine, Department of Medicine
Institute on Aging
Center for Bioethics
University of Pennsylvania
Philadelphia, PA

Tania Chao, B.S.
Program in Bioethics
College of Medicine
State University of New York Health Science Center
   at Syracuse
Syracuse, NY

Julia E. Connelly, M.D., F.A.C.P.
Professor of Medicine
Co-Director, Program of the Humanities in Medicine
University of Virginia School of Medicine
Charlottesville, VA

Tanya I. Edwards, M.D.
Assistant Professor of Family Medicine
Case Western Reserve University
University Hospitals of Cleveland
Cleveland, OH

Linda L. Emanuel, M.D., Ph.D.
Vice President, Ethics Standards Division
American Medical Association
Chicago, IL

Kathy Faber-Langendoen, M.D.
Associate Professor of Medicine
Medical Alumni Endowed Professor of Bioethics
Program in Bioethics
Department of Medicine, Division of Hematology-Oncology
State University of New York Health Science Center
   at Syracuse
Syracuse, NY

Maryanne Fello, R.N., B.S.N., M.Ed.
Assistant Vice President
Forbes Hospice, Cancer Services
Pittsburgh, PA

Susan Dorr Goold, M.D., M.H.S.A., M.A.
Assistant Professor
Division of General Medicine
Department of Internal Medicine
University of Michigan Health System
Ann Arbor, MI

Michael J. Green, M.D., M.S.
Assistant Professor, Departments of Humanities
   and Medicine
Penn State College of Medicine
Milton S. Hershey Medical Center
Hershey, PA

Amir Halevy, M.D.
Associate Professor of Medicine and Medical Ethics
Department of Medicine
Baylor College of Medicine
Houston, TX

Jay A. Jacobson, M.D.
Professor of Internal Medicine
Chief, Division of Medical Ethics
Department of Internal Medicine
LDS Hospital and University of Utah School of Medicine
Salt Lake City, UT

Jason H.T. Karlawish, M.D.
Assistant Professor of Medicine
Division of Geriatric Medicine, Department of Medicine
Center for Bioethics
Alzheimer's Disease Center, Institute on Aging
University of Pennsylvania
Philadelphia, PA

Alex J. Krasny, B.A.
Staff Associate
Ethics Standards Division
American Medical Association
Chicago, IL

John Lantos, M.D.
Associate Professor, Department of Pediatrics
Section Head, General Pediatrics
Associate Director, MacLean Center for Clinical Medical
   Ethics
University of Chicago
Chicago, IL

Gregory Luke Larkin, M.D., M.S.P.H.
Director of Research
Mercy Hospital of Pittsburgh
Emergency Medical Association of Pittsburgh
University of Pittsburgh School of Medicine
Pittsburgh, PA

Blaire S. Osgood, B.A.
Senior Staff Associate
Ethics Standards Division
American Medical Association
Chicago, IL

Lainie Friedman Ross, M.D., Ph.D.
Assistant Professor, Department of Pediatrics
Assistant Director, MacLean Center for Clinical
   Medical Ethics
University of Chicago
Chicago, IL

**Jeremy Sugarman, M.D., M.P.H., M.A.,
F.A.C.P.**
Associate Professor of Medicine and Philosophy
Director, Center for the Study of Medical Ethics
   and Humanities
Duke University Medical Center
Durham, NC

Daniel P. Sulmasy, O.F.M., M.D., Ph.D.
Sisters of Charity Chair in Ethics
The John J. Conley Department of Ethics
St. Vincents Hospital and Medical Center
New York, NY

Susan W. Tolle, M.D., F.A.C.P.
Professor of Medicine
Director, Center for Ethics in Health Care
Division of General Internal Medicine
Oregon Health Sciences University
Portland, WA

James A. Tulsky, M.D.
Associate Professor of Medicine
Duke University Medical Center
Director, Program on the Medical Encounter
   and Palliative Care
Durham VA Medical Center
Durham, NC

Contributors ◆

Gregg K. VandeKieft, M.D.
Assistant Professor of Family Practice
Michigan State University
East Lansing, MI

Peter J. Whitehouse, M.D., Ph.D.
Professor of Neurology
University Alzheimer Center
Case Western Reserve University
University Hospitals of Cleveland
Cleveland, OH

Benjamin Wilford, M.D.
Bioethics and Special Populations Research Program
National Human Genome Research Institute
Department of Clinical Bioethics
Warren G. Magnuson Clinical Center
National Institutes of Health
Bethesda, MD

Contents

Part

4

Preventive Ethics   223

Preface

The practice of primary care medicine is intertwined with a variety of ethical issues. Unlike the dramatic cases of ethical conflict, often involving technology, encountered in tertiary care medical centers, the ethical issues in primary care are often more subtle yet nevertheless complex. These issues take many forms. For instance, there are ethical issues related to the multiple allegiances in managed care, the appropriate use of consultation and referral, compliance and adherence to treatments, the use of alternative medicines, situations where there is suspected domestic violence, and pain control. Such issues can produce difficulties or confusion for patients, their friends and families, and their clinicians. Moreover, these issues can become problems in practice, making it difficult to determine the right course of action.

In fact, ethical problems are common in primary care. In a small study involving an outpatient practice, Connelly and DalleMura found that 21 percent of office visits involved ethical problems. Here, "the most common ethical problems for patients were costs of care (11.1%), psychological factors that influence preferences (9.6%), competency and capacity to choose (7.1%), refusal of treatment (6.4%), informed consent (5.7%)."[1] These problems stand in contradistinction to those reported by Lo and Schroeder, who catalogued the issues faced on an inpatient medical service. Paralleling those ethical issues that seem to garner substantial attention in the medical literature, Lo and Schroeder found that the majority of problems encountered in the inpatient setting were related to withholding tests or procedures (30%), informed consent (25%), and truth telling (20%).[2] Reports of physician surveys regarding the ethical issues experienced in primary care settings also suggest that different problems are encoun-

tered there compared to the hospital setting, yet it is difficult to interpret these data because of poor response rates in the studies.[3,4] In addition, data from these studies are over a decade old, which is of special relevance given the marked changes in the structure of practice of primary care that have occurred over this interval.

Although the true prevalence and range of ethical issues in primary care are unclear, these data suggest that the ethical issues in primary care have importantly distinctive features. Perhaps even more importantly, the ways in which they are manifested in practice are not well described. As Brody and Tomlinson have observed, "Because primary care is characterized by many repeated episodes of relatively mundane events instead of a few sharply defined crises requiring instant decisions, the way in which these ethical issues arise and the peculiar flavor they develop in a primary care setting may be more difficult to discern than the way in which ethical issues crop up in the intensive care unit."[5] Yet, descriptions are obviously a necessary first step in analyzing these issues. Consequently, to make *Ethics in Primary Care* relevant to contemporary medical practice, physicians who have done serious work in medical ethics were invited to prepare chapters on issues that seem to be prevalent in the practice of primary care. Their experience in clinical practice provided a means of developing a realistic portrayal of these issues. Some of these physicians also elected to collaborate with others (who are not necessarily physicians) in preparing chapters, thus providing additional and important perspectives.

Nonetheless, primary care medicine is also practiced by a variety of nonphysician clinicians, such as physicians' assistants and nurse practitioners. While it is likely that many of the issues faced by these clinicians will be similar or identical to those faced by primary care physicians, it is possible that differences based on training may emphasize different moral understandings. In addition, some of the theoretical arguments made in the book that are based on the professional obligations of physicians may not apply to all clinicians, since there may be unique considerations for those who endorse different professional traditions, such as nursing. Even so, as practice by teams becomes more customary in primary care than practice by individual clinicians, reliance on the moral systems familiar to single professionals may prove troublesome.

In this book, the term *ethics* is used to describe ways of examining different and perhaps competing moral claims in a given situation. In addition, the term *problems* is used broadly to depict the ethical aspects, issues, or implications inherent to particular types of occurrences in the practice of primary care. Thus, here the term *problems* need not necessarily connote conflicts easily recognized as problematic for those involved.

The main chapters in this book are divided into four parts. In Part 1 are problems in practice that may be inconspicuous. These include inappropriate requests for treatments and tests (e.g., when a patient requests antibiotics for a viral illness) as well as inappropriate requests for medical exemptions and privileges (e.g., a request for a "disabled" license plate for the sake of convenience rather than for a true disability). Other topics in this category include the ethical issues related to alternative medicine, compliance and adherence, preventive medicine, and genetic testing.

In Part 2 are problems related to systems of care. Here, some of the unique ethical issues related to managed care (e.g., the difficulties faced by clinicians who serve as gatekeepers, and gag rules that prohibit clinicians from sharing information with their patients) are described. There are also ethical tensions created by other systems of care including the ethical issues related to

conflicts of interest and obligation, referral and consultation, and home care and hospice.

In Part 3 are problems related to the process of care. These include truth telling, confidentiality, suspected abuse and neglect, the treatment of minors, refusal of treatment, pain control, and treatment at the end of life. Although these types of ethical issues may be more evident than those described in Parts 1 and 2, they require substantial creativity in knowing how best to respond to them as they arise in practice.

In Part 4 are methods of preventive ethics, that is, procedural considerations aiming in part to mitigate the advent of ethical conflicts. These include determining competency and decision-making capacity, obtaining informed consent, and doing advance care planning. A theme running through these chapters is that identification of the appropriate decision maker and giving that decision maker adequate information can help to forestall many ethical problems arising in practice.

Despite this broad array of problems, any specific selection obviously leaves some important topics unexamined. For example, some issues not included here include those associated with home care for nondying patients, access to care, provision of charity care, issues specific to non-physician providers, and discrimination in the clinic. Nonetheless, the approaches taken to related chapters should help readers respond to these unexamined problems as they occur in practice. In addition, the Appendix includes some resources in ethics to which readers might wish to refer.

Although the chapter authors had considerable liberty in their choice of examples, style, and theoretical approach, each chapter begins with representative clinical vignette(s) and then covers four general areas: (1) Scope of the Problem, (2) Background Theory and Context, (3) Toward Resolution, and (4) Closing comments. The vignettes are intended to pose selected issues related to the ethical problems discussed in each chapter. Although these vignettes are realistic, the names used in them are fictitious and are provided merely to facilitate discussion. The Scope of the Problem section generally includes an overview of the problem, definitions of terms, and, when available, data about the prevalence of the issue in primary care practice. The Background Theory and Context sections contain the theoretical arguments used in the chapter. The Toward Resolution section typically gives some practical advice regarding how to respond to common presentations of the ethical problem discussed in the chapter. Although every chapter has each of these sections, they receive variable amounts of attention. This diversity reflects the ethical problem being described, how much attention the problem has received previously, and the authors' priorities in addressing the problem.

Some readers might find it useful to read across chapters as well as within them. That is, to get a glimpse of the variety of ethical problems that arise in primary care, one might turn to the Scope of the Problem in all the chapters rather than working through each chapter independently. In contrast, those interested in theoretical issues might concentrate on the discussions of Background Theory and Context, whereas busy clinicians might opt to skip these on their initial reading. Alternatively, given a problem at hand, it might be worthwhile to read through the entire chapter focusing on that problem.

In reviewing the theoretical sections in this volume, it is helpful to know that different authors employ a variety of methods. This is perhaps not surprising, given that no singular (theoretical or practical) approach is currently endorsed by those with expertise in the field of medical ethics. For instance, some favor the use of principles (such as respect for autonomy, beneficence, nonmaleficence, and justice).[6] Others use a "clinical ethics" approach, invoking a specified set of considerations (indications for medical interventions, preferences of patients, quality of life, and contextual features).[7] Still oth-

ers use approaches that might be termed virtue-based, casuistic, narrative, and pragmatic. Although a comprehensive description of contemporary theoretical approaches to ethics is well beyond the intent of this book, the reference section of each chapter and the Appendix provide some direction for readers interested in pursuing these matters further.

Similarly, although *Ethics in Primary Care* offers descriptions of common ethical issues that arise in primary care as well as approaches toward resolving them, this volume does not attempt to construct a unified ethical theory for primary care. However, such important work might be facilitated by the various contributions in this volume. At minimum, it is apparent that a robust ethical theory of primary care would likely need to accommodate the unique value system intrinsic to primary care[8] as well as the changing notion of what constitutes primary care itself.

Even absent a comprehensive ethical theory of primary care, it is arguably essential for clinicians to be able to recognize and manage the range of ethical issues that arise in clinical practice. *Ethics in Primary Care* is intended to be helpful in performing these tasks.

Acknowledgments

I am grateful to several friends and colleagues who helped make possible *Ethics in Primary Care*. Laurence McCullough, Ph.D., encouraged my initial interest in this project. James Nelson, Ph.D., provided insightful comments on the conceptual approach described above. Paull Giddings gave useful editorial guidance. Suzanne Ellett worked diligently with the many contributors to this volume to produce a single manuscript. Finally, this book would not have been possible without the hard work of each of the contributing authors who accepted the challenge of working on issues that have largely not been explored in this way.

References

1. Connelly JE, DalleMura S: Ethical problems in the medical office. *JAMA* 260:812–815, 1988.
2. Lo B, Schroeder SA: Frequency of ethical dilemmas in a medical inpatient service. *Arch Intern Med* 141: 1062–1064, 1981.
3. Dayringer R, Paiva REA, Davidson GW: Ethical decision making by family physicians. *J Fam Pract* 17:267–272, 1983.
4. Robillard HM, High DM, Sebastian JG, et al: Ethical issues in primary health care: a survey of practi-tioners' perceptions. *J Commun Health* 14:9–17, 1989.
5. Brody H, Tomlinson T: Ethics in primary care: setting aside common misunderstandings. *Primary Care* 13:225–240, 1986.
6. Beauchamp TL, Childress JF: *Principles of Biomedical Ethics*, 4th ed. New York: Oxford University Press, 1994.
7. Jonsen AR, Siegler M, Winslade WJ: *Clinical Ethics: A Practical Approach to Ethical Decisions in Clinical Medicine*, 4th ed. New York: McGraw-Hill, 1998.
8. Smith HL, Churchill LR: *Professional Ethics and Primary Care Medicine: Beyond Dilemmas and Decorum*. Durham, NC: Duke University Press, 1986.

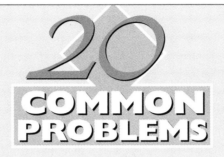

Ethics in Primary Care

Problems in Practice That May Be Inconspicuous

Allan S. Brett

Chapter

1

Inappropriate Requests for Treatments and Tests

John Smith is an otherwise healthy young man who presents with a 24-hour history of nasal congestion, throat irritation, and low-grade fever. Physical examination is normal except for the presence of nasal mucus. The clinician diagnoses a viral upper respiratory tract infection, reassures Mr. Smith that it is unlikely to be anything more serious, and suggests simple nonprescription remedies. Mr. Smith nevertheless insists on a prescription for an antibiotic.

Tom Johnson, 50-years-old, has a 20-year history of intermittent low back pain without radiation to the legs, muscle weakness, or sensory symptoms. Once or twice a year, he has a relapse that resolves after several days of rest and analgesic medication. He is now experiencing a typical relapse and visits his clinician. The physical examination—including a neurologic examination of the lower extremities—is normal. Mr. Johnson reports that he had normal plain x-rays of the lumbosacral spine many years ago. Now he requests magnetic resonance imaging, stating "maybe it's time to see what's really going on down there."

Mike McDougall, a 70 year-old man who recently selected a new clinician because his previous doctor retired, now comes for a general physical examination. He smoked heavily until age 65, then quit. He is currently asymptomatic, and his examination is normal. At the end of the visit, Mr. McDougall requests a chest x-ray to screen for lung cancer, stating, "My previous physician ordered a chest x-ray every year." Mr. McDougall regards this practice as prudent preventive care.

Scope of the Problem

More than ever before, clinicians practicing primary care are likely to encounter patients who request or insist upon specific interventions. In most instances, those requests appear sensible to health care providers and are rooted in generally accepted standards of medical practice. But in some cases, patients' requests lie near or beyond the limits of what many physicians believe they ought to provide.[1] When a clinician resists or refuses a patient's request for a specific intervention, the stakes are frequently higher than simply a moment of uneasiness. At a minimum, exploring and clarifying the disagreement may take considerable time; more importantly, the conflict may plant seeds of mistrust that undermine the relationship between the patient and clinician.

This chapter focuses specifically on patients' requests or demands for *conventional diagnostic tests or therapeutic interventions* that conflict with the clinician's judgment about what is necessary or appropriate in a primary care setting. Analogous tensions or conflicts occur in a variety of other situations discussed elsewhere in this book. For example, patients who use complementary or alternative medicine may seek the approval of their conventional clinicians (see Chap. 3), and the conventional clinician correspondingly may advise such patients about the potential benefits and harms of pursuing alternative remedies. But that clinician is usually not being asked to provide the alternative treatment, unlike the clinician who is being asked to order medications or diagnostic tests. Similarly, patients frequently ask clinicians to "stretch the truth" in completing paperwork for illness-related time off from work, disability evaluations, handicapped license plates, and the like (see Chap. 2); but in these cases, the conflict arises from an administrative role delegated by society to clinicians rather than medical decision making about diagnostic and therapeutic interventions. Finally, patients sometimes request specialist referrals considered unnecessary by the primary care clinician; in particular, this situation becomes ethically problematic in managed care settings, where the primary clinician may be a "gatekeeper" who is under pressure to limit referrals (see Chap. 7). However, that conflict derives from a particular organizational model of providing medical care and not simply from disagreements about the merits of a medical intervention.

It is worth commenting briefly on the language used by clinicians and the medical literature to describe interventions judged as not worthwhile. For example, the language of *futility* is fashionable in the recent bioethics literature, but this term is generally not used for common conflicts in primary care.[2] Rather, it typically connotes an emotionally charged debate about the value of life-sustaining therapies for critically or terminally ill patients or for patients with minimal or absent cognitive capacity (e.g., persistent vegetative state, anencephaly, advanced dementia, etc.). Thus, although we could in principle say that penicillin is a *futile* treatment for the common cold or that screening with chest x-rays is *futile* in attempting to reduce mortality from lung cancer, we rarely use this term in such instances.

More commonly in primary care, clinicians use terms such as *not indicated, contraindicated, inappropriate, unnecessary,* or *useless.* The connotations of these words overlap considerably but not entirely. For example, *not indicated* implies an approach that is outside standards of reference (e.g., published practice guidelines, clinical trials, expert opinion, etc.) supporting the clinician's judgment not to intervene. *Contraindicated* is a similar but stronger term, implying further that the intervention carries a finite and well-recognized risk of harm. A claim that an intervention is *inappropriate* is less likely to connote an explicitly stated profes-

sional standard; rather, common sense or case-specific clinical judgment suggests strongly that the intervention is of little value or potentially harmful. Labeling an intervention as *unnecessary* highlights the idea that, even if there is no plausible risk of harm, clinicians are not obligated to provide interventions with no plausible chance of benefit. The term *useless* has a similar but perhaps more pejorative connotation, implying that the patient requesting the intervention (or the clinician supplying it) is exercising poor judgment.

Although a detailed linguistic analysis of these terms would take us too far afield, the varied language suggests that clinicians use a variety of rationales and standards—implicitly or explicitly—when they consider and then reject requests for specific treatments or tests. Some of these rationales and standards will become apparent in the following pages.

Background Theory and Context

The Patient's Role in Clinical Decision Making

Most would agree that this problem—patients' requests for interventions deemed inappropriate by clinicians—is a relatively recent phenomenon. The idea that patients should participate actively in medical decision making has gained acceptance over the past few decades. Indeed, patient autonomy and self-determination are fundamental driving principles in modern bioethics, providing the moral underpinnings for a strong doctrine of informed consent (see Chap. 19). These principles challenge a previously dominant professional ethic in which the physician's judgment about what is best for the patient was overriding. Although a historical or sociological analysis of this development is beyond the scope of this chapter, two contextual aspects are worth noting briefly.

First, the idea that patients are entitled to direct their own medical care is part of a larger political context in which citizens increasingly assert "rights" to various social goods and protections. Thus, patients have become more like consumers of other goods and services: the patient/consumer makes the request and frequently expects the clinician/provider to comply.

Second, there is an unprecedented explosion of medical and health information available to the public through audiovisual, print, and electronic media. Such information is accessible to much of the population. In addition, the commercial side of medicine results increasingly in the marketing of services and medications directly to the public. The net result is a higher probability that patients will have firm convictions about what they want, even before setting foot in the clinician's office.

There are compelling reasons to take seriously patients' insistence on particular interventions and to come down on the side of satisfying patients' requests for interventions when the best course of action is uncertain. Patients demonstrate a wide range of personal values about their health and a wide range of preferences regarding health care. Most of these values and preferences lie within the scope of reasonable medical practice. Moreover, patients themselves are in the best position to draw upon relevant past medical experiences when new problems arise or new decisions must be made. Insights drawn from those experiences— including the patient's intuition about what interventions might or might not be worthwhile—may be of considerable value in guiding clinicians who are weighing diagnostic and therapeutic options. In a majority of cases, patients' requests for specific interventions can be incorporated comfortably into a model of shared decision making.

But there are limits to what patients can demand of clinicians, even if economic resources were unlimited. We can endorse patient autonomy and self-determination yet recognize that patients should not have access to any and all conceivable medical interventions of their choosing. Rights to goods and services are rarely if ever absolute; rather, they must be balanced against competing interests. In the particular case of medical care, there is no moral basis upon which to compel clinicians to provide goods and services they strongly believe to be useless or harmful. Patients' requests or demands do not carry decisive weight in clinical decision making unless the intervention is capable of producing at least a modicum of benefit, as seen from the perspective of the clinician and the values of the medical profession.[1]

Professional Integrity

The preceding position, enlisting professional values to support the clinician's refusal to yield to certain patient requests, can be described as an argument from professional integrity. The "professional integrity" position begins with the premise that medical practice embodies a set of scientific and humanistic principles, the goals of which are to benefit patients. These principles are expressed in both informal and formal professional standards of clinical practice and in professional role obligations. If clinicians were routinely expected to violate these beneficence-based standards and obligations simply because certain patients asked them to do so, the integrity of the profession would be threatened. Clinicians who repeatedly acted against their better judgment would ultimately become less effective, medical practice would become less predictable, and public confidence would decline. Even further, professional morale would suffer because clinicians would perceive some of these acts as violations of conscience.

The danger of the professional integrity justification is that it can be used to advance professional self-interest at the expense of patients' values. Therefore, it should be invoked only narrowly in circumstances where patients insist on interventions with no plausible medical benefit. Moreover, note that the professional integrity justification is not a simplistic claim that explicit professional standards are available to settle every case in which patients demand an intervention. Rather, the claim is that patients cannot expect clinicians to violate such standards where they exist or to violate personal conscience in cases where explicit standards do not exist. Finally, professional principles and standards are not generated solely from within the medical profession. Certain principles—for example, a professional responsibility to minimize waste and to expend medical resources efficiently—are rooted in the broader society's expectation of professional behavior.

It is important to recognize that the structure and regulation of medical practice in the United States clearly reflect a broad social mandate for clinicians to exercise independent professional judgment and to resist patients' requests for harmful or nonbeneficial interventions. For example, many drugs and most diagnostic tests cannot be obtained without the approval of a clinician; clinicians can be punished (through malpractice litigation) for actions that harm patients, even if requested by the patient; and, more generally, clinicians must meet standards endorsed by government agencies in order to be licensed. These mechanisms would hardly be necessary in a society that endorsed clinicians as passive advisers to patients or as passive suppliers of whatever patients requested. The situation is no different for other professions: lawyers are not expected to violate legal principles at the behest of their clients, teachers would not be expected to distort history in order to appease a parent's request to present revisionist views, and an architect or builder would not be expected to design a potentially unsafe home simply because the prospective homeowner asked for it.

Professional Standards and Practice Guidelines

In the discussion above, we referred to professional standards of practice as one possible source of the clinician's authority. Until recently, those standards were rarely articulated formally; rather, they represented the prevalent style of practice, sometimes described in textbooks or journals and sometimes existing only as an unwritten "common wisdom" among clinicians. Increasingly, however, standards are expressed in the form of so-called *practice guidelines*—formal statements or algorithms directing the clinician to address a specific clinical condition in a particular way. Such guidelines have now been generated for numerous diagnostic, therapeutic, and preventive interventions in medicine.

At first glance, practice guidelines would seem to be an ideal way to resolve disagreements between patients who demand specific interventions and physicians who resist them. That is, such guidelines presumably incorporate the best available research findings and represent the best medical practice and thus might be considered as an unbiased middle ground between arbitrary patient preferences and arbitrary clinician practices.

Unfortunately, the matter is not so simple, for several reasons. First, practice guidelines are still not available for many of the clinical scenarios that give rise to clinical disagreement. Second, there is widespread recognition that guidelines frequently fail to address the clinical nuances of specific cases; caveats or disclaimers, stating that a clinician's judgment may override a guideline, therefore commonly accompany practice guidelines. However, if clinicians are permitted to override guidelines on the basis of case-specific clinical judgment, one might argue that patients should also be permitted to override guidelines on the basis of case-specific personal preferences. Third, a myriad of government agencies, professional organizations, advocacy groups, insurance companies, and managed care organizations now generate practice guidelines. In some cases, those guidelines conflict with each other, reflecting the differing—and sometimes biased or self-interested—agendas of the groups that generated them. And fourth, some practice guidelines are driven by a population perspective or by cost-effectiveness considerations. That is, the guideline may incorporate an implicit judgment that an intervention is not justified because it benefits too few people, is too costly, or both. However, that underlying judgment may not be persuasive to patients in certain clinical circumstances.

For all of these reasons, practice guidelines do not provide an unambiguous solution for many cases in which clinicians believe patients' requests to be inappropriate. Nevertheless, in selected instances, practice guidelines can serve as a legitimate source of external support for the clinician's or patient's position.

Toward Resolution

Let us now return to the three vignettes presented at the beginning of this chapter. The first is a demand for treatment (an antibiotic for a viral respiratory infection), the second is a request for a diagnostic test (magnetic resonance imaging, or MRI, of the back, for a patient with long-standing, nonprogressive back pain), and the third is a request for a preventive intervention (a chest x-ray to screen for lung cancer). In the process of analyzing each of those cases, we will develop a general approach to their resolution.

The case of John Smith, who demands an antibiotic for a viral upper respiratory infection, (URI), is a commonly discussed prototype,[1,3] and with good reason. Primary care clinicians encounter this scenario repeatedly, and there is compelling evidence that clinicians frequently "give in" despite widespread publicity about the harms of inappropriate use of antibiotics.[4,5]

Ironically, therefore, clinicians perpetuate the problem by reinforcing the behavior of patients who insist on antibiotics. In my experience, clinicians offer three main defenses of this practice: (1) it takes too long to explain why antibiotics are ineffective; (2) there is a remote possibility that the patient has a bacterial, and thus presumably an antibiotic-responsive, infection; or (3) the patient will eventually get an antibiotic somewhere, so it might as well be prescribed here.

None of these arguments is defensible. First, spending the necessary time to educate patients is a professional responsibility. The clinician has a duty to attempt to correct the patient's mistaken belief that an antibiotic will hasten his or her recovery. Second, although the probability that this patient would benefit from antibiotics is not quite zero owing to a remote possibility that the diagnosis of viral URI is incorrect, it approaches zero. The probability of harm to the patient (in the form of a several percent probability of drug side effects) exceeds the near zero probability of benefit, and the likelihood of harm to society (by contributing to the development of widespread antibiotic resistance) is considerable. And third, clinicians should not abdicate their moral responsibility to exercise sound professional judgment simply because the patient may subsequently obtain an antibiotic from another practitioner who does not exercise sound judgment.

The viral URI case involving Mr. Smith illustrates that the existing pattern of practice in the community does not always reflect the highest professional standards. In this instance, the common practice of prescribing antibiotics for viral infections violates professional standards about the proper use of antibiotics. The professional standard reflects not only a rational assessment of the benefit-harm ratio for individual patients but also a public health perspective. Clinicians have a moral responsibility to address the growing public health problem of bacterial resistance, which is in part due to excessive use of antibiotics.

Because there are no reasonable arguments to justify a clinician's dispensing of antibiotics in this case, I conclude that the clinician has an obligation to withhold antibiotics. Note that this is a stronger conclusion than saying it is permissible to withhold antibiotics. The clinician should explain to the patient that the probability of harm exceeds the probability of benefit for the patient himself, that professionals are also obligated to act in the interests of public health (all other things being equal), and that the patient should notify the clinician if the clinical course happens to take an unexpected turn.

The second case, of Mr. Johnson, who makes a request for an MRI, is distinguished from the first case in that Mr. Johnson is requesting a diagnostic test rather than a therapeutic intervention. The ultimate goal of diagnostic testing is to reduce uncertainty about the cause of the patient's symptoms and thus improve the probability that the patient and clinician will select the most effective treatment. In considering a test, the clinician should anticipate the range of conceivable results of the test and note whether any of these results would influence the choice of treatment. In circumstances where there is no plausible chance that the outcome of the test will affect the subsequent management of the case, there is no rationale for the test.

There is considerable evidence that abnormalities such as disk bulges and protrusions are common findings on lumbosacral MRI in the general population, including persons with no history of back pain.[6] Thus, even if Mr. Johnson's MRI showed such an abnormality, we could not assume that it was the cause of his back pain, since he has no symptoms or signs consistent with pressure by a disk on a lumbosacral nerve. Because there is no plausible chance that the MRI will explain Mr. Johnson's intermittent back pain—and thus no plausible chance that treatment will change as a result of the test—there is no rationale for the test in this case. The analysis would obviously differ if the patient had unresolving pain, neurologic findings, or other changes in the clinical course; in

those circumstances, surgery might become an option, and the MRI might facilitate therapeutic decision making.

Diagnostic testing raises the additional issue of reassurance. That is, would the provision of reassurance be a sufficient reason to yield to a patient's request for a diagnostic test, even if one could not envision any test result that would change the treatment plan? After all, reassurance can provide psychological benefits for patients. I believe that in occasional cases (e.g., a patient obsessing about cancer as a possible cause of symptoms), reassurance for the patient can justify the performance of an otherwise unnecessary test. However, there is a considerable risk that testing merely to reassure the patient will backfire. For example, on lumbosacral MRI, the chance of an incidental disk "abnormality" with no clinical consequences may be as high as 50 percent.[6] Clinicians should thus warn patients about the possibility of incidental but inconsequential findings before ordering tests for the sole purpose of reassurance.

Finally, this case raises the issue of cost containment. Although a detailed discussion of the ethics of cost containment is beyond the scope of this chapter, I believe that there is still a consensus in the United States that ad hoc "bedside rationing" by individual clinicians is inappropriate unless both clinicians and patients have agreed to abide by rules permitting it. Thus, the decision as to whether or not to order the MRI should turn on the previous analysis about its role in medical decision making. If the MRI will not facilitate clinical decision making in a particular case, then the request for it should not be honored and additional arguments about its costliness are simply irrelevant. By this reasoning, the clinician in our case would also reject the patient's request for plain x-rays of the lumbosacral spine, even though the cost would be considerably lower than that of the MRI.

In summary, the clinician in this case has a strong obligation not to order the MRI. The clinician should explain that "to see what's really going on" is an inadequate rationale for a test if the results will not plausibly contribute to further decision making. On rare occasions, however, ordering a test in such circumstances might be permissible if the patient's need for reassurance is compelling.

The third case, involving Mr. McDougall, like the previous one, concerns a diagnostic test, but here its role is to screen for cancer in an asymptomatic person. Although the benefits of prevention ultimately are realized by individual persons, preventive strategies are usually conceived as applying to populations identified by age, gender, or risk factors (see Chap. 5). Perhaps more than in other areas of medical practice, specific criteria for preventive interventions have been articulated in practice guidelines, discussed earlier in this chapter.

For some types of cancer screening, practice guidelines conflict with each other, creating dilemmas for patients and clinicians.[7] For example, prostate cancer screening with the prostate-specific antigen (PSA) blood test is recommended by the American Cancer Society (an advocacy group) and not recommended by the U.S. Preventive Services Task Force (a government-appointed panel).[8] The American College of Physicians (a professional organization for internal medicine) has a neutral position, neither strongly endorsing nor rejecting the test.[9]

On the other hand, none of these groups recommends screening for lung cancer with chest x-rays, because large clinical trials have shown that, in the aggregate, such screening does not save lives or improve quality of life.[8] Therefore, in this case, the clinician's resistance to the patient's request for a chest x-ray is supported by explicit external standards that appear applicable to the patient.

The trouble with summarily rejecting the patient's request for a chest x-ray is that early detection and resection of a malignant solitary lung nodule undoubtedly does extend a patient's life, albeit on rare occasions. In large trials that found no average survival benefit for lung cancer screening, the occasional cases of extended life were presumably offset by other cases in which lives were shortened by the morbidity and mortality of surgical intervention in a population at high operative risk. However, it is conceivable that Mr. McDougall is at below-average operative risk and that the potential benefits of screening might outweigh the potential harms in his particular case. The problem, of course, is that we have no way to know whether this is true.

I believe that the clinician can reasonably refuse to order the test in this case, but that (unlike the situation in the previous two cases) he or she is not obligated to refuse. The clinician can justify a refusal by invoking a strong external consensus, articulated not only by government and professional organizations but also by lay advocacy groups. On the other hand, the clinician can justify ordering the test by the speculation that the lives of occasional persons might be saved by early detection, despite the negative results of clinical trials. Nevertheless, if the clinician does comply with a request for a screening x-ray, it should be made clear to the patient that a widely accepted standard is being violated. In addition, the clinician should alert the patient about the possibility of a false-positive result (i.e., a chest x-ray abnormality that leads to further invasive tests or major surgery but is ultimately found to be benign). A false-positive result, a common undesirable outcome of a screening chest x-ray, is to be weighed against potential benefits.

Closing Comments

Clinicians have strong obligations to respect the values of patients. In most cases, the preferences of patients for specific tests and treatments are consistent with the beneficence-based goals of medicine. Nevertheless, patients are not entitled to any intervention of their choosing, and clinicians correspondingly are not required to make every requested intervention available.

The integrity of medical practice is based not only on the satisfaction of patients' preferences but also on the rational and consistent application of a body of knowledge to specific cases. A patient may have a mistaken view that a non-beneficial or harmful treatment will be effective or that a diagnostic test will provide useful information; the clinician has no moral obligation to provide treatments or tests in response to mistaken views about their effectiveness or utility. Like patients, clinicians are moral agents whose values are not irrelevant in medical decision making.

There is no simple formula indicating when patients' preferences extend too far beyond the boundaries of reasonable medical practice, and no bright line separating appropriate and inappropriate requests. Thus, in deliberating whether to honor or reject patients' requests for interventions, the clinician must carefully consider the facts and context of each specific case. For this reason, in the cases presented above, I have paid considerable attention to clinical details, professional standards, applicable clinical research, and the logic of medical decision making. These factors, taken together, will frequently converge to justify decisions either to provide or withhold specific interventions. In cases where the relevant factors do not point in one direction or the other, patients' preferences should generally take precedence.

References

1. Brett AS, McCullough LB: When patients request specific interventions: defining the limits of the physician's obligation. *N Engl J Med* 315:1347–1351, 1986.
2. Truog RD, Brett AS, Frader J: The problem with futility. *N Engl J Med* 326:1560–1564, 1992.
3. Prendergast TJ: Futility and the common cold: how requests for antibiotics can illuminate care at the end of life. *Chest* 107:836–844, 1995.
4. Gonzales R, Steiner JF, Sande MA: Antibiotic prescribing for adults with colds, upper respiratory tract infections, and bronchitis by ambulatory care physicians. *JAMA* 278:901–904, 1997.
5. Nyquist A-C, Gonzales R, Steiner JF, et al: Antibiotic prescribing for children with colds, upper respiratory tract infections, and bronchitis. *JAMA* 279:875–877, 1998.
6. Jensen MC, Brant-Zawadski MN, Obuchowski N, et al: Magnetic resonance imaging of the lumbar spine in people without back pain. *N Engl J Med* 331:69–73, 1994.
7. Brett AS: The mammography and prostate-specific antigen controversies: implications for patient-physician encounters and public policy. *J Gen Intern Med* 10:266–270, 1995.
8. U.S. Preventive Services Task Force: *Guide to Clinical Preventive Services*, 2d ed. Baltimore: Williams & Wilkins, 1996.
9. American College of Physicians: Screening for prostate cancer. *Ann Intern Med* 126:480–484, 1997.

Michael J. Green

Inappropriate Requests for Medical Exemptions and Privileges

Ralph Potter, a 42 year-old businessman who is an occasional golfing partner of Dr. Osborne, comes to the medical office 2 days before he is scheduled to take a long airplane trip. For personal reasons, Mr. Potter wishes to reschedule his flight. He tells Dr. Osborne that the airline will not refund his ticket unless he has a medical excuse from a physician. Although he is not sick, Mr. Potter asks Dr. Osborne to write a note to the airline stating that he has an acute illness and is unable to fly.

Regina Swift is a 53-year-old patient with non-insulin-dependent diabetes. She recently lost her job as a teacher and no longer has health benefits. She tells her primary care clinician that she has run out of glipizide and metformin, both of which are needed to control her blood sugars. She says that without health insurance, she can no longer afford to purchase her medications. Since she was still employed last month, she asks the clinician to back-date a couple of prescriptions so that her previous insurance policy will pay for the medications.

Albert Holt, a 38-year-old construction worker, is new to the area. He presents to a physician's office reporting low back pain. Mr. Holt says he has had this low back pain on and off for many months and it has been evaluated in detail elsewhere. A physical exam is normal and a review of Mr. Holt's medical records does not reveal a reason for the pain. Mr. Holt is applying for disability compensation, and he wants the physician to fill out some forms to help him receive disability benefits. The physician does not believe that Mr. Holt is unable to work and suspects that he is not being completely forthright.

Alicia Kaplan, a 62-year old patient, has bunions on both feet. These have been chronic and stable and are mild in severity. One day, she tells her primary care clinician that a friend of hers with bunions received a "handicapped" sticker from her doctor that allows her to park her car in parking zones set aside for the handicapped. Mrs. Kaplan says it would make her life much easier if she too had such a sticker for her license plate. She asks the clinician to help her obtain one.

Scope of the Problem

In primary care settings, patients frequently ask clinicians to use their medical authority to help them get special exemptions or privileges from third parties. Sometimes these requests are straightforward and reasonable, as when a patient seeks a release from work during an acute episode of pneumonia. Other times, however, clinicians may consider the requests to be inappropriate for a variety of reasons. This chapter addresses the question of how to recognize and deal with these "inappropriate requests," concluding that to deceive others in order to help resolve such issues for patients is unwarranted.

Defining the Problems and Terms

According to the *Oxford English Dictionary*, something is "inappropriate" if it is "unsuitable to the particular case, unfitting, improper."[1] The process of determining whether a particular request is unfitting or improper is not always straightforward, however, in part because there is no consensus about what the goals of medicine ought to be. Although it seems appropriate for medicine to aim to prevent disease and injury, relieve pain and suffering, care for the ill, and avoid premature death,[2] questions arise about other goals. Is it the job of a clinician to make people happy? To ensure "customer satisfaction"? To solve a person's financial problems? To ensure access to medical care? Disagreement about these other goals can lead to significant confusion within the medical profession, as can disagreement about whether and how clinicians ought to act to help patients achieve them.

Some might argue that any time clinicians are asked to use their medical expertise and authority to serve social rather than medical ends, an inappropriate request is being made. For example, in a well-known speech before the Association of American Physicians in 1981, Donald Seldin claimed that medicine is a narrow profession, and problems faced by people "are medical problems and medical illnesses only when they can be approached by the theories and techniques of biomedical science."[3] By extension, the physician's only legitimate role is to make diagnoses and initiate treatments based on their expertise in science and pathology. Becoming involved in social, cultural, or personal issues is outside the physician's role and thereby inappropriate.

A broader view of medicine holds that these types of requests are not necessarily inappropriate, since clinicians would be unable to do their jobs well if the focus of their work were limited to addressing derangements of physiologic function. In the real world, clinicians must also contend with a variety of social, cultural, and political problems that affect patients' health. For example, of what use would it be to diagnose and treat childhood lead poisoning if the child then returns to the environment where lead poisoning is certain to recur? As noted by Perkoff, while conceiving physicians' role narrowly might make their work easier, it does not result in better doctors.[4]

In this chapter, I assume the broader view of medicine. The implication of this view is that the *types* of requests exemplified by the above cases are not necessarily inappropriate. Specifically, a patient may legitimately ask a clinician for a medical excuse to change an airline flight, to help obtain medications, to complete a disability assessment, or to acquire a handicapped parking sticker. The central challenge is to distinguish those particular instances that are appropriate from those that are not and to determine what a clinician should do when confronted with the inappropriate ones.

Kinds of Inappropriate Requests

Requests can be inappropriate in several different ways. First, the request may raise questions about boundaries to the clinician-patient relationship. For example, a patient who asks the clinician for money to buy medications for his wife or to borrow the clinician's car to drive her to the emergency room, may be transgressing some undefined but important social boundary. Second, a request may be inappropriate because it requires the clinician to act outside his or her area of medical expertise, as when an internist is asked to take over the medical care of an infant. Third, as discussed in Chap. 1, a request may be inappropriate when there is disagreement about what constitutes a necessary as opposed to desired medical intervention. An example would be a patient who says she needs to undergo magnetic resonance imaging (MRI) of the head to confirm a clinical diagnosis of a tension headache, or a patient who requests gastric stapling so he can lose 20 pounds. Finally, a request may be inappropriate because it requires a clinician to use deception to meet the patient's goals, as exemplified in the representative vignettes above.

Those requests that challenge boundaries or expertise are not necessarily of moral significance but may be primarily issues of medical etiquette and practice. Requests that raise questions about medical necessity or the need to deceive others may be morally inappropriate, since they are about conflicts of values, preferences, and obligations. Because of the central moral importance of the questions it raises, this chapter focuses exclusively on inappropriate requests that would require clinicians to use deception or misrepresentation of a medical condition in order to pursue a specific end desired by a patient. In particular, it addresses the question of how a clinician should respond to such requests, especially when there may be good reasons to acquiesce.

Prevalence

Little is known about either the frequency of inappropriate requests in primary care or clinicians' responses to them. However, judging from the titles of some recent journal articles, the issue appears to be of substantial concern to clinicians (see for example, "How Patients Stress, Con, and Intimidate Physicians to File Dubious Disability Reports,"[5] "The Detection of Deception,"[6] and "Defrocking the Fraud: the Detection of Malingering."[7])

Several empirical investigations may provide additional insight about how clinicians respond to these issues in medical practice. Novack and colleagues surveyed 407 practicing physicians to determine[8] how willing they would be to use deception. One scenario presented in their survey involved a woman whose insurance would not pay for a mammogram unless a breast mass were present or if there were other objective evidence of the possibility of cancer. Respondents were asked whether they would contend falsely that the mammogram was performed to "rule out cancer" rather than for screening, so

that the procedure would be reimbursed. Of the 199 who responded to this question, almost 70 percent indicated they would mark "rule out cancer" on the form. Of particular interest, Novack found that physicians indicated they were opposed to deception in general, but felt an overriding concern for their patients' welfare and would deceive if necessary to protect that welfare.

A second study was reported in a 1998 *Washington Post* investigative story on lying in medicine.[9] The article cites an informal survey conducted at a leadership conference of the American Medical Association in 1997. Of the 134 physician attendees who returned a questionnaire, more than a quarter said they had fabricated a medical finding to help a patient secure coverage for treatment during the past year, 60 percent said they had changed a diagnosis on the billing records to help someone get insurance coverage, and 70 percent said they had exaggerated the severity of a patient's condition to prevent early discharge from the hospital. A follow-up national study using a more rigorous methodology is currently under way.[10]

Third, Farber and colleagues surveyed 1000 physicians about their attitudes toward reporting patient-initiated insurance fraud to insurance companies.[11] Case vignettes of patients who used a relative's insurance to obtain health care were presented. Of the 307 physicians who responded, 15 percent indicated that *none* of the patients presented in the vignettes should be reported, while only 20 percent indicated that *all* should be reported. Further, the majority indicated that their willingness to report fraud would be influenced by factors such as the patient's wealth, severity of illness, or prior history of fraud.

These studies suggest that clinicians have a high tolerance for using deception in certain circumstances. Below, I will examine why this may be the case and whether such behavior is justifiable.

Background Theory and Context

Although survey findings are helpful for understanding how clinicians say they would act when faced with certain dilemmas, these data do not resolve normative questions about what clinicians *ought* to do in such circumstances. It seems clear that dealing with inappropriate requests in primary care can be awkward, yet it is not clear that awkwardness is a sufficiently good reason to misrepresent a patient's condition. But before dismissing efforts to placate a patient's inappropriate requests, it is useful to look at reasons clinicians might put forth in favor of using deception on behalf of their patients.

Reasons for Using Deception

There are a variety of reasons a clinician may be inclined to do as a patient asks in response to an inappropriate request. First, in these situations, it is often easier to say yes than to say no. Although a purist might declare that a virtuous clinician should simply refuse all requests that would compromise his or her personal integrity, in practice, doing so can have consequences that are difficult to endure. For example, Mr. Potter, the golfing buddy who is denied an airline excuse, may wonder why Dr. Osborne shows so little loyalty to his friends; Ms. Swift, the patient with diabetes, may be outraged that the clinician seems unconcerned with her well-being; Mr. Holt, the construction worker with back pain, may become angry that his doctor has so little compassion for his suffering; and Mrs. Kaplan, the woman with bunions, may change clinicians, telling her friends that her primary care clinician was not a patient advocate. Particularly in a litigious society such as ours,

clinicians want to please their patients, and they may perceive that using deception on their patients' behalf can go a long way toward achieving this short-term goal. The impulse to satisfy patients may be even stronger in settings where clinicians and patients must interact outside the office or where clinician compensation is influenced by patient satisfaction data, all which add to the motivation for clinicians to accommodate patients' requests.

Second, clinicians may believe that some of the policies set forth about work excuses, disability determination, access to medications, or parking sticker distribution are unfair. In the United States, millions of people lack access to affordable insurance to cover the cost of medical care—a situation many clinicians find morally unacceptable. In this context, if a policy is unfair, some clinicians may feel justified in skirting the rules, even if this involves the use of deception. For some, it represents an act of civil disobedience. A similar phenomenon occasionally occurs in criminal trials, when a jury's overriding distrust of the criminal justice system triggers them to acquit a defendant whom they believe committed a crime.

Third, clinicians may justify complying with an inappropriate request on the belief that doing so serves the medical interests of their patients. Perhaps Ms. Swift's short- and long-term health would be improved by having access to diabetic medications, Mr. Holt would have a more satisfying family life if he did not work in construction, and Mrs. Kaplan would have less foot pain if she had access to easier parking spaces. Although all requests are not equally compelling, when the health of a patient is at stake and a small deception may significantly improve a patient's physical and psychological well-being, some clinicians may feel justified (and even duty-bound) to use deception.

Fourth, a clinician may feel that misrepresenting a patient's condition to a third party would contribute to a therapeutic and trusting relationship with the patient. Once again, if the harms are small and the benefits great, using a little deception on behalf of a patient may be perceived as going a long way toward assuring a positive future relationship.

Underlying Ethical Issues

The above justifications are by no means complete arguments in defense of deception, but they do illustrate that clinicians in medical practice have conflicting obligations and divided loyalties. Balancing various competing duties can be difficult and the manner in which clinicians decide to act is often related to how they understand professional roles and responsibilities in relation to individual patients and to society. To further clarify these conflicts, it may be useful to examine some of the assumptions underlying deceptive actions. The fundamental ethical issues can be addressed by responding to three basic questions: Whom do clinicians serve? What are the limits to a doctor's obligations to patients? What other obligations do clinicians have?

WHOM DO CLINICIANS SERVE?

It has become almost reflexive to say that clinicians are duty-bound to serve the interests of patients above all others. Dating back to the times of Hippocrates, clinicians have been admonished not to permit self-interest or the interests of others to interfere with their primary responsibility to serve the patient.[12] The service of patients' interests is one of the core values on which the medical profession is based and is at the heart of this fiduciary relationship.

Although the interests of patients are central to the medical task, it would be wrong to assume that these are the only interests served by clinicians. As Leon Kass has pointed out,[13] there always have been other potential beneficiaries of physicians' services, including the

physicians themselves, insurers, and the public. Some of these are parties to whom physicians have binding obligations. Any attempt by a physician to benefit sick patients may be constrained and shaped by these other obligations.

Furthermore, depending on the particular task at hand, the patient may not even be the *primary* beneficiary of the clinician's service. For example, in the hypothetical case of Mr. Holt, who is applying for disability benefits, or Mrs. Kaplan, who wants a handicap parking sticker, the clinicians who are asked to complete these forms are actually being asked to act on behalf of another party, not the patient.[14] That is, in completing such forms, clinicians are investigators and recorders for third parties—roles that are often inadequately understood and that can involve divided loyalties and role conflicts for the clinician.[15]

When the interests of the patient and the third parties are congruent (for example, if a bus driver with an uncontrolled seizure disorder requests permission to avoid driving), there is no conflict between serving the interests of the patient and the third party. However, when the interests of the patient are at odds with those of third parties, conflict is inevitable. In the case of Mrs. Kaplan, while she may benefit from having a handicapped parking sticker, it would not be in the interests of society to provide such a sticker to someone who does not meet the criteria for obtaining one. If these stickers were distributed without regard to actual need, then people with legitimate claims to limited parking spaces might be denied access to parking, and this would be unfair. The clinician must decide, in such cases, which is more important—to make a patient's life easier by helping her obtain a parking sticker for which she does not qualify or to pursue a just allocation of stickers, which would involve making decisions about which patients do and do not deserve them.

The main point here is that patients and clinicians both need to understand that the clinician's obligations are affected by the role he or she assumes at given times. When a patient seeks the advice of a clinician for diagnostic or therapeutic purposes, the patient may presume that the clinician's recommendations and actions are based primarily on a judgment of what is best for the patient. On the other hand, such a presumption may be erroneous when a patient asks a clinician to complete a work-release or parking permit form. For, in this role, the clinician is acting as an agent of the work place or society and not necessarily as an advocate of the patient's best interests.

WHAT ARE THE LIMITS TO A DOCTOR'S OBLIGATIONS TO PATIENTS?

Although doctors may have obligations to third parties that are in conflict with their obligations to patients, some would argue that these other concerns should always be subordinate to the patient's interests. Pellegrino and Thomasma describe this view:

> The patient ordinarily assumes that the physician is his agent and will take all measures which may benefit the patient. The physician is expected to do everything possible for the good of the patient. . . . But the essential matter is the patient's expectation that the physician, and the hospital, will act in his behalf. This is, in fact, the moral center of medicine, the moment of clinical truth, that which makes medicine what it is. It is the point of convergence of the sciences and the arts of medicine. It is expressed in a decision to take this rather than that action for the good of *this* patient.[16]

This perspective is also reflected in the *American College of Physicians Ethics Manual*:

> The physician's primary commitment must always be to the patient's welfare and best interests, whether the physician is preventing or treating illness or helping patients to cope with illness, disability, and death. . . .The interests of the patient should always be promoted regardless of financial arrangements; the health care setting; and patient characteristics, such as decision-making capacity or social status.[17]

In asserting that a patient's health interests come first, several questions arise about the limits of a clinician's advocacy duties. For instance, should clinicians be bound to provide only what patients need medically (e.g., surgery for appendicitis) or also what they want or desire for other reasons (e.g., airline excuses, handicapped parking stickers, liposuction, tattoos, etc.)? If a patient will receive only marginal medical benefit from a procedure that is expensive, dangerous, or difficult to come by, is a clinician obliged to offer it as an option? If the clinician and patient disagree about what constitutes a medical need, who should decide? If it is a patient's desire that the clinician use deception to further nonmedical interests, should the clinician do so? These questions are not simple, and some are addressed in other chapters (see Chaps. 1 and 11). In analyzing these issues, it is reasonable to assume that a physician's obligation to any individual patient has limits. Determining where those limits lie, however, is subject to debate.

WHAT OTHER OBLIGATIONS DO CLINICIANS HAVE?

While a commitment to a patient's health is an important consideration, it is not the only one. Sometimes, other concerns take precedence over an individual patient's health—for instance, mandatory reporting of certain infectious diseases emphasizes the welfare of the public over that of individuals (see Chaps. 4 and 12). Furthermore, clinicians, like other moral agents, have fundamental obligations (sometimes known as *prima facie* duties) to be honest, to keep promises, and to be fair. To justify skirting these duties requires morally compelling arguments. For example, all would likely agree that a clinician should not be untruthful or break a promise when no conceivable benefit would occur and the damage to others would be significant. Further, most would agree that clinicians ought not deceive or break promises to serve their own self-interests. However, there may not be consensus about what clinicians ought to do in the event that they are asked by a patient to commit a small deception or breach of promise that would greatly benefit the patient without causing immediate harm to innocent third parties. Fundamentally, the issue comes down to this: Under what circumstances (if any) is a clinician justified in stretching the truth, bending the rules, or otherwise using his or her influence to help a patient?

Returning to the vignettes at the beginning of this chapter, each involves a patient who asks the clinician to engage in a deception, but for slightly different reasons. Mr. Potter wishes to benefit financially; Ms. Swift wants to avoid a serious medical complication; Mr. Holt desires an exemption from work responsibilities; and Mrs. Kaplan wants to make her life more convenient. The ethical issues raised by each are somewhat different, but only in Ms. Swift's case can a morally compelling argument be made that a clinician's obligation to the patient's health may outweigh the duty to be truthful.

Gaming the System

Morreim uses the expression *gaming the system* to address this issue.[18] She argues that despite myriad incentives to game the system in order to help patients, there are at least seven reasons clinicians ought to avoid the temptation to misrepresent the truth in their dealings with third parties:

1. It can harm the doctor-patient relationship. Lying, even when well intended, can lead to an erosion of trust between the clinician and patient, since lying inevitably undermines a person's credibility. Patients who observe that a clinician is willing to lie *for* them may legitimately wonder whether, under different circumstances, the clinician might be equally willing to lie *to* them.

2. It can harm the patients it intends to help. Even when the goal of "gaming" is to help a patient, doing so can paradoxically harm

those it intends to help. For instance, if a clinician were to exaggerate the extent of Mrs. Kaplan's debility in order to qualify her for a handicapped parking sticker, this would be documented in the medical record. If Mrs. Kaplan were to apply for health, life, or disability insurance in the future, the exaggeration could jeopardize her insurability.

3. It can harm other patients. In any system where resources are finite, unfairly benefiting one individual can harm another. For instance, if a patient is admitted to the intensive care unit as a result of deceptively substituting a diagnosis of "unstable angina" for its stable counterpart, a needier patient might be denied admission to intensive care at a crucial moment. Other patients might also be harmed if patterns of deception were discovered. For example, if airline executives come to believe that clinicians generally lie about medical illnesses so that passengers can alter their travel arrangements without cost, then the airlines could decide that clinicians should not be trusted to play a role in these matters, and some patients with legitimate medical excuses would not be able to reschedule their flights without penalties.

4. It can harm clinicians. When an individual clinician is untruthful, this can have a harmful effect on the entire medical profession. The trust that has been given to all clinicians would be undermined if the public were to view clinicians as deceptive or dishonest. This could play out in a number of ways. For example, if a clinician were to be involved in a legal proceeding, his or her credibility in the eyes of a jury would be severely eroded if it were thought that clinicians tend to misrepresent medical information.

These four arguments against the use of deception are based on utilitarian reasoning—such deceptions are considered ethically troubling because the overall harms of the action outweigh the benefits. But arguments that depend on the outcomes are not the only way to view such issues; there are other reasons to object to the use of deception that have nothing to do with undesirable consequences.

5. It offends veracity. Theologians such as St. Augustine and philosophers such as Immanuel Kant have argued that being untruthful, whether by overt lying or subtle deception, is always wrong. While St. Augustine objected to lying on the ground that God forbids lies and therefore liars endanger the liars' souls, Kant's objections are secular. He contends that truthfulness is a formal duty of all individuals, which must be upheld under all circumstances, because lying offends human dignity.[19] According to this reasoning, gaming is morally problematic even if motivated by good intentions, since it relies on duplicity and misrepresentation. Although clinicians may reject such absolute prohibitions against lying, there is a basic presumption that lying is generally unethical, whether or not it is motivated by good intentions.

6. It offends contractual justice. In addition to the moral obligation to be truthful, clinicians also have contractual obligations to various third parties (such as insurers, employers, and government agencies) that would be broken by making intentionally inaccurate statements. Even when the agreements are implied rather than overt, breaches of contract are problematic because they represent broken promises, and promises should be kept unless there are very compelling moral reasons to do otherwise.

7. It offends distributive justice. A final argument against misrepresenting a patient's condition is that the practice is unjust. If medical and other social resources are to be distributed fairly throughout society, we must have a system in which all members cooperate. If some members cooperate while others do not, then those who cheat the system gain unfair advantage by freeloading off those who adhere to the rules. Doing so undermines a system that is designed to be fair to all participants. Of course all systems are not fair. But gaming an unfair system is neither the only nor most ethical way to correct a perceived injustice. Alternatively, dissent in form of political activism, letters to medical journals, and speeches before learned societies would promote change and be open to public scrutiny without giving an unfair advantage to particular patients.

In summary, when approached with an inappropriate request, a clinician is faced with numerous competing obligations and responsibilities. These include the desire to please patients; a concern about unfair policies and rules, obligations to serve patients' best medical interests, the need to establish trusting relationships with patients, responsibilities to third parties, the duty not to engage in lying, and the responsibility not to harm patients. Data suggest that physicians are willing to use deception when they perceive that the overall benefits to patients outweigh the harms. On the other hand, some medical ethicists have argued that the long-term harms of deception outweigh any short-term benefits and that, regardless of the consequences, clinicians have a fundamental moral responsibility to be truthful, to keep promises, and to be fair.

Toward Resolution

Diagnosing an Inappropriate Request

As a practical matter, how is a clinician to proceed when confronted with what may be an inappropriate request? In general, the first step toward resolving an ethical problem is to recognize that one exists. As Lo showed a number of years ago, physicians underidentify ethical problems, and physicians who do not look are not likely to find them.[20] One simple way to identify an ethical problem is to pay attention to one's moral intuitions or to use what may be called the "sniff test." When a request "smells funny," elicits uneasiness, or just seems wrong, the clinician should take notice and think more carefully about the situation. Moral intuition has long been recognized as an important way to recognize ethical issues.[21] As articulated by Laurence Tribe,

> Wisdom often outpaces our ability to capture its essence in verbal formulas, and those who automatically dismiss deeply felt misgivings as insubstantial or as irrationally sentimental whenever we have not [yet] been able to capture those misgivings in a rigorous argument underestimate the profundity of human intuition—and overestimate the power of cold logic.[22]

A second way to identify an inappropriate request is to use the "village green" standard.* Whenever clinicians are considering complying with a questionable request, they should be willing to stand on the village green and do so publicly. If a clinician is not comfortable with openly sharing his or her behavior with colleagues or with openly explaining his or her reasoning to the administrative organization that is being gamed, chances are that either the request or the anticipated response to it is not appropriate.

A third way to identify and understand an inappropriate request is to reflect on which particular aspect of the request seems to be problematic. What specifically is being requested, and to what extent does the request require the clinician to violate a prima facie obligation such as honesty, promise keeping, or fairness? To

help clarify what is being asked, the clinician can integrate a series of questions into the medical interview:

- What is the nature of the problem you are having?
- What is your objective in having me do the requested action?
- If I do what you ask of me, would this be honest?
- Are there other ways to meet your goals that do not require me to be untruthful?

Asking patients to respond to such open-ended questions can not only provide valuable insight into how patients think, but will also transfer some of the burden of truth telling from the clinician back to the patient by requiring reflection about how the request may affect others. Some patients, upon realizing that they are asking someone else to be untruthful on their behalf, may withdraw or modify their requests.

After obtaining information from the patient, it may be helpful for the clinician to gather supplementary information. For example, the physical exam may help to determine whether the request is consistent with actual physical findings. In this regard, excellent guidelines for disability or impairment evaluations are available.[23–25] If the request does not seem to correlate with physical findings, the clinician should think about what makes the request inappropriate. Are boundaries between the clinician and patient being transgressed? Is the clinician being asked to assume a professional role that is outside his or her expertise? Is there a disagreement about what constitutes a needed intervention? Is the clinician being asked to misrepresent a patient's condition? Clarifying the nature of the problem can help with its resolution.

Responding to an Inappropriate Request

After clarifying the nature of the request and gathering relevant medical information, the clini-

---

* I am grateful to Norman Fost for his insight into this matter.

cian can proceed in a variety of ways. The following suggestions (modified from Lo)[26] may be helpful:

1. Document findings. Clinicians should document findings accurately, since lying in the medical record is not only unethical, but also prohibited by law and subject to legal penalty. Some have suggested that documenting the "literal truth" could help resolve the dilemma. For example, if it is not intended to mislead, stating that "Mrs. Kaplan reports that she has pain in her feet that makes it difficult for her to walk distances," might allow the physician to address Mrs. Kaplan's concerns while avoiding false statements. While such an approach may appear to resolve an ethical dilemma, this type of reporting has been criticized because no medical expertise is needed for a clinician to simply repeat what a patient says, and because it skirts, rather than addresses, the underlying problem.[15]

2. Determine alternatives to deception. Since it is important for clinicians to address their patients' concerns without using deception, doctors should attempt to find creative alternatives to misrepresenting a medical condition. For instance, a patient like Ms. Swift, who cannot afford to purchase her diabetes medications, can be given free samples. The clinician can appeal to the pharmaceutical manufacturer for free medications or help Ms. Swift apply for public assistance. Likewise, a patient like Mr. Holt can be referred to physical therapy to help him learn how to strengthen his back to prevent future injuries. While these alternatives may require additional time and effort from the clinician, they help achieve the goal of benefiting the patient while avoiding the pitfalls of deception. Of course, this also raises questions about the limits of a clinician's obligations to help a patient obtain expensive medications or prevent illness, a topic that is beyond the scope of this chapter.

3. Involve the patient. Clinicians need not bear the sole burden for resolving the ethical problems raised by inappropriate requests. Clinicians can tell patients of their desire to help while being firm about the obligation to be truthful. Clinicians should inform patients about potential role conflicts and the competing obligations this presents. Together, physicians and patients can explore alternative solutions that may help accomplish the patients' goals.

Primary care clinicians should be able to handle most inappropriate requests without outside assistance. But in difficult cases involving complex work-impairment problems, specialists in occupational and environmental medicine may be helpful. If there are questions about legal issues, a physician should consult with the appropriate legal counsel. If the physician remains uncertain about how to proceed, he or she may wish to ask a trusted colleague for advice. While this by no means guarantees a resolution to the problem, it might help. If still confused about what to do, one could consider seeking an ethics consultation or searching the relevant literature.

Closing Comments

Inappropriate requests for the use of his or her authority to obtain medical exemptions and privileges raise difficult ethical issues for the primary care clinician. While complying with such requests may offer the path of least resistance, doing so is problematic when it requires the clinician to deceive, misrepresent, or alter the truth. Clinicians have a *prima facie* responsibility to be truthful; to act otherwise requires strong moral justification. Saving a patient money, making his or her life more convenient, or helping to avoid an unpleasant task are not particularly compelling reasons to deceive, and the use of deception in these circumstances is inappropriate. On the other hand, many clinicians believe that the clinician's commitment to his or her patients' health is of such primary importance that, when this is at stake, it could justify acts of minor deception. There is no consensus about the use of deception in these circumstances. An alternative response is to openly oppose unfair policies that jeopardize a patient's health. This may incur some risk to the clinician, but it avoids the use of deception and subjects the policy (and the clinician's actions) to the scrutiny of peers.

Acknowledgments

The author is grateful for the comments of Drs. Bob Arnold, David Barnard, Norman Fost, John LaPuma, and Luanne Thorndyke, whose wisdom has helped make this a more compelling chapter.

References

1. Simpson JA, Weiner ESC: *The Oxford English Dictionary*, 2d ed. Oxford, England, Clarendon Press, 1989.
2. The goals of medicine: setting new priorities. *Hastings Cent Rep* 26:S1–S27, 1996.
3. Seldin DW: Presidential address: the boundaries of medicine. *Trans Assoc Am Physicians* 94: 75–84, 1981.
4. Perkoff GT: The boundaries of medicine. *J Chronic Dis* 38:271–278, 1985.
5. Brooks TR: How patients stress, con, and intimidate physicians to file dubious disability reports. *J Natl Med Assoc* 88:300–304, 1996.
6. Faust D: The detection of deception. *Neurol Clin* 13:255–265, 1995.
7. Resnick PJ: Defrocking the fraud: the detection of malingering. *Isr J Psychiatry Rel Sci* 30:93–101, 1993.
8. Novack DH, Detering BJ, Arnold R, et al: Physicians' attitudes toward using deception to resolve difficult ethical problems. *JAMA* 261:2980–2985, 1989.
9. Hilzenrath DS: Healing vs. honesty? For doctors, managed care's cost controls pose moral dilemma. *Washington Post* H:1,H:6–H:7, March 15, 1998.
10. Wynia M: Personal communication, October 14, 1998.
11. Farber NJ, Berger MS, Davis EB, et al: Confidentiality and health insurance fraud. *Arch Intern Med* 157:501–504, 1997.
12. Relman AS: What market values are doing to medicine. *Atlantic Monthly* 99–106, March 1992.
13. Kass LR: Ethical dilemmas in the care of the ill. *JAMA* 244:1811–1816, 1980.
14. Toon PD: Ethical aspects of medical certification by general practitioners. *Br J Gen Pract* 42: 486–488, 1992.
15. Holleman WL, Holleman MC: School and work release evaluations. *JAMA* 260:3629–3634, 1988.
16. Pellegrino ED, Thomasma DC: *A Philosophical Basis of Medical Practice: Toward a Philosophy and Ethic of the Healing Professions.* New York, Oxford University Press, 1981.
17. American College of Physicians: American College of Physicians Ethics Manual, fourth edition. *Ann Intern Med* 128:576–594, 1998.
18. Morreim EH: Gaming the system: dodging the rules, ruling the dodgers. *Arch Intern Med* 151:443–447, 1991.
19. Bok S: *Lying: Moral Choice in Public and Private Life.* New York, Vintage Books, 1978.

20. Lo B, Schroeder SA: Frequency of ethical dilemmas in a medical inpatient service. *Arch Intern Med* 141:1062–1064, 1981.

21. Ross WD: The knowledge of what is right, in *Foundations of Ethics*. London, Oxford University Press, 1939, pp 168–191.

22. Tribe L: On not banning cloning for the wrong reasons, in Nussbaum MC, Sunstein CR (eds): *Clones and Clones: Facts and Fantasies about Human Cloning*. New York, Norton, 1998, p 226.

23. Harber P: Impairment and disability, in Rosenstock L, Cullen MR (eds): *Textbook of Clinical Occupational and Environmental Medicine*. Philadelphia, Saunders, 1994, pp 92–103.

24. Mazanec DJ: The injured worker: assessing "return-to-work" status. *Cleve Clin J Med* 63: 166–171, 1996.

25. Velozo CA: Work evaluations: critique of the state of the art of functional assessment of work. *Am J Occ Ther* 47:203–209, 1993.

26. Lo B: *Resolving Ethical Dilemmas: A Guide for Clinicians*. Baltimore, Williams & Wilkins, 1995.

Peter J. Whitehouse
Tanya I. Edwards

Chapter

3

Complementary and Alternative Medicine

Jennifer Reynolds, age 37, has a 10 year history of rheumatoid arthritis. Initially her pain and swelling were controlled with over-counter anti-inflammatory agents, but over the last 3 years she has had to rely on stronger prescription drugs while battling their side effects. She has been increasingly concerned about the "battle" raging inside her body. Her rheumatologist describes the disease as her immune system attacking her joints while the medicines attack her immune system. This concept has never quite fit her viewpoint, and she has questioned her rheumatologist repeatedly about the reports that she has heard regarding the effectiveness of dietary changes, meditation, and herbs in treating her disease. She is discouraged from seeking "unproven treatments" and asks her primary care clinician for advice.

Bob Finch, age 45, has had fibromyalgia for 5 years. He has recently seen a Chinese herbalist who prescribed a tincture for him to use several times a day. He notes a significant improvement in his symptoms after the second week. His primary care clinician asks him to bring the preparation to the next office visit in order to assess the safety of the product. Mr. Finch brings a small brown vial with Chinese writing on the label.

Scope of the Problem

Interest in complementary and alternative medicine (CAM) has grown considerably over the past decade. A recent study revealed that patients are choosing CAM because the basic principles of these modalities are more congruent with their values and philosophy than is conventional medicine.[1] CAM may also be used because these treatments may offer hope or promise that is not provided by conventional therapy. Despite its growing popularity, however, the use of CAM poses a variety of challenges for primary care clinicians.

Prior to 1993, the best estimate of CAM usage in the American population was consistently around 5 percent.[2] In 1993, David Eisenberg reported that 34 percent of the U.S. population had used one or more forms of CAM in the previous year, spending an estimated $13.7 billion.[2] Visits to CAM practitioners outnumbered visits to all primary care providers that year!

Dr. Eisenberg repeated this survey in 1997, and found that the number of patients using CAM therapies had increased to 42 percent, with an increase in the total visits from 427 million to 629 million—still outnumbering all visits to primary care practitioners.[3] The estimated spending increased to $27 billion.

Despite such widespread use of CAM, patients tend not to disclose, specifically, although an estimated 15 million people took herbs *with* prescription medicine in 1997, seventy-eight percent reported not sharing this information with their physicians. These observations raise some important ethical issues for patients and clinicians. However, in order to work through these issues, it is necessary to first understand relevant terms, some of the forms of CAM, and research efforts directed at testing CAM.

Terms and Definitions

The many terms used to describe CAM suggest different roles for these and conventional modalities. *Alternative medicine* implies that either conventional or nonconventional therapies will be used, but not together. *Complementary medicine* denotes using nonconventional techniques in conjunction with first-line conventional approaches. *Holistic* is a term suggesting that mind, body, and spirit are intertwined and must all be considered in healing and prevention. Although this is a common theme of many "nonconventional" therapies, there are many to which this term would not apply. *Integrative medicine* implies that physicians will employ the *best* methods from a wide rage of healing systems. *Best* implies an evidence-based decision that is also culturally and philosophically congruent with healer and patient.

In his 1993 article, Eisenberg defines CAM as comprising interventions not taught widely in U.S. medical schools or generally available in U.S. hospitals,[2] yet this definition is rapidly becoming outdated. A recent survey of 125 U.S. medical schools (94 percent responding) found that 64 percent offered electives in CAM or included these topics in required courses.[4] This figure represents a doubling of those reported earlier.[5]

The Office of Alternative Medicine of the National Institutes of Health has defined alternative medicine as:

> a broad domain of healing resources that encompasses all health systems, modalities, and practices and their accompanying theories and beliefs, other than those intrinsic to the politically dominant health system of a particular society or culture in a given historical period.[6]

Although somewhat unwieldy, this definition helps us to understand that what is considered CAM in one culture or historical period may be mainstream in another.

Forms of Complementary and Alternative Medicine

The National Center for Complementary and Alternative Medicine (NCCAM) at the National Institutes of Health, considers seven major categories of CAM: (1) mind-body techniques; (2) manual healing; (3) alternative healing systems; (4) diet, nutrition, and lifestyle; (5) bioelectromagnetic applications; (6) pharmacologic and biological treatments; and (7) herbs (see Table 3-1). In order to understand the relevant

ethical issues raised by the use of CAM, it is important to know about the growing body of literature regarding these different modalities. For instance, are there potential herb-drug interactions? Are patients likely to get some benefit from their chosen therapy or are they being "ripped off?" Although it is beyond the scope of this chapter to provide a detailed review of the current literature regarding each of these modalities, we briefly describe some of the underlying premises of some of these approaches to healing.

MIND-BODY TECHNIQUES

The study of psychoneuroimmunology has shown the importance of the interaction between mental and physical phenomena. When either is out of balance, the other is also affected. For example, chronic stress results in the production of stress hormones as well as immune system depression, cardiovascular compromise, and a host of other possible consequences. Mind-body techniques can be used to decrease stress and the levels of stress hormones in the body[7] and can be useful in the treatment of a variety of medical conditions.[8–12]

MANUAL HEALING

The underlying premise of these healing modalities is based on the belief that dysfunction of one part of the body affects the function of other discrete, nonconnected body parts. Some forms of manual healing, including massage and spine manipulation, have been shown to be effective in selected situations.[13,14] Other forms of manual healing have also been evaluated.[15–22]

ALTERNATIVE HEALING SYSTEMS

Traditional healing practices emanate from many cultures. For most of these practices, scientific studies are not available. In these systems, health is typically based on the principles of internal balance and harmony. When harmony and balance break down, there is disease.

Table 3-1
Forms of Complementary and Alternative Medicine

MIND-BODY TECHNIQUES	MANUAL HEALING	ALTERNATIVE HEALING SYSTEMS	DIET, NUTRITION, AND LIFESTYLE	BIOELECTRO-MAGNETIC APPLICATIONS	PHARMACOLOGIC/BIOLOGICAL TREATMENTS	HERBS
Relaxation therapy	Massage therapy	Ayurveda	Macrobiotic diet	Magnet therapy	Chelation therapy	Echinacea
Meditative exercises Yoga Tai chi Qi gong Dance therapy	Spinal manipulation Trager Alexander	Traditional Oriental medicine Native American healing Curanderos	Megavitamins Cultural eating styles Mediterranean Asian	Transcutaneous nerve stimulation (TENS)	Shark cartilage	Garlic Ginger Ginkgo biloba
Music therapy	Feldenkrais	Ispiritismos				St. John's wort
Hypnosis	Biofield therapeutics Therapeutic touch	Traditional African healing				Saw palmetto
Prayer	Healing touch Reiki	Homeopathy Acupuncture				
Support groups						

For instance, Ayurveda is an eastern Indian form of healing with roots in Hindu philosophy. Traditional Oriental medicine consists of acupuncture, moxibustion, herbal medicine, cupping, therapeutic exercises, and dietary advice. Homeopathy is based on the principle of treating "like with like." For example, a substance that causes symptoms of illness in a well person can also be used, in minute doses, to cure similar symptoms when they result from illness. Of note, a meta-analysis of placebo controlled trials found homeopathy to be more efficacious than placebo for treating a variety of medical conditions, including seasonal allergies and postoperative ileus.[23]

DIET, NUTRITION, AND LIFESTYLE

This category includes macrobiotic diet, megavitamins, and "cultural eating styles" (e.g., traditional Asian or Mediterranean diets). While it is clear that Asian and Mediterranean diets are associated with a decrease in some types of cancer and cardiovascular disease, there is currently no evidence of efficacy for macrobiotic diet and megavitamin usage. Moreover, they have been shown to have potential adverse effects.[24,25]

BIOELECTROMAGNETIC APPLICATIONS

Magnet therapy is used for a variety of symptoms with some anecdotal reports being very positive; however, little systematic research is currently available. Transcutaneous electronic nerve stimulation (TENS) has been shown to be effective as an adjunct for the treatment of postoperative pain but is no better than sham stimulation for chronic low back pain.[8]

PHARMACOLOGIC/BIOLOGICAL TREATMENTS

This category includes an assortment of drugs and vaccines not yet adopted by conventional medicine, including chelation therapy and cartilage products. Both of these methods have been very controversial.[26–28]

HERBS

Herbs represent one of the fastest-growing market segments in pharmacies and mass-market retail outlets. A recent study noted that the use of herbs was the CAM modality that increased the most between 1990 and 1997.[3] Approximately 30 percent of American adults reported using herbs in 1996 and having spent over $3 billion on them in that year.[29] Major health insurance companies are beginning to consider including herbs in their formularies. As herbs are used more frequently, increased efforts will be required in evaluating the quality, safety, potential benefits, effectiveness, and appropriate therapeutic use of these entities.

Although herbs exert pharmacological effects in vivo, under the current U.S. regulatory framework they are considered foods, not drugs, and are therefore not regulated as stringently as drugs. Moreover, since herbal products are often not patentable, companies would never be able to recover the large costs of research required for approval by the Food and Drug Administration (FDA). Consequently, the 1994 Dietary Supplement Health and Education Act permits herbs to be sold as dietary supplements provided that therapeutic claims are not specified on their labels.[30] Unlike drugs, in the case of which safety and efficacy must be demonstrated prior to marketing, the FDA must prove that a botanical is *unsafe* before it can be removed from the market. Merely proving it ineffective does not warrant removal.

It is important to recognize that the use of herbal products is associated with issues related to safety, efficacy, side effects, and herb-herb/herb-drug interactions. Table 3-2 lists several common herbs along with the ways in which they are used and some relevant side effects and precautions.

National Research Efforts

The Office of Alternative Medicine at the National Institutes of Health was established in

Table 3-2
Medicinal Herbs[30]

Herb	Use	Side Effects/Precautions
Echinacea	Colds/flu Immune enhancement	Possible liver toxicity with long-term use
Garlic	Lower cholesterol Lowers blood pressure Inhibits platelet aggregation	May prolong bleeding time Not to be taken with warfarin
Ginger	Nausea	May prolong bleeding time Not to be taken with warfarin
Ginkgo biloba	Dementia	May prolong bleeding time Not to be taken with warfarin
St. John's wort	Depression	Not to be taken with other antidepressants
Saw palmetto	Benign prostatic hypertrophy	Not effective in tea form

1992 with an initial budget of $2 million. The office began funding academic "Centers of Excellence" to research various CAM modalities and established a CAM information clearinghouse. This office has enjoyed increased funding over the past 7 years and has recently been upgraded to the National Center for Complementary and Alternative Medicine, with an annual operating budget of $50 million. Within the NCCAM there are currently nearly 20 research centers with various emphases, including addiction, women's health, cancer, AIDS, pediatrics, and pain. Over time, experience garnered in these centers should help elucidate the proper role for CAM.

Background Theory and Context

Ethical Aspects of Complementary and Alternative Medicine

At first glance there may not appear to be any fundamentally new ethical issues raised by CAM that are not already of concern in orthodox Western or allopathic medicine. However, because of the historical and cultural contexts that surround CAM, sensitivity is needed to realize and address these issues. In some settings, as when a primary care provider is caring for a more and more culturally diverse population, these issues may be easier to recognize.[31]

Theoretical Approaches to Ethics

Ethics as a discipline is centuries old, whereas bioethics is a term that was coined only about 25 years ago.[32] The field of ethics focuses on human values and morals and how they are expressed in the rights and responsibilities that we share with others in society. Although there may be some candidates for near universals in ethical systems, such as the "golden rule" (i.e., to treat others as you would wish to be treated by them), ethical beliefs are elaborated in various ways in different cultures. Thus, most attempts to find universal ethical systems have been criticized from both multicultural and postmodern perspectives.[33] Both illness and its care occur in rich social environments and both are therefore affected by general cultural and ethical beliefs as well as by considerations involving health-related values. There have been many calls to engage social science and cultural studies in bioethics. The emergence of ethical issues surrounding CAM intensifies these calls and highlights the inadequacy of many current theoretical approaches to capture the ethical issues associated with CAM. These approaches are, of course, not mutually exclusive, and it is frequently appropriate to use a combination of approaches.

VIRTUE

Virtue ethics focuses on the character of individuals. We know in our own personal and professional lives that there are some individuals whom we believe to be morally wiser than others. Although clinicians and CAM providers can be judged on these personal characteristics, virtue ethics provides little guidance on how to handle difficult situations. Codes of ethics are associated with specific professions (such as the Hippocratic oath in the case of medicine). However the deprofessionalization of medicine and other professions may weaken the influence of such creeds on the ethical behaviors of clinicians.

PRINCIPLE-BASED

Perhaps the dominant form of ethical analysis currently used in the United States and western Europe is a principle-based approach. It examines ethical issues in terms of potentially competing theoretical principles such as autonomy, beneficence, nonmaleficence, and justice. The principle of *autonomy* focuses on the rights (and duties) of individual human beings in society. *Beneficence* addresses the responsibilities that health care providers have to patients. *Nonmaleficence* refers to avoiding harming patients. *Justice* relates to fairness in the distribution of resources—for example, in access to health care. A principle-based analysis of CAM[34] stresses the importance of helping patients achieve their own health-related goals in a culturally sensitive fashion but consistent with the knowledge base supporting the use of CAM.

DISCOURSE

An increasingly visible approach in biomedical ethics is discourse or communicative ethics. One begins an analysis using discourse ethics by identifying the practical issues faced by patients, families, and clinicians in a health care situation. The emphasis is on evaluating the quality of the communication and the power relationships among the parties in attempting to resolve ethical disputes. For example, in the care of patients with dementia, community dialogues have been used to address ethical issues and influence health care policy planning.[33,35]

In international bioethics (of relevance to CAM given its cultural diversity), the concept of a negotiated moral order has been proposed to replace the application of universal fundamental principles.[31] Such experiences with using discourse ethics makes clear that honest, sincere negotiation is key to ethical deliberations, whether they occur at the bedside, in the clinic, or in the community.

PRAGMATICS

Pragmatic bioethics follows the work of John Dewey and William James, which was based on scientific inquiry into naturalistic world settings and problems. It stresses the need to understand the cognitive processes involved in decision making and emphasizes that learning is critical to the maintenance of health. Like discourse ethics, pragmatic bioethics highlights the importance of cross-cultural communication.[36] Thus, discourse and pragmatic ethics may be particularly appropriate for understanding CAM, because interest in it has emerged largely from lay persons and client/patients rather than from conventional clinicians.

Aspects of Complementary and Alternative Medicine Relevant to Ethical Analysis

NATURALISM

Although there are many differences among forms of CAM, some common elements are found in many that likely contribute to its popularity. The first is that CAM is frequently viewed as more "natural" than conventional medicine. The conceptual frameworks of CAM, such as traditions of Oriental medicine, often relate to finding balance in the mind-body and balance between the mind-body and nature. If biological preparations such as herbs are used, they may be identified as being less artificial than drug products created by industry and closer to the natural state of chemical compounds. In con-

trast, conventional scientific medicine is seen as fighting nature to conquer diseases.[37]

INDIVIDUALISM

Many types of CAM emerge from societies in which the culture of individualism is less marked than it is in the West. Although we commonly employ the term *West*, we realize that geography does not determine cultural beliefs. Many Asian cultures, for instance, consider persons more in terms of social relationships than Western cultures do; group welfare is viewed as more important than individual autonomy. Thus, in discussions regarding ethical issues, the social nature of the self and relationships with the person's family and community are emphasized more than in "Western" traditions. For example, in Japan, attitudes toward persons with dementia are colored less by discussions of the individual's competence to make decisions and more by what is best for that person as a member of the family unit.[38]

SELF-CHOICE

CAMs permit more individual choice in health care. People who choose CAM can select which type of alternative approach, what practitioner, and what healing methods they prefer with greater independence than would be possible in most national health care systems. Personal responsibility for self-care is often emphasized in CAM.

SPIRITUAL ISSUES

A final characteristic that differentiates many forms of CAM from allopathic medicine is their attention to spiritual issues in health. Western scientific medicine tends to divorce religious and spiritual beliefs from the healing process—a result, perhaps, of the dominance of the scientific method. Religious and spiritual beliefs vary in different CAMs and may be more or less evident, particularly in forms that have been adapted for Western individuals, such as westernized acupuncture. However, Ayurvedic and Chinese forms of medicine include a rich spiritual belief system that influences concepts of health and attitudes toward it. This can be important, since spiritual beliefs may influence health outcomes.[39]

Toward Resolution

When a patient asks whether to adopt a particular CAM approach, the primary care clinician must address several practical and ethical issues related to knowledge about the proposed approach, the appropriateness of referral to a CAM practitioner, the existence of a conflict of interest, and financial implications of the CAM approach for patients.

Knowledge

In assessing whether the use of CAM is appropriate, the most critical element is the quality of the knowledge possessed by all parties. Clinicians first must ask themselves whether they have the knowledge to advise the patient about a particular CAM approach. For example, in the hypothetical case of Ms. Reynolds, presented at the opening of this chapter, both the rheumatologist and the primary care clinician need to assess their own knowledge. It is perhaps not wise for clinicians to place all CAM approaches into one large category which they discount, and dissuading patients from evaluating them. In the partnership between the patient and the clinician, much can be learned in the process of discussing an interest in CAM. Such knowledge can be helpful even if eventually CAM is not used. Clinicians will differ on how comfortable they are with this particular task. The evidence base for different CAMs varies and the skills of

different CAM practitioners also vary. Therefore, clinicians should have either adequate knowledge about CAM and/or should know where to refer a patient who desires this information.

A general problem with CAM is that the scientific evidence base supporting these approaches is smaller than that for Western allopathic medicine. Indeed, much of the evidence for CAM is based on testimonials. Although many such statements may be impressive, arguments based on the fact that people have claimed benefit from an approach should not be fully convincing to clinicians accustomed to using the results of controlled clinical research. Yet clinical trials, as well as basic science rationales can be found for some CAMs and more large-scale trials are under way. Where evidence exists for the effectiveness of CAM, clinicians must be careful to avoid a double standard—that is, requiring more evidence before using CAM than they would for conventional health care interventions. The current passion for evidence-based medicine emphasizes that perhaps 60 to 80 percent of allopathic medicine is not based on scientific evidence. In addition, we must consider whether it is fair to judge non-conventional approaches purely on the basis of Western scientific analysis. Perhaps a broader range of evidence is acceptable to support CAM. Certainly we should consider the approaches and evaluation procedures used within different forms of CAM.

Finally, there is an absence of comparison studies that allow one to select the best first-line treatment. For example, as in the case of Mr. Finch described at the beginning of the chapter, we have some evidence saying that acupuncture, massage, exercise, and antidepressants may all be helpful for fibromyalgia, but which is the best initial treatment is uncertain.

Referral

In many cases, primary care clinicians will be asked to evaluate a particular CAM practitioner or approach. Because of the diversity of CAMs, such tasks can be quite challenging (see Chap. 9). For example, as in the case of Mr. Finch, presented at the opening of this chapter, it can be difficult for even well-intentioned patients and clinicians to understand the full implications of using particular CAM approaches. Fortunately, accreditation boards now exist for many CAM disciplines. By referring to a practitioner who is licensed by the state or accredited by a professional board, clinicians are at least making some attempt to ensure that their patients will be dealt with in a reasonably competent fashion. There is little legal experience and case law in this area to guide the clinician in terms of possible risks associated with referral to CAM practitioners. Often, asking for written material provided by the CAM practitioner or calling the individual on the phone can provide some basic information about training and approaches. The cost of the CAM services should be made known to the patient.

Conflict of Interest

Part of the assessment of a CAM practitioner must also take into account the issue of conflict of interest (see Chaps. 8 and 9). Many CAM practitioners support themselves by both selling products and employing them in their practice. This is not unique to CAM, as U.S. physicians can own diagnostic equipment; in Japan, physicians actually dispense medications and earn a percentage of their personal revenue doing so. Of relevance, conflict of interest itself is not inherently bad.[40] Life is full of situations where two potentially competing goals coexist—for example, the financial well-being of the practitioner and the well being of their clients. Nevertheless, in assessing the appropriateness of using CAM it would be prudent to ensure that there is no overriding conflicts of interests that would undermine the health of the patient.

Financial Aspects

The financial aspects of CAM also raise certain ethical issues. Prices on similar products vary considerably, largely as a function of marketing rather than a demonstration that one product is more effective than another. Further, it is important to note that although chemical compounds from different sources can be biologically identical, variations may exist in preparations (especially in CAM products), including impurities or other unidentified agents.

Some managed care organizations and insurance plans are beginning to include CAM benefits. However, most consumers pay out of pocket for CAM, posing such choices as whether to pay for prescription medications or CAM.

Closing Comments

In summary, the growing interest in CAM is a phenomenon of considerable importance. This is not so much based on scientific evidence as on the fact that these approaches may be more appealing than conventional medicine for a number of reasons. They support patients' interests in promoting their own self-care and in developing images and ideals of health that are broader than conventional models emphasize. However, it is also true that a considerable amount of money is spent on CAM where the evidence for the effectiveness of such therapies is limited and the opportunities for charlatanism are considerable. Thus it is important for primary care clinicians to be aware not only of CAM but also of the ethical conflicts that the use of such approaches may pose.

References

1. Astin JA: Why patients use alternative medicine: results of a national study. *JAMA* 279:1548–1553, 1998.
2. Eisenberg DM, Kessler RC, Foster C, et al: Unconventional medicine in the United States: prevalence, costs, and patterns of use. *N Engl J Med* 328:246–252, 1993.
3. Eisenberg DM, Davis RB, Ettner SL, et al: Trends in alternative medicine use in the United States, 1990-1997: results of a follow-up national survey. *JAMA* 280:1569– 1575, 1998.
4. Wetzel MS, Eisenberg DM, Kaptchuk TJ: Courses involving complementary and alternative medicine at U.S. medical schools. *JAMA* 28:784–787, 1998.
5. Daly D. Alternative medicine courses taught at US medical schools: An ongoing listing. *J Alt Comp Med.* 2:315–317, 1996.
6. Panel on Definition and Description: CAM Research Methodology Conference, April 1995—defining and describing complementary and alternative medicine. *Alt Ther Health Med* 3:49–57, 1997.
7. Massion AO. Meditation, melatonin and breast/prostate cancer: hypothesis and preliminary data. *Med Hypoth.* 44:39, 1995.
8. Spencer JW, Jacobs, JJ: *Complementary/Alternative Medicine: An Evidence-Based Approach.* St. Louis, Mosby, 1999.
9. Garfinkel MS, Singhal A, Katz WA, et al: Yoga-based intervention for carpal tunnel syndrome: a randomized trial. *JAMA* 280:1601–1603, 1998.
10. Lai JS, Lan C, Wong MK, et al: Two year trends in cardiorespiratory function among older tai chi chuan practitioners and sedentary subjects. *J Am Geriatr Soc* 43:1222–1227, 1995.
11. Jin P: Efficacy of tai chi, brisk walking, meditation, and reading in reducing mental and emotional stress. *J Psychosom Res* 36:361–370, 1992.
12. Wolf SL, Barnhart, HX, Kutner NG, et al: Reducing frailty and falls in older persons: an investigation of tai chi and computerized balance training. *J Am Geriatr Soc* 30:345–351, 1996.
13. Field T: "Touch Therapy Research", in Eisenberg DM (ed): *Alternative Medicine: Implications for Clinical Practice and State of the Science Symposia* (Eisenberg). Cambridge, MA, Harvard Medical School, 1999.
14. Haldeman S: "Chiropractic: Clinical Practice and the State of Science," in Eisenberg DM (ed): *Alternative Medicine: Implications for Clinical Practice and State of the Science Symposia* (Eisenberg). Harvard Medical School. 1999.
15. Witt PL, MacKinnon J: Trager Psychophysical Integration: a method to improve chest mobility of patients with chronic lung disease. *Phys Ther* 66:214–217, 1986.
16. Dennis RJ. Functional reach improvement in normal older women after Alexander technique instruction. *J Gerontol A Biol Sci Med Sci* 54:M8–M11, 1999.
17. Laumer U, Bauer M, Fichter M, Milz H: Therapeutic effects of the Feldenkrais method "awareness through movement" in patients with eating disorders. *Psychother Psychosom Med Psychol* 47:170–180, 1997.
18. Perry J, Jones MH, Thomas L: Functional evaluation of rolfing in cerebral palsy. *Dev Med Child Neurol* 23:717–729, 1981.
19. Weinberg RS, Hunt VV: Effects of structural integration on state-trait anxiety. *J Clin Psychol* 35:319–322, 1979.
20. Rosa L, Rosa E, Sarner L, et al: A closer look at therapeutic touch. *JAMA.* 279:1005–1010, 1998.
21. Olson K, Hanson J: Using Reiki to manage pain: a preliminary report. *Cancer Prev Control* 1:108–113, 1997.
22. Bullock M: Reiki: a complementary therapy for life. *Am J Hosp Palliat Care* 14:31–33,1997.
23. Linde K, Clausius N, Ramirez G, et al: Are the clinical effects of homeopathy placebo effects? A meta-analysis of placebo-controlled trials. *Lancet* 350:834–843, 1997.
24. van Dusseldorp M, Schneede J, Refsum H: Risk of persistent cobalamin deficiency in adolescents fed a macrobiotic diet in early life. *Am J Clin Nutr* 69:664–671, 1996.
25. Dordain G, Deffond D: Pyridoxine neuropathies: review of the literature. *Therapie* 49:333–337, 1994.
26. Chappell LT, Janson M: EDTA chelation therapy in the treatment of vascular disease. *J Cardiovasc Nurs* 10:78–86, 1996.

27. Elihu N, Anandasbapathy S, Frishman WH: Chelation therapy in cardiovascular disease: ethylenediaminetetraacetic acid, deferoxamine, and dexrazoxane. *J Clin Pharmacol* 38:101–105, 1998.

28. Miller DR, Anderson GT, Stark JJ, et al: Phase I/II trial of the safety and efficacy of shark cartilage in the treatment of advanced cancer. *J Clin Oncol* 16:3649–3655, 1998.

29. Johnston BA: One third of nation's adults use herbal remedies. *Herbalgram* 40:49, 1997.

30. Tyler VE: What pharmacists should know about herbal remedies. *J Am Pharm Assoc* NS36:29–37, 1996.

31. Baker R: A theory of international bioethics: multiculturalism, postmodernism, and the bankruptcy of fundamentalism. *Kennedy Inst Ethics J* 8:201–231, 1998.

32. Potter VR, Whitehouse PJ: Deep and global bioethics for a livable third millenium. *Scientist* January 5, 1998, p. 9.

33. Post SG, Ripich DN, Whitehouse PJ: Discourse ethics: research, dementia and communication. *Alzheimer Dis Assoc Disord* 8:58–65, 1994.

34. Sugarman J, Burk L. Physician's ethical obligations regarding alternative medicine. *JAMA* 280:1623–1625, 1998.

35. Post SG, Whitehouse PJ: Fairhill guidelines on ethics of the care of people with Alzheimer's disease: a clinical summary. *J Am Geriatr Soc* 43:1423–1429, 1995.

36. McGee G: *Pragmatic Bioethics.* Nashville,TN, Vanderbilt University Press, 1999.

37. Whitehouse, P: The ecomedical disconnection syndrome. *Hastings Cent Rep* 29:1:41–44, 1999.

38. Deal PE, Whitehouse PJ: Concepts of personhood in Alzheimer's disease: considering Japanese notions of a relational self in Long SO (ed): *Caring for the Elderly in Japan and the United States: Practices and Policies.* In press.

39. Larson D, Swyers J, McCullough M (eds). *Scientific Research on Spirituality and Health: A Consensus Report National Institute for Healthcare Research.* Rockville, MD, The John Templeton Foundation, October 1, 1997.

40. Kodish E, Murray T, Whitehouse PJ: Conflict of interest in university-industry research relationships: realities, politics, and values. *Acad Med* 71:1287–1290, 1996.

Jay A. Jacobson

Compliance and Adherence

James Ford, 54 years old and married, had previously been in good health. Other than some shortness of breath with stair climbing and a morning cough, he had no specific complaints when he had his first visit with his general internist, Dr. Berg. His past medical history and review of systems were unremarkable except that Mr. Ford smoked cigarettes. His father had died in his early sixties of a heart attack. Mr. Ford works as a used-car salesman and does not have health insurance. His physical examination disclosed a blood pressure of 160/100 and abdominal obesity. The rest of his examination was essentially normal.

Dr. Berg recommended a weight-loss program that included diet and exercise as well as smoking cessation. He ordered a complete blood count and lipid studies. At the second visit, a month later, Mr. Ford had no new complaints. His weight and blood pressure were unchanged. He said that he had tried to stop smoking, but he was unsuccessful. However, he was doing more walking each day. Dr. Berg noted that Mr. Ford's lipid profile was abnormal, with significant elevations of total and low-density-lipoprotein cholesterol. He repeated his previous recommendations and prescribed lovastatin for hyperlipidemia and hydrochlorothiazide for hypertension. At his third appointment, Mr. Ford's weight had decreased by 4 lbs and his blood pressure was somewhat improved at 150/90. Dr. Berg ordered repeat lipid studies and prescribed enalapril, for better control of blood pressure.

Just before seeing Mr. Ford for the fourth time, Dr. Berg reviewed his laboratory results from the previous visit and noted that the lipid values were unchanged. He also saw from the nurse's notes that the patient's weight and blood pressure were unchanged as well. He asked Mr. Ford whether he was having any difficulty with his medication. Mr. Ford, who seemed somewhat embarrassed, said that after the second visit he went to the pharmacy to fill his prescriptions, but when he learned how much the lovastatin cost, he decided to get only the hydrochlorothiazide, which he had been taking on most days.

Danny Merchant, 24 years old and single, works as a consultant for a large communications company and has been a patient of Dr. Black's for several years. Mr. Merchant has had some minor musculoskeletal problems and upper respiratory infections. The problem that caused him the most concern, however, was genital herpes. His first episode, 3 years ago, included penile lesions, inguinal adenopathy, fever, and malaise. These symptoms seemed to respond to acyclovir, but they recurred about 2 months later and he came into the office again. Dr. Black diagnosed recurrent genital herpes and prescribed acyclovir twice a day for chronic suppressive therapy. He advised Mr. Merchant to use condoms so as to avoid transmitting his infection. Mr. Merchant reported about two recurrences per year after that, but from his prescription refill calls, Dr. Black realized that his patient was not taking his acyclovir as prescribed.

At today's appointment, Mr. Merchant reports that he has been doing well and announces that he will be getting married in 3 months. Almost immediately, Dr. Black is concerned about Mr. Merchant's fiancé. Has she been told about the herpes infection? What measures are being planned to minimize the risk of transmission? Dr. Black wonders how to ascertain answers to these questions most appropriately.

Scope of the Problem

Noncompliance is common in the practice of medicine. It occurs everywhere. It is costly and it can be dangerous for patients and others. By understanding noncompliance, clinicians can achieve better outcomes for patients and lessen the confusion that sometimes clouds the care of patients who are repeatedly noncompliant.

Defining the Problem

The clinical vignettes above offer examples of patients who are not taking medications as prescribed or who may not be following medical recommendations. This type of behavior has been called *noncompliant.* Such clinical scenarios are commonplace in an office-based practice. In a hospital setting, *noncompliant* is a label often applied in situations such as when a young diabetic patient is repeatedly admitted for diabetic ketoacidosis or when an intravenous drug user is admitted for treatment of repeated bouts of endocarditis.

The term *noncompliant* generally denotes failure to follow an order or instruction or a behavior that does not conform to a policy or law. It does not suggest or even imply that patients with regard to their clinicians—unlike soldiers with regard to their officers or employees with regard to their employers—have no right to choose which instructions or recommendations to follow. To encompass this important element of patient choice and not imply disproportionate clinician power or control over these choices, new terms have come into use to describe how patients behave with respect to prescriptions and medical recommendations. These include *adherence, concordance,* and *cooperation.* Whatever terminology we may choose, the failure to comply with a medically

recommended regimen is a complex problem. It may reflect a rational, valid, or even medically astute choice by the patient. It may not reflect the patient's preferences and may even be out of the patient's control for physiologic, psychological, or economic reasons. It may stem from a misunderstanding about instructions or the clinician's failure to state clearly what is recommended and to use strategies that foster and promote adherence. Nonadherence can and often does result from a combination of these circumstances.

Nonadherence—that is, a patient's failure to follow a medical regimen that he or she has tacitly or explicitly agreed to follow—is important for several reasons: it can have health consequences for patients; it can be confusing for clinicians when undetected and frustrating when recognized; and it can lead clinicians to make unnecessary or inappropriate diagnostic or therapeutic recommendations. At another level, it can adversely affect the clinician's regard for the patient and his or her concern about and interest in the patient's health. Some clinicians, third-party payers, and health care institutions may feel that resources are "wasted" on nonadherent patients.

Nonadherence can also be expensive. If there are adverse medical consequences, the cost of these may be borne by the patient, employers, or third-party payers. Within managed care systems, there may be economic consequences for clinicians whose patients are nonadherent and who thereby require more acute or specialized care to address their medical problems.

Finally, nonadherence can be dangerous to patients and to others, even those the patient would least wish to harm. Patients with communicable diseases who do not follow therapeutic or preventive regimens may endanger their most intimate contacts, as in Mr. Merchant's case, or unknown and unsuspecting individuals, as in the case of a patient with untreated or inadequately treated tuberculosis. It is alarming to note that in a study of outpatients given oral drug therapy for tuberculosis, only 50 percent had positive urine tests for their drugs.[1] In the treatment of tuberculosis, poor adherence with daily therapy and/or failure to complete a full course of therapy increases both the likelihood of treatment failure and the emergence of multiple drug-resistant strains. This has serious consequences for the patient and for exposed contacts who become infected. Nonadherence with regimens that correct or prevent conditions that impair the patient's ability to drive safely not only threatens the patient who may be driving but also his or her passengers, other drivers, and pedestrians. If patients who take sedatives or drugs that produce drowsiness as prescribed, but do not follow the recommendation not to drive while the drugs are acting, they, too, pose a threat to themselves and others.

Prevalence

Nonadherence is a very widespread behavior and is thought to be the most common cause for treatment failure. Investigations have reported rates from 4 to 92 percent.[2] Average adherence with long-term drug regimens is 50 to 65 percent.[3] Not surprisingly, the rates vary depending on the patient population, how nonadherence or noncompliance is defined and measured, and what behavior is recommended or treatment prescribed. The lowest rates of adherence are seen with preventive health care, diet, and appointment keeping.[4]

Medical appointments are not the only ones to which individuals fail to adhere. Nonadherence with appointments is now so prevalent outside of medicine that airlines routinely overbook flights, restaurants often request a phone number to confirm reservations, and hotels usually require a deposit or a guarantee from a customer who reserves a room. These businesses focus on how nonadherence affects them and take steps to protect their interests. Medicine sometimes takes the same focus but must be especially concerned with how nonadherence affects patients.

The vignettes presented at the opening of this chapter include a variety of conditions and recommendations for which adherence has been studied. Mr. Ford has several addressable risk factors for coronary artery disease, lung disease, and lung cancer. Adherence rates with the recommendation to stop smoking or to lose weight are generally quite low. Adherence to a prescribed drug regimen for asymptomatic hypertension ranges between 20 and 80 percent and averages about 50 percent.[5] In Mr. Merchant's case, involving recurrent herpes, two strategies were recommended: antiviral treatment to prevent recurrence and condom use to minimize the risk of transmission. Adherence to antiviral therapy for recurrent herpes may be comparable to adherence to short-term regimens of oral antibiotic therapy, where mean rates were found to be 80, 69, and 38 percent, depending on whether the drugs were to be taken once, twice, or three times per day.[6] Compliance with condom use for preventing herpes or the even more serious HIV infection has not been specifically reported, but it seems unlikely that it would be higher than the compliance rate of 50 to 75 percent with condom use for contraception. Compliance with condom use is simply not as amenable to measurement as is prescription drug use, where measurement of drug levels in body fluids avoids the problems of recall and the pressure to report expected and recommended behaviors.

Background Theory and Context

The Phenomenon of Nonadherence

Nonadherence is hardly a new problem for medicine, but it has certainly been more widely recognized in recent years.[7–10] For much of medicine's history, physicians provided or performed treatments or procedures themselves, often in patients' homes. Whether it was the administration of an herbal remedy, a purgative, or bleeding, the doctor was directly involved. Even when medical care moved to doctors' offices, physicians often dispensed the medicines they prescribed. However, the emergence of apothecaries and then pharmacists made medication use a phenomenon that occurred largely outside the purview of the doctor, making nonadherence more likely and more difficult to recognize.

The development of many new, effective therapies has led to an astounding increase in prescribed drugs. Unfortunately, these agents often require multiple daily doses; many are expensive; and some have unpleasant side effects. Patients are usually expected to obtain them and take them without direct medical supervision. Thus, the opportunities and reasons for nonadherence have grown. The report of an apparent 50 percent nonadherence rate with antituberculosis therapy in 1957 was surprising,[1] but the more than 4000 articles on nonadherence that were listed in the *Index Medicus* by 1988 attest to the frequency, significance, and the persistence of this behavior.[8]

Despite ample evidence that nonadherence is a common problem, many clinicians regard it as a form of deviant or aberrant behavior. They have labeled nonadherent patients as "forgetful" and "careless."[7] Clinicians also seriously underestimate the rate at which nonadherence occurs. In one study, doctors judged that 95 percent of their patients took medications as prescribed all of the time or usually, while only 75 percent of their patients reported doing so.[8–10] Other studies indicate that even patient self-reporting overstates the objectively measured rate of adherence.[9] Not only do doctors overestimate adherence for patients in general but their predictions of individual adherence to a particular drug regimen, digoxin for example, are no better than chance.[8]

Social scientists and clinicians who have systematically investigated nonadherence tend to construe it as a behavior with different causes and explanations. Several categories, by themselves or in combination, explain nonadherence. These include misunderstanding, inability to comply, refusal to comply, and not understanding why a drug is prescribed.[4]

In seeking associations or risk factors for nonadherence as opposed to explanations for it, systematic investigations have refuted several presumptions. Poor and poorly educated patients, for example, are no more or less adherent than wealthier or better-educated patients. Studies of other patient characteristics, such as age and gender and physician sociodemographic characteristics, have found that these also tend to be weak and inconsistent predictors of adherence.[9]

Theoretical Considerations

In distinction to these findings, based on the social sciences, some argue that patients have a moral obligation to comply with prescribed instructions. This obligation is derived from the doctor-patient relationship in terms such as the following: "When the doctor performs a service, the patient is obligated to reciprocate . . . by complying with the medical recommendations once he leaves the doctor's office." In an article quoting that view, the author disagrees, arguing that "the doctor was almost certainly giving his services for money, so the patient's only obligation was to pay or be insured."[8]

From a consequentialist or utilitarian perspective, it might at first appear that nonadherence leads to bad results and is therefore wrong. That is, adherence would be expected to lead to more "good" than nonadherence. However, many factors require examination of that conclusion. First, even if a patient makes an authentic, informed choice to be nonadherent, it is not necessarily the case that the choice reduces the "good" that could be achieved by way of adherence. Missing an occasional dose of an antihypertensive drug or even all the doses of an antibiotic that was inappropriately prescribed for a viral upper respiratory infection may not result in harm. It is also possible that, in the case of a nonindicated or marginally effective agent, partial or complete nonadherence may have more positive consequences than adherence would with respect to costs saved and adverse reactions avoided. Patients who are nonadherent may choose to be so because they consider it better to experience the untreated or partially treated state than the fully treated state, even though they acknowledge some benefit of treatment. Examples include patients who prefer to be in some pain, but fully alert and without nausea, to having a painful condition fully treated with a narcotic that produces these side effects. A smoker with metastatic lung cancer might choose to continue smoking because he values the short-term pleasure it affords and concludes that it will cause little or no additional harm. In general, if patients value something more than complete adherence to treatment, judging them ethically wrong may be incorrect, especially if the net good of nonadherence has been miscalculated.

From a rule-based perspective, patients do not seem to have an obligation to comply that devolves from their role as patients. Rather, if they promise to comply, then the rules of promise keeping would seem relevant. Even here, though, caution should be exercised in judging actions. It seems that it is not perhaps nonadherence per se that is at issue but rather the breaching of a promise or an untruthful statement about a given behavior.

In some ways, nonadherence with medical recommendations may be more ethically problematic for clinicians than for patients. It is clinicians, after all, who have the duty to inform patients about the reasons for their recommendations and how their recommendations or prescriptions are to be followed. If subsequent nonadherence is attributable to misunderstanding or lack of information, it would seem that the clinician has breached this duty. Similarly, one would expect that it would be clinicians, not patients, who would take responsibility for enhancing adherence to medical recommendations. Patients might be excused for indicating that they would adhere to a complex multidrug, multidose regimen even though they were concerned about predictable but as yet unexperienced side effects. Clinicians, on the other hand, might be regarded as negligent if they did not address the probable occurrence of nonadherence and take actions to minimize it.

Toward Resolution

Recognizing the Problem

Clinicians can observe signs. They depend upon patients to learn about symptoms. There are signs and symptoms that should raise a clinician's concerns about nonadherence. A patient's lack of financial resources may be evident from the context in which the patient is seen (e.g., a clinic for indigent patients) or from demographic information in the medical record (e.g., unemployed, uninsured). In Mr. Ford's case, his uninsured status was recorded in his records. If Dr. Berg had noted this, he might have anticipated the patient's difficulty in purchasing lovastatin. Signs apparent in the course of a visit include evidence of sensory or cognitive impairment. Decreased hearing or mental function can interfere with understanding, as can limited comprehension of medical language. Decreased vision or arthritic fingers can also interfere with the ability to comply with a prescribed treatment.

The usual physical examination and appropriate laboratory tests may also provide clues to nonadherence. A physical finding or laboratory abnormality that is not improving on therapy may be a sign that the patient is not following a recommended regimen.

In Mr. Ford's case, brown-stained fingers and teeth would be a sign of continued smoking. The patient's unchanged weight and blood pressure could be signs of non-adherence to the recommendations about diet, exercise, and anti-hypertensive therapy. The unchanging lipid levels could be a sign of nonadherence to the prescription for lovastatin.

Information on symptoms related to adherence may come from the patient spontaneously or in response to routine or selectively focused questions. Some may report a new symptom, and they may or may not relate it to their regimen or comment on its effect on their adherence.

Diagnosing Nonadherence

Clinical judgment is an unreliable way to diagnose the phenomenon of nonadherence. Clinicians are prone to presume nonadherence and to be less understanding of it when patients are stigmatized by social or cultural circumstances or a particular disease condition (e.g., chemical dependence). The diagnosis of nonadherence should not be presumptive, but rather systematic and sequential. At the time of making a recommendation or giving a prescription, the clinician should ascertain the patient's understanding and ability to comply. This could have saved considerable time in Mr. Ford's case, where, if Mr. Ford had known about the cost of lovastatin and Dr. Berg had recognized Mr. Ford's difficulty paying for the drug, alternative approaches could have been considered sooner. When patients show no predictable therapeutic changes, it is again time to consider nonadherence. Clinicians should ask directly, but without being judgmental or threatening, about adherence. For example, clinicians might politely ask patients simply to state, in the case of prescription drug use, what medicines they are taking

and when they are taking them. Introductory remarks can be helpful; for example, "People often have difficulty when taking their pills for one reason or another. Have you ever missed any of your pills?"[9] If patients acknowledge this, they may be prepared to report at what rate they adhere, although patients may overestimate their rates of adherence (according to one study, by about 17 percent).[9] Patients may also disclose why they are having difficulty with adherence. If Dr. Black had asked Mr. Merchant about how he was doing with taking his acyclovir as prescribed, even mentioning what he had learned from looking at the prescription refill records, Mr. Merchant might have indicated that it was hard to remember to take the drug twice a day. Dr. Black could then have switched to a single-daily-dose regimen.

Poor therapeutic response and self-reported nonadherence identify a bit more than half of the cases of nonadherence.[9] Unannounced pill counts are inexpensive and may be more accurate than self-reports, but a patient's practice of combining prescribed pills into one bottle, sharing medicine with a family member, or confusion about dosing may complicate the interpretation of a pill count.[9] Measuring serum levels of a drug should only be necessary when self-reports and therapeutic response are significantly discrepant. Such measurements can then be helpful regardless of results. Clinicians can recognize nonadherence as the probable cause of therapeutic failure, but they must be careful not to alienate patients by the way they respond to this result. Nevertheless, results may reflect adherence and suggest that the prescribed drug is ineffective, thus leading to a change in therapy.

Getting Help

Some situations that involve nonadherence lead to considerable frustration and, in turn, prompt consultation. In my institution, the ethics committee or a clinical ethicist has been asked to assist with several cases that have been labeled "compliance problems" or even "problem patients" by the primary physician. These cases include patients with juvenile onset, insulin-dependent diabetes who have had recurrent admissions for diabetic ketoacidosis and intravenous drug users with a second or third episode of bacterial endocarditis that may require valve replacement. In such cases, referring physicians seem convinced that the patients would not comply with recommendations (diet and insulin use in the first type and abstaining from intravenous drug use in the second type). The clinicians seemed to regard nonadherence in these cases as willful, wrong, and blameworthy. Furthermore, their inclination was to withhold specific treatments (hospitalization in the first type and surgery in the second). Their arguments frequently were that (1) the patient's behavior is self-destructive, therefore medical intervention is unwarranted and therapy inappropriate, and (2) subsequent nonadherence will negate or reverse the benefits of treatment, so that pursuing treatment would be futile.

Many specialists could be asked to consult on these problematic cases. Psychologists, psychiatrists, diabetologists, substance-abuse specialists, social workers, and case managers may all have something to contribute and all would certainly have a different understanding of what the problems and potential solutions were. As ethics consultants, my colleagues and I have generally tried to bring recognized ethical principles, clinical skills, and additional specially trained professionals together to help with these cases.

Our clinical evaluation of the patients and knowledge of the contemplated interventions indicated that these interventions would very likely be of considerable benefit at least in the short term (i.e., correction of the ketoacidosis and elimination of bacterial endocarditis) and the long term (i.e., reduction of the attendant morbidity and mortality). We also took note of what had been done and what had not been done to investigate and address the causes of nonadherence. In analyzing these cases, we assumed that nonadherence was not a *prima facie* reason to eliminate an obligation to treat patients, especially those with a life-threatening condition. Thus we generally agreed that pursuing treatment was not futile because some short-term medical goals would likely be achieved, and although poor future adherence was possible, relatively little had been done to address it directly, suggesting that adherence might be improved. Finally, even future nonadherence would not negate the benefit of a present intervention or even necessarily render future interventions futile.

Planning an Intervention

Intervening with nonadherence can be preventative or reactive. As with all potentially dangerous conditions, it is helpful to identify those at risk and take steps to minimize the risk. When the condition occurs, it is important for clinicians to diagnose it quickly, determine the cause, and address it appropriately. Thus, whenever possible, clinicians should take measures to enhance adherence. Knowledge about adherence behaviors may help clinicians elicit better information about patients' adherence to medical regimens. This knowledge also suggests a variety of simple measures to enhance adherence. These include making sure patients understand what their medicines are, what they are for, and when and how to take them. Written instructions and patient-demonstrated understanding are both helpful. Clinicians should recommend the shortest regimen possible and the one that requires the fewest doses per day. For all patients, but especially for those with limited ability to pay, the least expensive yet effective interventions should be selected. Obviously, for some patients, this consideration will override duration and dosing features. If a once-a-day drug is prohibitively expensive, then a multiple-dose affordable agent may be the only regimen to which the patient can adhere. Clinicians should specify easy-to-use packaging that is conducive to adherence, even if this means dispensing drugs to elderly or disabled patients in containers that are not childproof but are accessible to those patients. Reminders, either incorporated in packages like dated dispensers or cards for the drug cabinet or refrigerator, are helpful. Involving one of the patient's family members can be a way to reinforce and remind the patient about adherence. It also provides the clinician with a therapeutic ally in the home and another evaluator and reporter of adherence, adverse effects, and therapeutic benefits.

A number of interventions could have proved useful for the patients described at the beginning of this chapter. Dr. Berg could have indicated at the first visit with Mr. Ford that adherence to smoking cessation, diet, and exercise programs would be difficult but important for specific reasons that he could list. He could also ask questions about the patient's lifestyle and interests that would enable him to make more specific suggestions. He could have directed Mr. Ford to resources such as dieticians and support groups. He could have discussed smoking-cessation aids and their costs. It might have been helpful to invite the patient's wife to the second visit and to enlist her support and assistance.

Specific questioning might also have identified particular problems with adherence. Recognition of financial difficulties with one lipid-lowering agent could have led to the substitution of another agent (such as cholestyramine) or added emphasis on diet and exercise. Continuing to ask about adherence at each visit and expressing pleasure at successful efforts and encouragement for not yet successful ones might have promoted adherence.

As mentioned above, Dr. Black could have made adherence easier for Mr. Merchant, who had recurrent herpes, by prescribing a once-a-day dose of suppressive therapy initially or as soon as there was evidence that adherence was a problem. For this patient, however, and for other patients with communicable diseases, adherence is important not only for their personal benefit but for their contacts as well. Dr. Black did advise Mr. Merchant about what measures to take, but reminders at each visit or prescription refill might have been helpful. Although protection of others may be a concern for clinicians taking care of patients like this, the responsibility also belongs to the patient, the public health system, and potentially the criminal and civil justice systems.

Adherence and Public Health

When nonadherence poses a health risk to others, public health measures are frequently indicated. For instance, some jurisdictions require that some or all communicable and particularly sexually transmitted diseases be reported (see Chap. 12). Such reports may identify contacts and inform them of their risk. Reminding patients of required reporting can be a significant incentive for patients to change behavior that puts others at risk and/or to tell them about the infection and their risk. In some cases of highly communicable and/or highly dangerous and difficult-to-treat infectious diseases, the law provides more forceful responses to nonadherence because of the threat it poses to others or the harms that have resulted from it. These include observed therapy and/or confinement for tuberculosis and criminal penalties for willful transmission of HIV infection. Parents who refuse immunization of their children for measles may be required to accept immunization for them or keep them at home until they are no longer at risk and/or pose no risk to others. These severe impositions on personal choice and liberty should be reserved for cases where the threat to others is substantial, not otherwise avoidable, and where less Draconian measures have been tried and have failed.

Closing Comments

Studies of nonadherence have shown that it is a common, complex, and to some degree predictable and reducible phenomenon. Yet it is remarkable that patients adhere even 50 percent of the time to expensive, unpleasant, hard-to-remember treatment regimens that often produce no discernible short-term benefit and may or may not save them from a low-probability event in the distant future.

In thinking about the phenomenon of nonadherence, it may be constructive to think about it in terms of the clinician's role, the patient's role, and society's role. The clinician's role is to make the patient's choice informed and not to make adherence any more difficult than it has to be. The patient's role is to make choices between value-laden alternatives. Society's role should be to equitably limit or distribute medical regimens for patients who want to adhere to them and who will benefit from them.

References

1. Dixon WM, Stradling P, Woolton DP: Outpatient PAS therapy. *Lancet* 2:871–872, 1957.

2. Meichenbaum D, Turk DC: *Facilitating Treatment Adherence: A Practitioner's Guidebook.* New York, Plenum Press, 1987, pp 21, 44–45.

3. Haynes RB, Dantes R: Patient compliance and the conduct and interpretation of therapeutic trials. *Contr Clin Trials* 8:12–19, 1987.

4. Fletcher RH: Patient compliance with therapeutic advice: a modern view. *Mt Sinai J Med* 56:453–458, 1989.

5. Costa FV: Compliance with anti-hypertensive treatment. *Clin Exp Hypertens* 18:463–472, 1996.

6. Sclar DA, Tartaglione TA, Fine MJ: Overview of issues related to medical compliance with implications for the outpatient management of infectious diseases. *Infect Agents Dis* 3:266–273, 1994.

7. Cramer JA, Mattson RH, Prevey ML, et al: How often is medication taken as prescribed? *JAMA* 261:3273–3277, 1989.

8. Wright EC. Non-compliance—or how many ants has Matilda? *Lancet* 342:909–913, 1993.

9. Stephenson BJ, Rowe BH, Haynes RB, et al: Is this patient taking the treatment as prescribed? *JAMA* 269:2779–2781, 1993.

10. Melnikow J, Kiefe C: Patient compliance and medical research: issues in methodology. *J Gen Intern Med* 9:96–105, 1994.

Daniel P. Sulmasy

Preventive Medicine

Fred Nelson, age 65, has had three-vessel coronary artery bypass surgery. One day he walks into his doctor's office and says, "My wife told me I should get one of those PSA tests she heard about on TV." Ought Mr. Nelson be screened for prostate cancer? What standard of evidence is ethically required before he is offered a screening test? Does he have a right to demand it? If it is to be done, what should he understand before he gives informed consent for testing? Are his age and history of coronary artery disease contraindications to testing? Would it be just to withhold a screening test on the basis of age? How will testing be reimbursed? What issues of justice are raised by differences in access to testing among different patient groups?

Scope of the Problem

Prevention is an essential aspect of primary care. Much of doing primary care involves giving treatment, screening, and offering advice about prevention. Yet despite centuries of preventive medical practice, preventive medicine has attracted little attention in the field of bioethics.[1,2] Perhaps this is because prevention does not elicit the same excitement as the ethical problems seen in intensive care units. Nonetheless, television newscasters report constantly on new preventive findings, and patients ask about them; congress debates measures to prevent teenage smoking, and mayors ask about the morality of needle exchange programs to prevent HIV infection.

As in Mr. Nelson's hypothetical case depicted above, the ethical issues in prevention also confront clinicians on a daily basis. Yet these clinical issues are rarely recognized as ethical issues. In this chapter, many of the ethical issues in prevention are described. It is important to start with the basic question of whether there is a moral obligation to pursue preventive health care measures in the first place, and why. And if there is such an obligation, it is essential to determine whether there are any ethical limits to the pursuit of prevention.

Background Theory and Context

Moral Grounding

Although it might seem obvious that it is morally praiseworthy to prevent illness, one needs to know what justifies prevention in the first place in order to assess whether any particular preventive intervention is ethically justified. In this section, five ethical notions regarding prevention are introduced: utilitarianism, "the rule of rescue," avoiding harm, stewardship of the body, and holism.

UTILITARIANISM VERSUS THE RULE OF RESCUE

Some would ground the morality of preventive health measures in a utilitarian moral framework. *Utilitarianism* is a theory holding that an act is morally justified if and only if it improves the net ratio of good to bad consequences for all those affected by the act. Thus, utilitarians argue that prevention is justified because it produces great social benefit. Utilitarians call into question the priority of what has been called "the rule of rescue." Once someone has suffered illness or injury, particularly if the condition is life-threatening, society is willing to justify huge expenses to "rescue" that person but seems unwilling to expend a similar amount to prevent illness and injury.[3] Utilitarians criticize this rule as irrational, arguing that a life is a life and that there is no moral difference between "statistical lives" and the lives of those who can readily be identified as sick and in need of intervention.[4,5]

But simple utilitarian arguments may underestimate the ethical complexity of prevention. There does seem to be something morally compelling and even logical in responding to the needs at hand and in the discounting of possible future needs. The compelling nature of "rescue" cannot simply be dismissed as irrational. Those who are now sick do seem to have a just claim on society and on clinicians. The obligation of beneficence toward those who are now sick is founded in the traditions of Hippocratic medicine and in the dynamic of the relationship between the sick person and the clinician who asks the sick person, "How can I help you?"

AVOIDING HARM

It is unarguable that clinicians have a moral duty to avoid harming patients. However, the Hippocratic dictum "to help, or at least do no harm"[6] has far more weight in the preventive situation than it does in that of actual illness. For example, once it is clear that someone has a fatal illness, very toxic therapies with only a slight chance of cure become morally acceptable simply because the possibilities for harm from the intervention pale in the face of the impending harm at hand. Harming people who are now well in the interest of saving them from a possible illness in the future seems intolerable. For example, even though thousands of lives were saved by vaccination during the "swine flu" influenza epidemic of the 1970s, it was considered absolutely intolerable that the vaccine caused a grave neurologic illness in a relative handful of persons.[7]

STEWARDSHIP OF THE BODY

Despite these complexities, however, there is an unmistakable moral mandate for prevention, and this might also be established on nonutilitarian grounds. Prevention, in one form or another has been a part of medical practice for several millennia.[8,9] One nonutilitarian way of establishing a moral basis for a duty to prevent illness and injury lies in what might be called a principle of stewardship of the body. A healthy body is valuable, and the duty to maintain a healthy body flows from this.

A healthy body is of value in three ways.[10] First, our health is valuable to ourselves. We need healthy bodies to do the sorts of things we want to do. Second, our health is valuable to others, whether family, friends, or society at large. We can only help others if we ourselves are healthy. Third, many persons will see their bodies as valuable gifts from a Creator. Such persons will be motivated to care for their bodies out of gratitude. The bottom line is that all persons seem to have a duty, under ordinary circumstances, to care appropriately for their bodily health. By extension, the ordinary presumption in medical ethics is to preserve life and to prevent illness.

HOLISM

The value of the human body derives not simply from what one can do with it but also from the fact that it is a constitutive element of the human person. Bodies are integral to persons, and persons alone are worthy of the respect demanded by the value called human dignity. Body parts and functions exist for the sake of the whole. Disruptions of the integrity of this unified entity can be tolerated only for the sake of the whole. This gives rise to a *principle of holism* stating that the functions and parts of the body have value in service to the whole person.

Holism is the underlying moral principle that justifies such things as amputations. One would not ordinarily think it morally justifiable to cut off a healthy patient's leg just because he or she asked for it. Autonomy alone does not justify it. However, if it is necessary, for instance, to remove a gangrenous limb in order to save a patient's life, the principle of holism justifies the act. It is reasonable and proper to examine preventive health care interventions under the extension of this principle of holism. Measures that promote the fully integrated function of the embodied person should be permitted. Measures that detract from the fully integrated function of the embodied person should be viewed with suspicion.

Types of Risk Factors

Preventive measures are directed toward a wide variety of risk factors that might affect the likelihood that an individual will develop disease, disability, or death. If these risk factors can be avoided, modified, or eliminated, such ills might be prevented.

There are three general categories of risk factors, and the ethical issues involved in assessing them vary.[11] The first category comprises *behavioral* risk factors, such as diet, exercise, and smoking. The second set of risk factors is *environmental*, including water purity, air pollution, mosquito control, radiation, and secondhand smoke. The third set of risk factors is *genetic*. Some persons are predisposed to illness on the basis of their genetic makeup, such as a familial predisposition to breast cancer or familial hyperlipidemia.

Some risk factors are undoubtedly mixed, and some combinations of risk factors can be particularly potent. However, the ethical issues involved in assessing risk factors are not the same for all types of risk factors and all types of interventions. For instance, interventions aimed at behavioral risk factors raise questions about the spectrum between *persuasion* (trying to convince patients to comply) and *coercion* (forcing patients to comply). Questions also arise about the extent to which persons can be held accountable for their risky behaviors through higher taxes or higher insurance premiums or the withholding of treatments from persons who engage in behaviors that cause disease. If so, which behaviors and which diseases should be so classified? For example, should bypass surgery be precluded for active smokers? Should smokers pay higher taxes or health insurance premiums?

Environmental interventions raise questions about justice. Who should pay for cleaning up pollutants? What is the proper degree of trade-off between safety and cost in inspecting the meat supply?

Genetic interventions raise even more complex questions. Should germ-line cells (sperm and eggs) be manipulated to prevent genetic disorders? Can healthy early embryos be "selected" for further development into fetuses? All of these interventions are preventive, yet each gives rise to a unique set of ethical questions.

Types of Interventions

Different types of interventions are also used in preventive health care,[12] and each is associated with different ethical questions. The two classifications of types of interventions considered in this chapter are (1) primary prevention versus secondary or tertiary prevention and (2) screening versus risk-factor modification.

PRIMARY, SECONDARY, AND TERTIARY

Some measures are designed to prevent the occurrence of disease. This is called *primary prevention*. Other measures are designed to intervene after the disease has first developed (at an early, asymptomatic stage), aiming to cure it or prevent it from becoming clinically manifest. This is called *secondary prevention*. Once the disease has become symptomatic, one aims to ameliorate the manifestations of the disease or to keep the disease from getting worse. This is called *tertiary prevention.*

I suggest that, as a general ethical rule for screening, primary prevention requires more evidence of effectiveness and more evidence of long-term safety than does secondary or tertiary prevention. I base this on the principle of avoiding harm.

In primary prevention, people do not yet have disease, and many never will. Therefore, the likelihood of benefit for any one individual in a population will be small, even though for a few unknown individuals the benefits will be substantial. To get a sense of this, epidemiologists often calculate the *number needed to treat*—that is, the total number of healthy persons who must take the treatment in order to prevent one heart attack, save one life, or achieve some other health benefit. With all other things being equal, the lower the number needed to treat, the greater the moral claim for its use.

One must be much more certain that benefits will accrue before implementing a primary prevention policy than a secondary prevention policy. One must also be much more certain that there are no long-term detrimental side effects. Following the principle of avoiding harm, a primary preventive intervention for the general population must be *very* safe.

SCREENING VERSUS RISK-FACTOR MODIFICATION

One must also distinguish between screening interventions and interventions designed to modify risk factors. Screening is usually secondary prevention. It usually aims at identifying patients who already have disease, but the hope is to detect it at an early stage, when it will be easier to treat and perhaps even curable. Mammography is an example of this type of screening. Screening can also be done for a risk factor that predisposes to disease, and this sort of screening could be considered primary prevention. Another example would be screening for

high cholesterol or high blood pressure. The goal of these measures is the prevention of heart attacks and strokes by the identification of persons with risk factors.

I want to suggest that risk-factor modification, as a general moral rule, requires more justifying evidence of safety and efficacy than disease detection. This is because risk-factor modification requires intervention in persons who are not yet diseased. Such interventions are bound to have side effects. It may also turn out that modification of the risk factor does not prevent the disease. The risk factor itself may simply be an early manifestation of the disease and not a cause. Or it may be an *epiphenomenon*—something associated with the true cause but not the true cause itself.

This is not to say that screening does not also require justification by establishment of its safety and efficacy. Screening may simply detect disease at an earlier stage, and treatment may or may not be good enough to truly affect the outcome. Or screening might be too sensitive and detect subclinical disease that will never manifest itself clinically. If so, persons might be subjected to the risk of side effects of both screening and treatment without any real benefits. Not all screening is ethically good preventive medicine.

Ethical Issues in Primary Prevention

In evaluating the ethical issues in a proposed effort at primary prevention, it is important to address several empirical questions and moral considerations.

EMPIRICAL QUESTIONS

Assume that there is a risk factor x associated with disease y for which a preventive intervention, has been proposed. A series of empirical questions must be asked in assessing the moral warrant for any proposed preventive health care intervention (see Table 5-1).

Table 5-1

Primary Prevention: Empirical Questions of Moral Concern

1. How good is the evidence that the alleged risk factor actually causes the disease to be prevented?

2. How good is the evidence that the disease is detrimental, and to whom?

3. How good is the evidence that the proposed preventive intervention will actually control the alleged risk factor?

4. How good is the evidence that controlling the alleged risk factor will influence development of the disease to be prevented?

5. What is the likely net effect of the proposed preventive intervention upon the individual and upon society?

HOW GOOD IS THE EVIDENCE THAT THE ALLEGED RISK FACTOR ACTUALLY CAUSES THE DISEASE TO BE PREVENTED? The mere demonstration that an epidemiologic association exists is not evidence of causation. For example, early epidemiologic studies suggested that coffee consumption was strongly associated with cancer of the pancreas.[13] Until the finding was disproven, many took this as a reason to urge those who drank coffee to refrain from drinking it.[14]

HOW GOOD IS THE EVIDENCE THAT THE DISEASE IS DETRIMENTAL, AND TO WHOM? Not all diseases are equally burdensome and equally worthy of enormous social efforts at prevention. Acne vulgaris and the common cold impose health burdens that should not be trivialized, that is true. But cancer, heart disease, AIDS, tuberculosis, and malaria can claim moral precedence for the time, energy, and resources of preventive efforts. This is so by virtue of the nature and magnitude of their consequences. In general,

rare diseases and diseases of minimal consequence command less moral claim for preventive efforts than common diseases of major consequence.

However, this does not preclude specific preventive efforts for specific subgroups known to be at high risk for rare diseases of important magnitude. Screening for phenylketonuria is a good example,[15] since screening can identify, inexpensively and rapidly, infants who have the disease, and dietary measures can then be employed as primary prevention to avoid the disease's consequences.

However, in general, it can be said that there is less moral claim for primary preventive efforts aimed at *everyone* if the disease affects only a few people—unless that effort is a program to screen a population in order to identify a subpopulation at risk and then attempt risk-factor modification for that subpopulation. For example, giving all infants penicillin at birth because some might be born with congenital syphilis would be inappropriate.

HOW GOOD IS THE EVIDENCE THAT THE PROPOSED INTERVENTION WILL ACTUALLY CONTROL THE ALLEGED RISK FACTOR? It is a necessary condition for controlling disease y by changing risk factor x that intervention p should change x. Although this seems obvious, there are countless examples of preventive programs that have been attempted without meeting this minimum standard. Exercise programs to lower blood pressure must be proven to lower blood pressure if they are to prevent strokes. Mosquito-control programs must be shown to control mosquito populations if they are to prevent malaria. Millions of tons of pesticides and countless ditches have been dug without significant impact on mosquito populations and consequently no significant impact on malaria.

The moral rule that I suggest is that if the intervention has not been demonstrated to affect the risk factor, no matter how good the theoretical evidence that it "should" work, one

ought not waste health care resources or subject people to the risks of such an untested
intervention.

**HOW GOOD IS THE EVIDENCE THAT CONTROLLING THE
ALLEGED RISK FACTOR WILL INFLUENCE DEVELOPMENT
OF THE DISEASE TO BE PREVENTED?** Surprisingly
often, this step is passed over, since it is much
easier to demonstrate that an intervention can
control a risk factor than it is to show that this
intervention actually prevents disease. Risk factor x may be causally associated with disease y
but may account for only a small degree of the
variance in the expression of the disease, so that
controlling x would not substantially diminish
the burden of disease y. Or, risk factor x may be
insensitive to manipulation, so that modification
of this risk factor with intervention p would not
change x enough to diminish the disease burden of y. Therefore, for instance, one may
believe that stress reduction can prevent heart
attacks but be unable to reduce stress enough to
make any difference. Or the role stress plays
might be so minimal that diminishing it would
make no appreciable difference.

It might also be the case that the risk factor is
a genuine causal factor for the disease but that it
acts as a cause only when some other factor is
present or absent. So, for instance, deficiencies
of a given vitamin might be causally linked to a
particular disease. It might also have been
demonstrated that giving people high doses of
the vitamin raises its levels in their blood. If,
however, it turned out that deficiencies of this
vitamin caused the disease only when there was
a deficiency of some other unknown vitamin
found naturally in the same foods as the known
vitamin, the disease could not be prevented
merely by identifying a risk factor, establishing
causality, and changing the risk factor through
the intervention. At the very least then, this
intervention would be wasteful and might
engender a false sense of security. Furthermore,
it might even be harmful to increase the levels
of the one vitamin without increasing the other.

It would seem morally inappropriate to promote
such a preventive strategy.

**WHAT IS THE LIKELY NET EFFECT OF THE PROPOSED
INTERVENTION ON THE INDIVIDUAL AND ON SOCIETY?**
Far too often, prevention enthusiasts settle for
evidence of efficacy rather than effectiveness.[16]
Efficacy means that intervention p worked in the
controlled experimental conditions of a clinical
trial. *Effectiveness*, on the other hand, means
that intervention p has also been tested in the
way it was intended to be used—as a widespread practice in the community with all sorts
of variations in facilities, nurses, clinicians, and
patients. Sometimes, for instance, it is the diligent attention to detailed clinical care occuring
in a clinical experiment that actually results in
the effect and not the proposed intervention
itself. When the intervention goes out on the
mass market, people will not be cared for as
diligently as are research subjects. Therefore, in
general, the moral warrant for proceeding with
the prevention scheme is greater if it is based on
proven effectiveness rather than mere efficacy.

NET OUTCOMES More importantly, in assessing the
outcome of an intervention, one is interested in
data about the *net* outcome—the burdens as
well as the benefits. The effects of an intervention include not only its effects on the disease
process at hand but also on other body systems.
So, for example, it is important to know more
than the effect on "cardiovascular morbidity and
mortality." One must take account of all possible
effects, good and bad (especially the unexpected and unintended effects). For example,
aspirin is efficacious for the primary prevention
of heart attacks, but it also causes gastrointestinal bleeding and an increases the risk of hemorrhagic stroke.[17]

And the measured effects should include the
full range of effects, including quality of life and
the psychological impact of the intervention
itself. For example, some antihypertensive drugs
can cause impotence and depression.[18] Even

screening can have side effects. For instance, it has been shown that patients want to be informed (*before* they consent to screening) about the possibility that they might worry about the meaning of the results of a PSA screening test for prostate cancer, especially in case of a borderline result. On the other hand, surveyed "experts" never considered this an important aspect of informed consent.[19] There is increasing concern that patients who undergo screening will suffer from the "burden of information." This is especially so for tests for which there is no effective treatment, such as Alzheimer's disease.[20] Might these patients be better off not knowing their risk?

ABSOLUTE VERSUS RELATIVE RISK   The magnitude of the benefit for individuals should be soberly appraised. Sometimes, the way in which the data are presented can be difficult to understand. In general, presenting what is called the *relative risk reduction* is most useful for understanding the effect of the intervention on common diseases in large populations. However, for individual patients, what is called the *absolute risk reduction* is more important. For example, the relative risk reduction over 10 years for healthy men who take an aspirin every other day to prevent heart attack is 44 percent.[17] This sounds impressive. However, the absolute risk reduction is only 1.9 percent. This is because very few of these men will suffer heart attacks over this time period. A 44 percent reduction in relative risk corresponds to a risk of 4.4 percent for men who do not take aspirin versus 2.5 percent for men who do take aspirin. Now, from the standpoint of public health, an absolute risk reduction of 1.9 percent in a cohort of 10 million men means that 190,000 heart attacks will be prevented over 10 years. This is certainly impressive. Yet, consider looking at this question by calculating the number needed to treat: about 50. That is, 50 men must take aspirin every other day for 10 years to prevent one heart attack. And consider a particular patient. If

he does not like the taste of aspirin and knows that he also increases his risk of hemorrhagic stroke and bleeding from the stomach by taking aspirin, how strongly should he be encouraged to take aspirin in order to reduce his risk of a heart attack over the next 10 years from 4.4 to 2.5 percent? Would it be neglectful of his duties of stewardship of his body if he were not to do so? Are the risks associated with taking aspirin justified by the principle of holism—i.e., risking a stroke for the sake of saving the heart? At the very least, it would seem difficult to argue that taking aspirin is a duty of strict obligation.

LONG-TERM VERSUS SHORT-TERM   For preventive interventions, the burden of proof in demonstrating the safety and long-term benefit of the intervention ought to be higher. The consequences of the preventive intervention may manifest themselves years down the line, both for good and for ill. Showing that patients did better in the first week after the intervention is not as useful as knowing that they did better 5 or 10 years after the intervention. For some interventions, this has been proven. Mammography had the potential to cause side effects (even cancer) because of the use of radiation. With contemporary mammographic techniques, this risk has been greatly reduced. The long-term benefits of screening mammography for women over 50 years of age are clear.[21] However, controversy still surrounds the interpretation of the data for 40- to 50-year-old women.[22,23]

COST   The cost of a preventive intervention should also be taken into account. Once again, cost seems to have more moral weight in prevention than in treating those who are already ill. It would be inappropriate for society to offer preventive measures so costly that no resources would remain for the care for those already identified as sick.

One should be wary of simple utilitarian solutions to this problem. One could easily justify preventive health care measures on the basis of net gains in productivity or quality-adjusted life-years (QALYs) at the expense of the chronically ill, the elderly, and the poor, whose quality of life tends to be rated low by the general population and whose life-years tend to be shorter anyway.[24] There is an ever-present danger of using a crude utilitarian calculus to turn prevention into a social conspiracy on the part of the young, wealthy, and well against the elderly, poor, and sick.

OTHER MORAL CONSIDERATIONS

JUSTICE It is important to consider how the benefits of the preventive intervention are likely to be distributed within society. This raises questions of social justice. For example, formal cost-benefit analysis leads to the conclusion that the most lives saved per preventive health care dollar would result from a program to promote medication compliance among patients who have already been diagnosed as having hypertension, rather than trying to discover and treat undiagnosed hypertensives. However, justice concerns can be raised on the ground that those already diagnosed are predominantly wealthy and white, while the undiagnosed, who are predominantly poor persons of color, would be left to languish.[25] Issues of social justice also form part of a moral critique of preventive health care measures.

SIMPLICITY Preventive interventions ought to be simple, relatively noninvasive, and widely acceptable to the population. Relatively complex and invasive procedures, such as flexible sigmoidoscopy for colon cancer screening, have been recommended by experts in preventive medicine for years. Why has this test not seen widespread usage?[26] Perhaps this is so because it violates this rule regarding screening tests. People feel very understandably reluctant to have a test like this, which is invasive, somewhat embarrassing, and carries some degree of risk.

Secondary and Tertiary Prevention

I have been discussing the ethical issues involved in examining the consequences of a primary prevention measure in detail and will only touch upon the similar set of questions that should be asked in evaluating secondary or tertiary preventive measures. Once one understands the complexity of analyzing a primary prevention measure, the approach to a secondary or tertiary measure follows.

The moral analysis of secondary preventive measures follows similar lines to those detailed above regarding primary prevention. Although limitation of space precludes a detailed analysis, it should be easy to apply these principles to secondary prevention.

1. How well does test z detect the early presence of disease y?
2. How good is the evidence that y is detrimental, and to whom?
3. How good is the evidence that screening test z actually detects early cases of disease y or that intervention p actually modifies risk factor x?
4. How good is the evidence that early detection of y saves lives, or that treatment of risk factor x with intervention p effectively ameliorates disease y?
5. What are the consequences of screening test z or intervention p in the fullest possible sense and with longest reasonable follow-up?

Tertiary prevention involves interventions to modify risk factors once an individual has been identified as already suffering from a disease. For example, one might try to lower the cholesterol of a patient who has sustained a myocardial infarction. The basic principles for evaluating the impact of the intervention apply. However, since the disease already affects the patient symptomatically, the principle of avoiding harm, while still a consideration, loses some of its special salience. In any event, a very broad range of effects of a proposed preventive intervention ought to be taken into account before one decides that there is a moral warrant to proceed with the intervention, either at the social level or at the individual level.

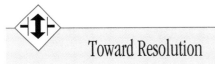

Toward Resolution

A Framework for the Ethical Evaluation of Preventive Medical Interventions

Preventive interventions raise a wide variety of ethical questions. Prevention is at once medical and social; private and interpersonal. The varieties of preventive interventions further complicate the picture. Accordingly, the ethical evaluation of preventive interventions is far more complex than might first be imagined. But to aid in tackling problems of this sort, I propose a systematic way to organize the ethical evaluation of preventive interventions in health care. Specifically, I propose five categories for consideration (see Table 5-2). Each is discussed in turn.

THE PREVENTIVE INTERVENTION ITSELF

One should begin by evaluating the preventive intervention itself as an intentional act. One must be very clear about exactly what the proposed preventive act is, what sort of preventive measure it is, and what it is intended to accomplish. Is it screening or risk-factor modification? Primary, secondary, or tertiary? Aimed at behavioral, environmental, or genetic risks? Precisely what is proposed, and what is the aim of the measure?

One important aspect of the evaluation of a preventive intervention is whether the act is truly preventive or whether it is an act of enhancement. That is, is the act preventing a defect (such as giving folate to pregnant women to prevent neural tube defects in the fetus) or is it designed to enhance (such as giving growth hormone to short-statured children who are not suffering from any known form of dwarfism or other defect, but whose parents simply want taller offspring). The morality of genetic enhancement is a very complex issue that will become even more significant as knowledge from the human genome project becomes available (see Chap. 6). Precise delineation of the difference between prevention and enhancement can sometimes be difficult, but specifying this difference is an important task to undertake in evaluating preventive interventions. Someday physicians may be able to perform intrauterine gene therapy, for instance, to correct genetic forms of familial hypercholesterolemia. This would be a wonderful preventive achievement. But intrauterine gene therapy could also be used to enhance. Inserting genes associated with extremely high intelligence would raise more moral problems than correcting hypercholesterolemia.

Table 5-2

Issues to Consider in Evaluating the Moral Aspects of a Preventive Intervention

1. What are the moral aspects of the intervention itself, as an intentional act?
2. What is the motive for the intervention?
3. What are the consequences of the intervention, both for the individual and for society?
4. What are the issues of freedom and interpersonal relationships involved in the intervention?
5. What are the morally relevant circumstances under which the intervention is to be undertaken?

THE MOTIVES BEHIND THE INTERVENTION

There are at least two agents in most preventive health care interventions—the preventor and the preventee. In general, the former is a health care professional or a society. But it is also possible for a single individual person to assume both roles, acting unilaterally to prevent disease in himself or herself. The motives of the agents bear importantly upon the moral evaluation of proposed preventive interventions. It is also useful for clinicians to know the most morally appropriate ways to motivate patients to participate in preventive measures.

The motivation for a person to seek preventive health care can arise out of the principles of stewardship and holism in a completely positive way. One cares for one's body because doing so is itself a good and also necessary for the concrete acts that make the body most fully human—for example, acts of intellect, imagination, or love. There is a healthy sense, then, in which one has duties toward oneself for preventive health care. One may also engage in preventive measures out of the motive of true charity—to care for one's family or to preserve one's health for the sake of service to others.

Health care professionals and societies can also have many good and positive motives for engaging in preventive health care—for the good of individual patients, for the good of others close to the patient (such as a patient's children), for the promotion of a better society, and for the motive of good stewardship of health care resources (which ought never to be squandered). Those who promote preventive health care measures are often motivated by all of these.

But one must frankly realize that preventive health care interventions can be undertaken on the basis of motives that are far less noble. Inappropriate motives may move both the preventor and the preventee.

BIOLOGICAL PERFECTIONISM   Prevention can be undertaken as a form of biological perfection-ism. In many Western nations, for example, preventive health care has become an obsession.[27] In some quarters, prevention has taken on a quasireligious character. For instance, one now encounters health-food rituals of an almost pharisaic nature: steak becomes "sinful" and chocolate cake becomes "decadent."[28] This sort of motivational attitude violates the principle of holism. It makes bodily well-being the point of life, which is an unbalanced approach. Prevention can become an end in itself or even a form of idolatry, a danger that Maimonides was able to foresee in the Middle Ages.[29]

SLOTH AND GLUTTONY   At the other extreme, persons can be slothfully or even selfishly negligent about their health. Some people neglect their bodies, and this sort of imbalance is equally improper. Others regularly overeat purely for pleasure. This, of course, is gluttony. Such actions are also morally inappropriate, since they violate the principles of stewardship and holism.

SOCIETY'S MOTIVES   Health care professionals and societies, as described above, often initiate preventive health care programs from the noblest of motivations. But the motives of those who encourage or provide preventive health care services are not always so pure. Rather, prevention may become a tool of oppression.[30] A government or employer may enforce preventive health care measures solely in order to create a healthier work force and increase productivity for the sake of profits. Prevention may be a tool for maintaining a healthier military with which to carry out acts of international aggression. Prevention of stress-related illness though the regular use of relaxation techniques during the workday might be urged without ever questioning the morality of the working conditions that lead to such stress. Social motives for undertaking preventive health care practices must be very carefully measured.

THE CONSEQUENCES OF THE INTERVENTION

It is also crucial to measure carefully the consequences of various preventive interventions and to account for all the steps in the chain of evidence that lead to a recommendation for or against such an intervention. As discussed above, when a person is not yet sick, it is critical that what is proposed in the name of preventing disease not be harmful.[31] In addition, as also discussed above, the burden of proof will generally be higher for primary preventive measures than it will be for secondary or tertiary preventive measures and higher for risk-factor modification than it will be for case finding and treatment. Nonetheless, the burden of proof for any such intervention should be upon those who propose it to show that it really is helpful in the long run.

One should also be careful to assess the consequences not only for the individual considering the preventive intervention but also those for the society as a whole. The necessary data will differ according to the type of intervention under consideration, whether primary, secondary, or tertiary.

Issues of Freedom and Interpersonal Relations

Ultimately, the knowledge that decisions about prevention have an effect upon others raises questions about freedom and interpersonal relationships in preventive interventions. States have traditionally justified compulsory preventive measures on the basis of their responsibility to protect and promote the common good. But how much freedom should individuals enjoy in making decisions about preventive health care? What limits can be set on the preventive measures a state might take to compel preventive measures in the name of the common good?

There are five broad categories of stands that health care professionals or other social institutions such as governments can take with respect to the freedom of individual patients regarding preventive health care decisions: (1) coercion, (2) promotion, (3) indifference, (4) discouragement, and (5) prohibition. From an ethical perspective, different stands will be appropriate for different preventive interventions.

COERCING PREVENTIVE PRACTICES

Individual clinicians should never be allowed the power to decide unilaterally to coerce any individual into a preventive health care decision. Such power should properly be reserved to the state, and ultimately, in a democratic society, this means that it is a decision for the society as a whole. Not even a collective professional judgment—for example, by a medical organization—should be allowed to assume a coercive role, no matter how noble the goal. Coercion should be allowed only when a society decides that the burdens imposed upon others through the failure of individuals to comply with the preventive intervention are very significant. Even then, such decisions should be made only with trepidation.[32]

The most common examples involve contagious diseases. Governments have long required compulsory vaccination and quarantine. These are extremely significant encroachments upon individual freedom and should never be undertaken lightly. In general, compulsory interventions are warranted only if the common good is truly served, so that benefit accrues to all individuals to a greater extent when all participate. Vaccines fit this model well. Quarantine might in some cases also fit this model, especially for highly infectious diseases such as smallpox. Whether tuberculosis fits this model is debatable, but some jurisdictions in the United States retain the power to incarcerate individuals who refuse treatment for this disease.

In general, there is greater warrant for a coercive preventive measure if there is a benefit for the individual being forced to comply as well as a benefit for others. With all other things being equal, the greater these individual benefits, the greater the warrant. Contact tracing and partner notification for certain infectious diseases fit this model more or less well, depending upon the disease. The question of whether case reporting for HIV infection should be mandatory is an excellent example of a controversial case. When treatment was less effective, there was less moral warrant. Now that there is effective treatment, partner notification has the potential to benefit those who have shared needles or sex with the person known to be infected. This increases the moral warrant for mandatory case reporting as a preventive measure. However, while this is an important consideration, it is far from sufficient justification. The matter remains controversial.[33]*

Other considerations include exhausting all other means. Risks to individuals so compelled and the encroachment on their liberty must be as minimal as possible. In general, less demonstrated benefit should be required to *restrict* behaviors than to completely *outlaw* them. And, in general, less demonstrated benefit should be required to restrict behaviors of potential harm to others, while more demonstrated benefit should be needed to force individuals to undergo testing, treatments, or behavioral measures designed to enhance their health or the health of the public.

Although vaccination programs are an excellent example of a situation in which promotion of the common good seems to justify compulsory intervention, quarantine is a different matter. The extent of the contagion must be very great, the consequences of the infection must be profound, and all other means must have been exhausted before such a step is undertaken. On these grounds, therefore, Cuba's preventive

strategy of lifetime quarantine of HIV-infected persons seems unwarranted.[34]

Compulsory seat belt laws are of benefit to the individual so compelled, are of economic benefit to a society that supports health care through the state, but are an infringement on individual liberty. The moral warrant for such laws is therefore a bit more ambiguous. Still, most prudent persons consider the benefits sufficient to justify this minor degree of infringement on individual liberty. Laws requiring physical exercise by all citizens are even less warranted, because the benefits seem really to accrue more to the state than to the individual and the infringement on liberty seems greater.

PROMOTING PREVENTIVE PRACTICES

Many situations exist in which preventive measures are of clear benefit to individuals but may be of little benefit to the rest of society (other than by improving the aggregate health of the public). If these benefits are substantial and the risks are minimal, then these interventions should be actively promoted but not compelled.

The extent to which such interventions should be persuasively promoted will depend upon a consideration of all of the other ethical issues discussed above, especially a frank assessment of the potential benefits and harms from the perspective of the individual rather than the population. The ability to express benefit in terms of absolute risk reduction rather than relative risk reduction, becomes very useful in discussing the degree to which an individual should be encouraged to undertake the preventive intervention.

Where possible, it seems wise to target subpopulations at particular risk before recommending a preventive intervention, rather than subjecting the entire population to the risks of the intervention when many will have little chance of benefit.[35] For example, rather than treating everyone with borderline high choles-

---

*In June 1998, for example, the New York State Assembly passed what could become the first mandatory HIV partner notification law in the U.S., raising many questions about the moral status of such laws.

terol, it makes more sense to treat those with other known risk factors, such as diabetes, high blood pressure, and a family history of heart disease.

In general, it also requires less moral warrant to promote healthy practices that are part of common human experiences than is required to promote medical interventions. Encouraging people to consume fewer calories, exercise regularly, avoid smoking, wear seat belts, and avoid excessive sun exposure is far easier to justify than encouraging people to take cholesterol-lowering medications.

Finally, it must be understood that the patient's informed consent is required for any preventive intervention that has not been made legally mandatory.[36] Strategies to promote preventive measures cannot employ tactics that are manipulative or coercive.

PREVENTION TOSS-UPS

For some interventions, the data about risks and benefits will be of such a nature that clinicians ought only inform patients as fully as possible and then allow them freely to make the decision without being strongly encouraged one way or another. In some instances, this will be because the data are well established but the balance of incommensurable risks and benefits is such that it should really be up to the patient freely to decide, on the basis of his or her own evaluation of the relative weight of these risks and benefits. Consider estrogen-replacement therapy: the prevention of osteoporotic fractures and the reduction in heart attacks and strokes must be weighed against the fact that replacement doses of estrogen can sometimes cause nausea, headaches, or edema, the renewed onset of menses, the risk of uterine cancer, and uncertainty regarding the risk of breast cancer.[37] In such situations, the decision rightly belongs to the patient.

In other cases, the data are simply insufficient to meet the outcomes criteria set forth above.

For example, as in the case of Mr. Nelson described in the beginning of the chapter, PSA screening for prostate cancer falls in this category. It is simply not currently known whether programs of early detection of prostate cancer will ultimately save more lives, since this cancer is often slow-growing and relatively innocuous, and many men die at ripe old ages of other causes, harboring small prostate cancers that were never detected in life and never bothered them at all. Screening for prostate cancer is not without risks—of creating anxiety, of false-positive test results, and of the chain of events set off by the decision to screen. The rule of avoiding harm has a very important role to play in such cases. It seems premature to recommend massive screening programs for prostate cancer with PSA, but patients should be allowed to make informed choices, and this preventive intervention should neither be encouraged nor discouraged.[19]

DISCOURAGING PREVENTIVE PRACTICES

Some potential preventive practices are of limited social value but might be of value to some individuals and are not so harmful that they should be banned outright. *Discouragement* will be the appropriate moral stand to take for quite a few preventive measures. For example, even the most enthusiastic experts would not recommend PSA screening for men below the age of 40. Might a patient in such an age group demand such a test? Might there be clinicians who would recommend such testing on a regular basis? Certainly it would seem so. Moreover, the trouble of tracking down and banning such a practice seems too great, and the harm to patients too small, to justify an outright ban.[38] In such cases, discouragement of the practice through patient and clinician education, guidelines, and similar means might help to discourage such use of these preventive measures (see Chap. 1).

Whether third-party payers should underwrite such an intervention is another matter. It would seem that, where there is a clear consensus among experts that the intervention has no benefit, it would be morally permissible for third parties not to underwrite the cost of such a measure. However, if there is only a small beneficial effect, there will often be controversy about whether that level of beneficial effect is important.

PROHIBITING PREVENTIVE PRACTICES

Some preventive measures ought to be banned outright. These include those that seem directly to violate the fundamental principles upon which prevention is grounded—stewardship and holism. These would include, in my view, euthanasia as a means of "preventing" the onset of Alzheimer's disease. Other practices, however, might also be banned outright because they might help some individuals, but only at the price of significant harm to others. An example might be a preventive measure that had a rare but significant side effect of violent behavior toward others. In some cases, one might consider the risk to the individual to be too great to allow use of the intervention, no matter how much the individual might fear the disease in question. For example, a patient with significant symptomatic ventricular tachycardia might refuse to accept an implantable defibrillator and insist on drugs that are actually known to make this condition slightly worse.[39] In such a case, the treatment the patient is demanding is actually harmful, and the physician ought not to supply the medicine even if it were persistently demanded (see Chap. 1).

Circumstances

In the end, one must tailor almost all of these recommendations regarding prevention to the circumstances surrounding the case. Between compulsion and prohibition, there is an entire spectrum of degrees of force of recommendation for and against preventive interventions. It would be very foolish to pretend that recommendations could not be altered along this spectrum by the circumstances of individual cases. The particulars of the case must always be accounted for in ethical decision making. As Aristotle observes, ethics is concerned with action, "and action is about particulars."[40] In clinical practice, there will never be a substitute for this sort of practical wisdom.

Closing Comments

I have offered a framework for evaluating the morality of proposed preventive health care interventions based upon three major principles: stewardship, holism, and avoiding harm. It is my hope that this chapter will stimulate further investigation of these issues and that the framework I have provided will assist clinicians and ethicists in the analysis of many of the particular ethical issues raised by preventive medicine that are very much an integral component of primary care.

References

1. Pellegrino ED: Health promotion as public policy: the need for moral groundings. *Prev Med* 10: 371–378, 1981.
2. Weed DL, Coughlin SS: Ethics in cancer prevention and control, in Greenwald P, Kramer B, Weed DL (eds): *Cancer Prevention and Control.* New York, Marcel Dekker, 1995, pp 497–507.
3. Jonsen AR: Bentham in a box: technology assessment and health care allocation. *Law Med Healthcare* 14:172–174, 1986.

4. Hadorn DC: Setting health priorities in Oregon: cost-effectiveness meets the rule of rescue. *JAMA* 265:2218–2225, 1991.

5. Morreim EH: Of rescue and responsibility: learning to live with limits. *J Med Philos* 19:455–470, 1994.

6. Hippocrates. "Epidemics" I.xi, in *Hippocrates*. Vol. I. Jones WHS, trans. Cambridge, MA, Loeb Classical Library, Harvard University Press, 1931, p 165.

7. Safranek TJ, Lawrence DN, Kurland LT, et al: Reassessment of the association between Guillain-Barre syndrome and receipt of swine influenza vaccine in 1976–77: results of a two-state study. *Am J Epidemiol* 133:940–951, 1991.

8. Hippocrates: "Regimen in health," in *Hippocrates*. Vol. IV. Jones WHS, trans. Cambridge, MA, Loeb Classical Library, Harvard University Press, 1931, pp 43–60.

9. Weiss RL, Butterworth CE (eds): *The Ethical Writings of Maimonides*. New York, New York University Press, 1975, pp 34–41.

10. Pellegrino ED: Autonomy and coercion in disease prevention and health promotion. *Theoret Med* 5: 83–91, 1984.

11. Brett AS: Ethical issues in risk factor intervention. *Am J Med* 76:557–561, 1984.

12. Riegelman RK, Povar GJ: *Putting Prevention into Practice*. Boston, Little, Brown, 1988, pp 67–68

13. McMahon B, Yen S, Trichopoulos D, et al: Coffee and cancer of the pancreas. *N Engl J Med* 304: 630–633, 1981.

14. Zheng W, McLaughlin JK, Gridley G, et al: A cohort study of smoking, alcohol consumption, and dietary factors for cancer of the pancreas. *Cancer Causes Control* 4:477–482, 1993.

15. Tiwary CM: Proposed guidelines for screening of metabolic and endocrine diseases of dependent neonates of the U.S. Armed Forces, derived from a survey of state guidelines for neonatal screening of metabolic diseases. *Clin Pediatr* 26:349–354, 1987.

16. Diamond GA, Denton TA: Alternative perspectives on the biased foundations of medical technology assessment. *Ann Intern Med* 118:455–464, 1993.

17. Steering Committee of the Physicians' Health Study: Final report on the aspirin component of the ongoing Physicians' Health Study. *N Engl J Med* 321:129–135, 1989.

18. Webster J, Koch HF: Aspects of tolerability of centrally acting anti-hypertensive drugs. *J Cardiovasc Pharmacol* 27(suppl 3):S49–S54, 1996.

19. Chan ECY, Sulmasy DP: What should men know before giving informed consent for prostate-specific antigen screening for prostate cancer? *Am J Med* 105:266–274, 1998.

20. Roses AD: Genetic testing for Alzheimer disease: practical and ethical issues. *Arch Neurol* 54: 1226–1229, 1997.

21. Kerlikowske K, Grady D, Rubin SM, et al: Efficacy of screening mammography: a meta-analysis, *JAMA* 273:149–154, 1995.

22. Sickles EA, Kopans DB: Mammographic screening for women aged 40 to 49 years: the practitioner's dilemma. *Ann Intern Med* 122:534–538, 1995.

23. Smigel K: NCI proposes new breast cancer screening guidelines. *J Natl Cancer Inst* 85:1626–1628, 1993.

24. La Puma J, Edward F. Lawlor EF: Quality-adjusted life-years: ethical implications for physicians and policymakers. *JAMA* 263:2917–2921, 1990.

25. Stason WB, Weinstein MC: Allocation of resources to manage hypertension. *N Engl J Med* 296:732–739, 1977.

26. Ferrante JM: Colorectal cancer screening. *Med Clin North Am* 80:27–43, 1996.

27. Meador CK: The last well person. *N Engl J Med* 330:440–441, 1994.

28. Sulmasy DP: *The Healer's Calling*. New York, Paulist Press, 1997, p 77.

29. Weiss RL, Butterworth CE (eds): *The Ethical Writings of Maimonides*. New York, New York University Press, 1975, pp 34–41.

30. Skrabanek P: Preventive medicine and morality. *Lancet* 1:143–144, 1986.

31. McCormick J: Health promotion: the ethical dimension. *Lancet* 344:390–391, 1994.

32. Skrabanek P: The physician's responsibility to the patient. *Lancet* 1:1155–1157, 1988.

33. Steinbrook R: Battling HIV on many fronts. *N Engl J Med* 337:779, 1997.

34. Bayer RR, Healton C: Controlling AIDS in Cuba: the logic of quarantine. *N Engl J Med* 320:1022–1024, 1989.

35. Avins AL, Browner WS: Improving the prediction of coronary heart disease to aid in the management of high cholesterol levels. *JAMA* 279:445–449, 1998.

36. Skrabanek P: Why is preventive medicine exempted from ethical restraints? *J Med Ethics* 16:187–190, 1990.

37. Grady D, Rubin SM, Petitti DB, et al: Hormone therapy to prevent disease and prolong life in postmenopausal women. *Ann Intern Med* 117:1016–1037, 1992.

38. Aquinas T: *Summa Theologiae* I-II, Q. 96, a. 2, in Parry S (ed): *Treatise on Law.* Washington, DC, Regency Gateway, 1987, pp 90–93.

39. The Cardiac Arrhythmia Suppression Trial (CAST) Investigators: Preliminary report: effect of encainide and flecainide on mortality in a randomized trial of arrhythmia suppression after myocardial infarction. *N Engl J Med* 321:406–412, 1989.

40. Aristotle: *Nichomachean Ethics* 1114b.16. Irwin T, trans. Indianapolis, IN: Hackett, 1985, p 158.

Benjamin S. Wilfond

Genetic Testing

Jill Smith, 35 years old, is worried about Huntington disease. Her mother died of it 3 years ago and Jill was her mother's caregiver. Ms. Smith tells her primary care physician, Dr. Martinez, that she wants to be tested to see whether she is going to get the disease. How should Dr. Martinez respond?

Sally Jordan, 36 years old, is 12 weeks pregnant. She discusses the possibility of amniocentesis for chromosome abnormalities with her physician, Dr. Brown. Ms. Jordan isn't sure that she wants to have the test and asks Dr. Brown for advice. What should Dr. Brown tell her?

Johnny Larson, 7 years old, has had recurrent pneumonia. A sweat test is done and he is diagnosed with cystic fibrosis (CF). Dr. Morgan explains the recessive inheritance pattern to Johnny's parents and suggests that the parents inform each of their siblings that they may also be carriers. Johnny's father, Bob, tells Dr. Morgan that he has not talked with his sister in years and doesn't intend to call her now. What should Dr. Morgan do?

Johnny also has a sister, Gail, who is 3. She has asthma and Dr. Morgan recommends a sweat test, since there is a 1 in 4 chance that she has CF. The test is negative; however, when Dr. Morgan explains that Gail has a 2 in 3 chance of being a carrier, Mr. Larson asks to have Gail tested for carrier status. He reasons that Gail is more likely to be sexually responsible as a teenager is if she knows that she is carrier. What should Dr. Morgan do?

Scope of the Problem

Genetic testing invokes both some of the potential promises and some of the potential fears of modern medicine. It raises the prospect, although often overstated, of being able to predict the future health status of persons and the possibility of intervening in such a way as to alter that future.[1–4] It also raises the specters of eugenics and discrimination.[5,6] Although the concept of genetic testing is not new and the ethical issues it raises have much in common with those raised by other aspects of medicine, current advances in genetics highlight a number of ethical issues. The specific issues regarding genetic testing addressed in this chapter focus on those falling within the context of the clinician-patient relationship: Under what circumstances should clinicians recommend or not recommend genetic tests? What information is important to include as part of the informed consent process of genetic testing? What obligations are there to inform family members or third parties about the results of genetic testing? And what unique considerations arise in prenatal and pediatric genetic testing?

Genetic testing has long been part of medical practice. For instance, biochemical analysis can sometimes determine a genetic diagnosis and even autosomal recessive carrier status. Examples include measurement of the enzyme hexosminadase to diagnose Tay-Sachs disease and serum electrophoresis to diagnose alpha$_1$-antitrypsin deficiency. Although imprecise, a family history is also a predictor of disease and raises most of the same ethical issues as do direct genetic tests. In addition, practically all diseases have both genetic and environmental dimensions. For example, serum cholesterol, although a biochemical marker and clearly subject to environmental influences, is determined by genes and can indicate specific genetic conditions—namely, hyperlipidemias. Thus, primary care clinicians are regularly involved in genetic testing.

Nevertheless, advances in DNA technologies have increased the spectrum of genetic diseases that may be detected. This includes the ability to detect genes than may predict future genetic diseases, such as Huntington disease,[7] and the ability to detect susceptibility to diseases such as breast cancer,[8] Alzheimer disease,[9] emphysema,[10] and hemochromatosis.[11] The possibility of being able to detect genetic markers associated with the risk for developing complex, multifactorial diseases such as asthma or heart disease, as well as behavioral and psychiatric conditions, further complicates genetic testing.[12]

There are a number of aspects of genetic testing, such as those illustrated by the cases above, that, while not unique to genetics, converge to create reasons for special attention. First, the information related to genetic testing is often very complex and probabilistic, which can pose difficulties in communication during the process of informed decision making in the setting of brief office visits. Second, many of the potential risks of genetic tests are psychosocial, including anxiety, self-esteem, stigmatization, and discrimination in insurance and employment. This might result in either exaggerations or minimizations of the perception of the risks. Third, there may be familial implications of test results that create challenges for interactions among family members. For instance, some patients may wish to keep test results private. Finally, the influence of genetic information on reproductive decision making can be tough for health care professionals to discuss with their patients.

Background Theory and Context

Genetic Counseling

For several decades, genetic testing has been provided largely in conjunction with genetic counselors. Genetic counselors generally have master's level training in genetics and clinical counseling and often work in collaboration with medical geneticists.[13] Yet, as genetics is becoming more integrated into medical practice, primary care practitioners are more likely to directly face the issues related to testing with their patients. To prepare for this, it is helpful to understand how genetic counselors have approached genetic testing.

In the 1970s, most genetic counselors spent their time discussing recurrence risks for families who had a child with an inherited medical problem. Because these discussions centered on reproductive choices and because of the legacy of the eugenic movements in the United States, the United Kingdom, and Germany, genetic counselors developed a "nondirective" approach to such counseling. That is, genetic counselors have attempted to avoid influencing the reproductive decisions of their clients, focusing rather on the provision of information and the facilitation of decision making.

In recent years, genetic counselors have become more involved in areas such as cancer and neuropsychiatric genetics, yet they have maintained the position that for the most part, the patient's decision to have a genetic test that is not being done for clear medical benefit should not be influenced by the views of the clinician. On the other hand, in clinical practice, clinicians routinely make recommendations to patients. These apparently discrepant approaches are reconcilable. First, in clinical practice, nondirectiveness may not be achievable or desirable. It may not be achievable, because all interactions convey messages shaped by the information presented and how the information in framed.[14] Nevertheless, in some settings, as for reproductive decision making and other "course of life" decisions, a respect for self-determination would support an approach that strives toward nondirectiveness.[15] Furthermore, where there are clear medical benefits, it seems desirable for clinicians to make recommendations about a test or intervention. Regardless, clinicians must be explicit about the potential use of interventions, realizing that some patients may value these interventions differently.

Informed Consent

The complexity of genetic testing calls for a broad view of informed consent, which, for genetic testing, should involve a process of education and deliberative interaction with the provider.[16] Information without comprehension is inadequate. Before deciding about having a genetic test, persons should understand the implications of being tested. This should include a discussion of the potential benefits and risks of the test and an assessment of comprehension (see Chap. 19). Clinicians can help patients to determine for themselves whether the likely benefits outweigh the risks.

PRESYMPTOMATIC TESTING

The development of testing for presymptomatic Huntington disease included extensive pretest education and consent.[17] Since there is no effective intervention for Huntington disease, the potential benefit from testing would rest in reducing uncertainty as to whether one was at risk of developing the disease and enabling one to make better decisions about career, finances, or other life plans. How a person would respond to these results may be very personal. Among people at risk for Huntington disease who have had testing, adverse reactions in both affected and unaffected persons have been observed.[18] Thus, one of the challenges for clinicians who might counsel patients at risk for diseases such as Huntington disease is to help them consider how they might respond to the information and whether this information is most likely to be helpful to them. For example, although some individuals might think that testing for Huntington disease might allow them to prepare financially for the future, the potential for insurance or employment discrimination poses the risk that testing might actually make their financial situation more tenuous. When given this information, few people at risk for Huntington disease decide to have the test.[19]

When testing is done for disease susceptibility, such as BRCA1 testing to determine if a woman is at increased risk of developing breast and ovarian cancer, it can be difficult to convey the ambiguity of test results.[20] For example, mutations in BRCA1 increase one's risk but do not mean that one will develop cancer. Similarly, not having a mutation does not mean that one will not develop cancer. Additionally, while certain interventions may offer the potential of reducing the risk of cancer, they still do not provide guarantees against developing cancer.

PRENATAL TESTING

When genetic testing is used in the context of reproductive decision making, concerns about how clinicians might influence decisions are heightened. In contrast to testing patients for conditions that may affect their health, prenatal testing raises issues—such as the morality of abortion—that some clinicians may be uncomfortable discussing. Indeed, some studies report that clinicians often do not mention that one of the potential outcomes of prenatal testing is needing to make a decision about abortion.[21]

However, in obtaining informed consent for prenatal testing, it is important to include a discussion of abortion, since some people who are not interested in abortion may not want to assume the risk of miscarriage associated with amniocentesis or face considering whether to have an abortion based upon the results of testing.

In prenatal testing, it is possible that a clinician's own views might influence how a particular condition is described, even when the clinician's intention is to remain nondirective. For instance, a description of Down syndrome that portrays the potential medical complications may have a different impact than a description that focuses on the positive potential for such children and their families.[22] Further, there may be a tendency for clinicians to think of decisions about prenatal diagnosis as medical decisions based on risk rather than personal decisions based on how one views one's role as a parent. This is not surprising, since many clinicians have limited experience with children and families with disabilities and may make unwarranted assumptions about the difficulties of caring for child with a disability.

IMPLICATIONS FOR FAMILY MEMBERS

Another consideration in genetic testing is that the results will have implications for family members. Sometimes the results for one person will give precise information about other family members (e.g., testing adult children for dominant conditions, or testing identical twins). At other times, test results may mean that siblings or other family members might also be at risk, as with the determination of carrier status.

In some circumstances, genetic testing may identify misattributed parentage. While the actual population incidence of this is not clear, it is often estimated conservatively at 5 percent.[23] Although many geneticists do not routinely disclose this information, sometimes the results of genetic testing are interpretable for patients only when they receive an explanation about parentage.

Privacy and Confidentiality

Many persons are concerned about the privacy of genetic test results as well as medical information in general. This is due in part to the fact that the release of medical information can result in the potential for discrimination in employment or insurance. Although problems of discrimination are not unique to genetic testing, the stakes are high for society as well as for individuals, since all of us likely carry genes that might place us at risk for discrimination if confidentiality were breached. For example, a woman may be reluctant to undergo BRCA1 testing out of fear that increased insurance rates might result if this information were disclosed by a clinician. This concern is not easily solved by simply obtaining assurances from the clinician that such information will not be disclosed without consent. Even if the clinician does not disclose this information, the patient may be asked about such testing directly, or an insurance company or employer may learn of it on the basis of the patient's disclosure to a third party. Although a number of states have passed legislation to prevent insurance discrimination, the protections are incomplete and largely untested.[24] Additionally, it remains unclear whether the Americans with Disability Act will protect individuals before the onset of symptoms.[6]

Although the relevance of these issues may depend on the patient's specific employment and insurance circumstances, these issues have evoked much public interest. There are reports of genetic testing resulting in problems with insurance; however, their incidence is not well defined.[25] Yet it is possible that a perception of these risks may discourage testing, even if this problem is not likely to occur.

A clinician may also recommend that a person inform other at-risk family members; but occasionally, for complex personal reasons, an individual may not want to do this. Does the clinician have a responsibility to warn family members that they may be at risk for carrying a mutation that increases their risk of disease, or that their children have a risk of having a disease? The legal status of a duty to warn in this setting is contested,[26,27] and there may be a presumption in favor of confidentiality unless several conditions are met. The first condition is whether the harm that will occur without disclosure is serious. The second is whether the harm is likely to occur. The third is whether informing the person is likely to result in the harm being avoided. Unlike the paradigms used for determining whether to disclose the risks for homicide or HIV transmission, most circumstances of genetic testing are not likely to meet these criteria.

Testing Children

Testing children when there is no direct medical benefit of testing, such as testing for carrier status or for adult-onset conditions, raises unique issues related to the limits of parental authority and the role of children in decision making.[28] Some have argued that it is the parents' right to seek such information about their children and have suggested that clinicians should assist in arranging the tests.[29] One claim here is that these decisions are a parent's expression of self-determination. Another claim is that parents are most likely to make a decision consistent with the interests of the child. However, concerns about the potential adverse impact of such testing, foreclosing of future decision-making options, and invasion of privacy suggest that children should not be tested. There are a number of considerations in resolving these views.

The first consideration is whether the harms outweigh the benefits of testing. When testing children, these harms and benefits may be quite speculative. There may be potential benefits to children of knowing their carrier status, particu-

larly since they already know that they are at increased risk and may already believe that they are carriers.[30] Thus, clarification of this uncertainty may be beneficial. On the other hand, positive test results may cause anxiety or stigmatization or may adversely affect family relationships.

This uncertainty of benefit is particularly important when the intended benefit derives from anticipated behavioral change, as in the hypothetical case of the Larsons, described at the opening of this chapter, who hopes that testing will discourage his daughter from becoming sexually active as a teenager. Although this may be a desirable goal, there is little evidence that testing would have this effect on adolescent behavior, and it is plausible that it might have unintended negative consequences.

A parent with a child at risk for Huntington disease may want to use testing to direct the child in educational or career decisions. Another possible use of such information would be to help the parents make further reproductive decisions. For example, parents may want to know whether their young child has Huntington disease to help the parents decide whether to have more children. Although these may be potential benefits for the family, they are not necessarily in the interest of the child.

Given the uncertainty of benefits and harms, some argue that it should be up to parents to decide about testing. Others suggest there should be a presumption to avoid potential harms.[31] There are some additional considerations that seem to tip the scales toward a presumption to defer such testing until adulthood, or at least until the child has adequate decision-making capacity to decide about testing. First, testing in childhood forecloses future choices in adulthood.[32] Many adults decide not to be tested for Huntington disease or BRCA1.[33] Children who are tested will not be afforded an opportunity to make these choices.

The second consideration is based on the observation that some adults wish to be tested but do not want to share this information with their parents. For example, an adult who is a carrier of Tay-Sachs disease may not wish her parents to know this because they have different views on abortion and reproductive decision making.[34] If such testing is done in a child, he or she will never have the chance to exercise the choice of not revealing this information to his or her parents.

The third consideration regards the involvement of the child in the decisions concerning genetic testing. A child's capacity to make decisions evolves over time, and rather than arbitrarily assume this happens at a defined age, an individualized approach seems warranted. In some cases, an adolescent, particularly from a family with individuals affected by a genetic disease, may have both adequate decision-making capacity and an interest in testing. However, given the potential impact and irrevocability of the decision, a high threshold for decision-making capacity for these specific decisions may still be reasonable. Such a determination of decision-making capacity involves a detailed assessment of the child (see Chap. 18).

Toward Resolution

When asked about genetic testing, clinicians should consider whether the complexity of the issues involved are ones that they have both the time and information to adequately address or whether it would be best to refer such patients elsewhere. For example, most testing for Huntington disease is done at specialized clinics staffed by neurologists and genetic counselors. On the other hand, many obstetricians provide prenatal genetic testing. As genetic testing becomes commonplace it is more likely that clinicians will receive requests from patients or receive information about new genetic tests marketed by laboratories. For example, in the

past 5 years there have been commercial offerings of genetic susceptibility testing for breast cancer and Alzheimer disease. As with pharmaceuticals, it may be prudent for clinicians to rely on independent sources of information about these tests instead of depending solely on information from the companies that market them. Thus, the diffusion of genetic testing into routine practice will require clinicians to keep up to date on advances in genetic technology and the proper ways of undertaking genetic testing.

When a patient receives results of genetic testing, genetic counseling must be provided. There are a number of complex issues to be discussed. For example, even for those who test negative, issues such as survivor guilt and change of self-image or life expectations need to be addressed.

In the second hypothetical case described at the beginning of this chapter, if an abnormality is found in Sally Jordan's amniocentesis, she will need detailed information and counseling to decide what to do. In addition to Down syndrome (trisomy 21), there is a range of conditions that may be detected, from XYY, which does not typically have clinical manifestations, to trisomy 13, which is always associated with profound mental retardation. The provision of counseling to help families make decisions about terminating a pregnancy can be challenging. Occasionally, expectant parents may choose termination for an apparently "normal variant" such as XYY, while others may choose to continue pregnancies for trisomy 13. It may be difficult for clinicians to see patients make choices that they consider less than ideal, but respect for self-determination suggests that clinicians should continue to support such personal decisions.

Genetic counseling may also be useful after the diagnosis of a genetic condition in a child or adult, as in the third case vignette described above, involving CF. In cases such as these, information about the risk of CF in subsequent children, and carrier risks in siblings of the parents and in their other children, should be discussed. It is also important to realize that individuals with genetic conditions will also be facing their own reproductive decisions as adults and that they too may benefit from discussions of these issues.

The first step in providing genetic testing is to ensure that the clinician is adequately informed about the potential benefits and the risks of the test as well as how to interpret the results; he or she should also have accurate information about the diseases and the effectiveness of any interventions. Dr. Martinez, in the first case above, who is considering testing Ms. Smith for Huntington disease, would need to understand the relationship between the number of trinucleotide repeats[35] and the likelihood of being at risk of Huntington disease as well as the risk of sui-cidal behavior among individuals who are tested.[36] In testing for cancer-susceptibility genes, there may be additional concerns about the probability of getting cancer and the availability and effectiveness of preventive interventions such as prophylactic mastectomies or oophorectomies.[37]

The second step is facilitating decision making so patients can make authentic and informed decisions. This goes beyond just providing information. It involves engaging patients about complex personal issues that they may not have considered fully. Ms. Smith, at risk for Huntington disease, may be asked before testing whether she thinks she will be found to carry the gene. She should be asked to consider how she will feel if she finds out that she will certainly develop Huntington disease and how she would feel is she did not carry the gene. It is essential to know that there have been adverse reactions in some patients who were found not to carry the gene, because they always assumed they did, and the new information changed how they viewed their lives. Rather than both Dr. Martinez and Ms. Smith assuming that a negative result for Huntington disease would be good news, this issue should be explicitly addressed. Similarly, concern about health insurance prob-

lems may depend on Ms. Smith's current and anticipated occupational status. This may be more of a concern if she is self-employed or anticipates changing jobs.

Similarly, Ms. Jordan may wish to consider what she thinks she would do if prenatal diagnosis showed that her fetus had Down syndrome. Ms. Jordan might want to consider what it would mean for her and her family to have a child with a chromosomal abnormality. We all have different conceptions of parenthood and value children differently. Rather than assume that all families have similar views, these issues should be discussed. Further, some people who would not consider abortion may still be interested in prenatal diagnosis to allow them to prepare emotionally for a child with special needs.

Whenever possible, it is best to try to anticipate relevant issues before testing. In some cases it may alter the patient's decision about being tested, but at the very least, it might help prepare patients for unanticipated issues. This may not be as relevant when the primary reason for testing is direct medical benefit. For Johnny and Gail, the sweat tests were obtained to make a diagnosis that would allow appropriate interventions if they had CF. These direct medical benefits for Johnny may override the potential psychosocial concerns about the diagnosis or implications for family members and thus may not be as important to address with Johnny's father, prior to diagnostic testing. However, it is still important to provide counseling afterward about the implications of the results.

After the detection of Huntington disease, Down syndrome, or CF, there are many psychosocial issues to be addressed in genetic counseling. Ms. Smith will need to consider how a positive test for Huntington disease should affect her life plans. Ms. Jordan will need to make a decision about her pregnancy. Johnny's father will need to decide about informing his relatives and testing Gail to see if she is a carrier. The primary care clinician has a role in helping patients address such issues. Although these are more social decisions than medical decisions, they are based on medical information, and the clinician may be in a position to help patients address them. The challenge for the clinician is to minimize the influence of his or her own views in these matters and to help patients make decisions that express their personal values.

There may be a greater role for advice when the decision will have a direct effect on others. The decisions that Mr. Larson faces about whether to inform his estranged sister or test his daughter will directly affect others. His sister may also be a carrier, and this information may affect her reproductive decisions. The clinician can explain these implications and even offer Mr. Larson suggestions on how to present the information to others. However, it does not seem that the likelihood, seriousness, and impact of this information rise to level that would warrant a breach of confidentiality by Dr. Morgan by directly informing the sister.

The situation is slightly different with testing Gail, Mr. Larson's young daughter. Although this case warrants providing directive advice, Dr. Morgan should still not test Gail, even if Bob is not persuaded. Dr. Morgan should explain his concerns about the lack of direct benefit and Gail's future autonomy and privacy. Clinicians who care for children have a fiduciary responsibility to these patients that results in an obligation to avoid doing things clearly not in the interests of children.

Closing Comments

Ethical issues related to genetic testing are bound to become more commonplace, and it will be important for primary care clinicians to keep up to date on advances in genetic testing

technology. A number of guiding principles can assist clinicians who are asked to consider genetic testing in their patients. One is that the informed consent process should be robust and give explicit attention to the potential psychosocial risks of testing. Since these issues are complex, time should be taken to explore the potential medical and social ramifications for each patient. Further, because the concepts of probability, risk, and uncertainty are interpreted in varying ways, it is important to verify the patient's understanding of the specific issues involved. The familial implications of genetic testing should also be explored prior to testing. In the prenatal setting, extra care should be taking to allow for voluntary decision making and to avoid subtle recommendations about testing. In treating children, it may be reasonable to be more directive with parents, particularly when it seems that testing may not be in the interest of the child. Finally, it is important to consider referring patients to genetic counselors if clinicians do not feel that they have the time or experience to address properly the many complex issues associated with genetic testing.

References

1. Holtzman NA: *Proceed with Caution: Predicting Genetic Risks in the Recombinant DNA Era.* Baltimore, Johns Hopkins University Press, 1989.
2. Andrews LB, Fullerton JE, Holtzman NA, Motolsky AG (eds): *Assessing Genetic Risks: Implications for Health and Social Policy.* Washington, DC, National Academy Press; 1994.
3. Holtzman NA, Watson MS (eds): *Promoting Safe and Effective Genetic Testing in the United States: Final Report of the Task Force on Genetic Testing.* Bethesda, MD, National Human Genome Resarch Institute, 1997.
4. President's Commission for the Study of Ethical Problems in Medicine and Biomedical and Behavioral Research. Screening and Counseling for Genetic Conditions: *The Ethical, Social, and Legal Implications of Genetic Screening,*

Counseling, and Education. Washington, DC, US Government Printing Office, 1983.

5. Kevles D: *In the Name of Eugenics: Genetics and Uses of Human Heredity.* Berkeley, CA, University of California Press, 1985.

6. Rothstein MA (ed): *Genetic Secrets: Protecting Privacy and Confidentiality in the Genetic Era.* New Haven, CT, Yale University Press, 1997.

7. Nance MA: Huntington disease: clinical, genetic, and social aspects. *J Geriatr Psychiatry Neurol* 11:61–70, 1998.

8. Brody LC, Biesecker BB: Breast cancer susceptibility genes. BRCA1 and BRCA2. *Medicine* 77: 208–226, 1998.

9. Post SG, Whitehouse PJ, Binstock RH, et al: The clinical introduction of genetic testing for Alzheimer disease: an ethical perspective. *JAMA* 277: 832–836, 1997.

10. Eriksson S: Alpha$_1$-antitrypsin deficiency: lessons learned from the bedside to the gene and back again—historic perspectives. *Chest* 95:181–189, 1989.

11. Burke W, Thomson E, Khoury MJ, et al: Hereditary hemochromatosis: gene discovery and its implications for population-based screening. *JAMA* 280:172–178, 1998.

12. Marteau T, Richards M (eds): *The Troubled Helix: Social and Psychological Implications of the New Human Genetics.* Cambridge, England, Cambridge University Press, 1996.

13. Baker DL, Schuette JL, Uhlman WR (eds): *A Guide to Genetic Counseling.* New York, Wiley-Liss, 1998.

14. McNeil BJ, Pauker SG, Sox HC, Tversky A: On the selection of preferences for alternative therapies. *N Engl J Med* 306:1259–1262, 1982.

15. Geller G, Tambor ES, Chase GA, et al: Incorporation of genetics in primary care practice: will physicians do the counseling and will they be directive? *Arch Fam Med* 2:1119–1125, 1993.

16. Geller G, Botkin JR, Green MJ, et al: Genetic testing for susceptibility to adult-onset cancers: the process and content of informed consent. *JAMA* 277:1467–1474, 1997.

17. Quaid KA, Brandt J. Folstein SE: The decision to be tested for Huntington's disease. *JAMA* 257: 3362, 1987.

18. Wiggins S, Whyte P, Huggins M, et al: The psychological consequences of predictive testing for Huntington's disease. *N Engl J Med* 327:401–405, 1992.

19. Binedell J, Soldan JR, Harper PS: Predictive testing for Huntington's disease: I. Predictors of uptake in South Wales. *Clin Genet* 54:477–488, 1998.

20. Burke W, Daly M, Garber J. Botkin J: Recommendations for follow-up care of individuals with an inherited predisposition to cancer: II. BRCA1 and BRCA2. *JAMA* 277:997–1003, 1997.

21. Marteau TM: Towards informed decisions about prenatal testing: a review. *Prenat Diagn* 15: 1215–1226, 1995.

22. Lippman A, Wilfond BS: Twice-told tales: stories about genetic disorders. *Am J Hum Genet* 51: 936–937, 1992.

23. Le Roux MG, Pascal O, Andre MT, et al: Nonpaternity and genetic counseling. *Lancet* 340:607, 1992.

24. Hudson KL, Rothenberg KH, Andrews LB, et al: Genetic discrimination and health insurance: an urgent need for reform. *Science* 270:391–393, 1995.

25. Billings PR, Kohn MA, de Cuevas M, et al: Discrimination as a consequence of genetic testing. *Am J Hum Genet* 50:476–482, 1992.

26. McAbee GN, Sherman J, Davidoff-Feldman B: Physician's duty to warn third parties about the risk of genetic diseases. *Pediatrics* 102:140–142, 1998.

27. Olick RS: Physician's duty to warn third parties about the risk of genetic diseases (letter). *Pediatrics* 103:855, 1999.

28. American Society of Human Genetics Board of Directors and the American College of Medical Genetics Board of Directors: Points to consider: ethical, legal and psychosocial implications of genetic testing in children and adolescents. *Am J Hum Genet* 57:1233–1241, 1995.

29. Sharpe NF: Presymptomatic testing for Huntington disease: is there a duty to test those under the age of eighteen years? *Am J Med Genet* 46:250–253, 1993.

30. Fanos JH, Johnson JP: Perception of carrier status by cystic fibrosis siblings. *Am J Hum Genet* 57: 431–438, 1995.

31. Clarke A (ed): *The Genetic Testing of Children.* Oxford, England, Bios, 1998.

32. Davis DS: Genetic dilemmas and the child's right to an open future. *Hastings Cent Rep* 27(2):7–15, 1997.

33. Lerman C, Narod S, Schulman K, et al: BRCA1 testing in families with hereditary breast-ovarian cancer: a prospective study of patient decision making and outcomes. *JAMA* 275:1885–1192, 1996.

34. Davis D: Discovery of childrens carrier status for recessive genetic disease: some ethical issues. *Genet Test* 2:323–327, 1998.

35. Bruland O, Almqvist EW, Goldberg YP, et al: Accurate determination of the number of CAG repeats in the Huntington disease gene using a sequence-specific internal DNA standard. *Clin Genet* 55:198–202, 1999.

36. Almqvist EW, Bloch M, Brinkman R, et al: A worldwide assessment of the frequency of suicide, suicide attempts, or psychiatric hospitalization after predictive testing for Huntington disease. *Am J Hum Genet* 64:1293–1304, 1999.

37. Wilfond BS, Rothenberg KH, Thomson EJ, Lerman C: Cancer susceptibility testing: ethical and policy implications for future research and clinical practice. *J Law Med Ethics* 25:243–342, 1997.

Part

2

Problems Related
to Systems
of Care

Howard Brody
Gregg K. VandeKieft

Chapter
7

Managed Care

Dr. Wales is a family physician in a small city of about 100,000 population in the Midwest. About a third of her practice is enrolled in True-Care, a network-model HMO. Although Dr. Wales thinks highly of most of her local subspecialist colleagues, one exception is the local pair of neurosurgeons, who do all of the operations for lumbar disk problems. She has no hard data to support this view (and is not sure just how such data could be obtained), but Dr. Wales feels that if she or a member of her family needed a disk operation, she would go to the larger city 70 miles away.

Dr. Wales sees Mr. Ireland, who has had increasing muscle weakness in one leg and whose magnetic resonance imaging (MRI) scan has just confirmed the clinical impression of a routine herniated disk at L5-S1. She knows that True-Care (Mr. Ireland's insurer) will not pay for routine surgery out of the area, and she also knows that Mr. Ireland has limited financial resources.

Should Dr. Wales tell Mr. Ireland what she thinks about the local neurosurgeons—knowing, practically speaking, that these may be his only option and that what she says would simply make him more worried without offering him any realistic alternative? Should she fill out the referral form to reflect the possibility that Mr. Ireland's case is quite unusual or complicated (even though this is not true), in hopes that True-Care will then approve payment for an out-of-area referral? Or should she simply ask if Mr. Ireland wants to proceed with surgery and, if he does, refer him to the local team?

Scope of the Problem

Managed care represents the most significant shift in American primary care physicians' financial and organizational incentives since the advent of health insurance in the 1930s and 40s. Following the availability of insurance, physicians became accustomed to a fee-for-service system where there was a financial temptation to provide unnecessary or unwanted services. Yet, overnight it seemed, a variety of changes in the funding of health care created new incentives that tempted clinicians to withhold potentially beneficial but expensive services from patients. This change has raised ethical questions that the field of medical ethics is only beginning to address.

Managed care in the United States today is such a heterogeneous phenomenon that a single formal definition would be difficult and poten-tially misleading. However, one helpful definition is: "A managed care organization combines health care insurance with the delivery of a broad range of integrated health services for a population of plan enrollees, financing the services prospectively from a predicted, limited budget."[1]

In this chapter we place the ethical issues facing the primary care clinician within the context of the full range of ethical issues presented by managed care. We next try to fine-tune the ethical analysis by sorting out some of the many issues raised by clinicians when managed care is mentioned, trying to decide which are true ethical concerns and which represent emotional reactions to changes in the status quo. We next look in detail at the gatekeeper role of the primary care clinician, arguing that some role of this sort is inevitable, and then ask what ethical rules might best govern this role. Finally we investigate a specific but instructive issue in the organization of managed care plans: gag rules.

Background Theory and Context

Ethical Issues in Managed Care

Although it is natural to imagine that the primary care physician and patient are the two parties to the transaction that matter most, the issues are much more complicated than that. Managed care affects a complex system of relationships among:

- The patient
- Primary care clinicians (including physicians, nurse practitioners, physician's assistants, etc.)
- Specialist physicians
- Other health professionals (such as mental health, physical therapy)
- Institutions such as hospitals and home health agencies
- Payers (usually large employers)
- Managed care plans, their administrators, and staff
- Other patients enrolled in the managed care plan

In addition, government and the legal system are also becoming increasingly involved.

At the most general level, many of the ethical issues raised by managed care are those of justice in the distribution of health care resources. This means that we cannot resolve all of the issues by appealing to the principle of respect for patients' autonomy, because the questions involve which among many competing patients, each of whom may be fully autonomous, has the *greater* right to a particular scarce resource. That is, managed care is one way of allocating health care, so a discussion of the justice of managed care arrangements must occur within the context of the broader discussion of the ethics of the allocation of resources.

Managed care did not simply appear, nor is it a plot designed solely to annoy clinicians. It is at least a somewhat calculated response to a major social problem, the escalating cost of health care, in a setting where political decisions have been made not to challenge the capitalist nature of the system of paying for health care. The fee-for-service system was seen as being responsible in large part for out-of-control health care costs.

Merely stating that managed care is unethical and should be eliminated presupposes that the fee-for-service system was inherently preferable and less predisposed to ethical conflicts. Such an assumption should not be accepted at face value. Those who proclaim the fee-for-service system's ethical superiority over managed care should, at the least, acknowledge frankly that the fee-for-service system was responsible for ethical problems and conflicts of its own. Simply calling for the elimination of managed care begs at least two questions: (1) What system should be put in its place to deal with the real problems of the affordability of health care? (2) How is that system ethically superior to managed care?

Managed care is open to criticism to the extent that it fails to solve some of the broad policy problems in health care, especially if, instead, it seems to be making the problems worse. For instance, a major question of justice in the United States today is the number of uninsured persons who lack access to decent medical care.[2] Some free-market advocates argued that with managed care, costs would go down, insurance would become more affordable, and more Americans would be insured without the government having to step in. However, the data so far suggest the opposite: the number of uninsured is actually rising as managed care takes over a bigger proportion of the U.S. health care market.[3]

Managed care plans are both providers of health care and businesses. (So, of course, is a private physician's office in a fee-for-service system.) One of the important features of the ethics of managed care is how these functions are intertwined—how business decisions affect the provision of care and vice versa. Distinct ethical questions arise regarding how the business aspects of managed care are run, and many of these questions require a combined approach using business ethics as well as medical ethics.[4] To take just one example, serious questions can be raised about whether for-profit managed care plans fall into a completely different ethical category from nonprofit plans.[5–9]

Finally, one can raise ethical questions about the impact that managed care plans may have on specific medical problems and categories of patients. For instance, commentaries have recently appeared focusing upon the way managed care deals with chronically ill children,[10] mental health,[11] and patients with relatively unusual but very expensive health needs.[12]

In this chapter, we focus on one subset of ethical issues in managed care commonly raised under the heading of "the primary care clinician as gatekeeper." This expression indicates that the patient cannot simply get insurance coverage for whatever services he or she wants without the clinician's approval. Gatekeeping of one sort or another has always been part of primary care. Even under a fee-for-service system, patients could not go to the drugstore and buy morphine without a prescription, and if the patient needed a note from the physician to excuse a work absence, the physician had to decide whether to write one or not. The problem of gatekeeping attributed to managed care is tying the gatekeeper role to financial incentives designed to favor withholding services.[13] In the older system, patients whose physicians would *not* write a prescription might be very angry, but at least they had good reason to believe that these physicians, however wrongheaded, were trying their best to serve patients' interests. After all, physicians who kept their patients happy by writing prescriptions whenever they were wanted could probably be assured a steadier flow of fees. But, in a man-

aged care arrangement, such patients do not have similar reason to trust clinicians who will not write prescriptions, knowing that these clinicians might very well be putting more money into their own pockets by withholding the medication.[14]

The Real Ethical Questions

During the 1990s, the response of clinicians to managed care has been largely negative, or at least the negative voices have been the loudest. If one listens to these voices, one can only conclude that managed care is an unmitigated ethical disaster. Our own position is that managed care poses important ethical challenges for medicine but is not *necessarily* unethical; indeed, done the right way, it could provide an ethically superior form of care. To defend our position and explicate what we think are the real ethical concerns, we must first clear away a lot of misconceptions and rhetoric.[15]

One common source of misconceptions is a readiness to overgeneralize, which the very term *managed care* tempts us to do. A clinician who had a bad experience with Acme HMO, Inc., in Flat Rock, Ohio, in the summer of 1994 might go around saying "managed care is bad," as if all plans in all places at all times are substantially similar. In fact, the diversity of managed care in the United States today is so great that it could be questioned whether the term itself is not a misnomer, obscuring as much as it reveals. If plan A in one town and plan B in the next are both capitated and put the clinicians at risk financially, for instance, then it may look on the surface as if the two plans were substantially similar. Yet if plan A pays primary care clinicians a generous sum for each enrolled patient per month while plan B pays a predictably inadequate sum, the ethical implications of working within those two plans are vastly different.

Another problem is clinicians' tendency to sentimentalize the old fee-for-service system just because it was familiar and tended to reward physicians generously both in money and in control over the workplace. Yet as described above, fee-for-service medicine had its own set of ethical problems, even if familiarity obscured them. And whatever its benefits might have been, the bottom line is that the old fee-for-service system simply became unaffordable.

A third problem is to assume that managed care is ethically inferior because it may reward underservice. This stance reflects the popular American attitude that more is always better. In fact, it can be shown that some patients do better with fewer medical services being provided for them or with less expensive services.[16] Virtually all studies comparing managed care with fee-for-service medicine among comparable patients in the era from 1985 to 1995 showed that either there was no difference in health outcomes or that managed care patients were actually healthier.[17] Managed care is ethically problematic because it inserts a financial incentive that may conflict with what is best for the patient, but no one has yet invented a scheme for financing health care that rewards clinicians when and only when they do exactly what benefits each patient.

Fourth, many clinicians' complaints about managed care amount to complaints about new trends toward reducing clinicians' autonomy. Clinicians are increasingly being monitored, being asked to adhere to clinical practice guidelines, and so forth. This is an uncomfortable change for those trained in the earlier era of physician freedom. But is it an ethical problem for patient care? Certainly, some reductions in clinicians' autonomy limit the ability of the clinician to serve as a patient advocate. And, as a general rule, excessive micromanagement is arguably a bad way to practice medicine (and a bad way to run a business too). But what if adherence to practice guidelines means that clinicians are more likely to remember to provide preventive services like mammograms and Pap tests? And what if close monitoring of clinicians' practices means that almost all patients

are given beta blockers following myocardial infarction (which are proven to be lifesaving but which as many as 50 percent of patients in some studies today do not receive despite an absence of contraindications)? Can we honestly say that these particular losses in physician autonomy are ethically wrong from the patients' point of view?

To address in a sound way the real ethical challenges posed by managed care, we must get past some things we regard as nonissues. From 1965, when Medicare and Medicaid started to pay physicians reasonable if not generous sums for caring for the poor and elderly, until managed care started to make an impact around 1990, American medicine went through a very unusual phase. During that period, physicians could divert huge sums of other people's money to pay for expensive medical care for sick patients.[18] They could do this merely on their own say-so, having to provide minimal or no evidence that the patient was really sick and that, more importantly, the treatment provided a real benefit. Moreover, physicians were also allowed to take a hefty cut of the proceeds for their own incomes. (Although physicians' incomes accounted for only about 10 percent of total health care costs, decisions controlled by physicians accounted for 80 percent, leading to the adage "The most expensive piece of medical equipment is the physician's pen.") In retrospect, this combination of maximum earning potential, maximum power, and minimum accountability was not a sustainable system. Primary care physicians, to be candid, were seldom placed so as to be able to take real advantage of such a system; the excesses that brought the system down in the end were much more the work of procedure-oriented subspecialists. But all clinicians have to live with the consequences. And it seems inevitable to us that, even if managed care were to be wiped off the earth tomorrow, whatever system replaces it will still demand a much higher level of clinician accountability than ever existed in the "good old days."

Toward Resolution

Primary Care Clinicians: Gatekeepers, Patient Advocates, or Both?

The primary care clinician is supposed to serve as a patient advocate, and the incentives of the gatekeeper potentially interfere with fulfilling that obligation.[18] An obvious response to this observation is that primary care clinicians should similarly not be gatekeepers within managed care. So the first question that must be answered is whether it is an option not to function as a gatekeeper. If the answer to that question is no, the next question is how one might most appropriately balance the duties of patient advocacy with gatekeeping responsibilities.

Many critics of clinician gatekeeping assume that one ethical option is simply not to assume the role of gatekeeper at all.[19] These critics often use the term *bedside rationing* to summarize what is wrong with being a gatekeeper.[20] This term implies that even if medical care needs to be rationed, the person to do it is not the clinician taking care of the individual patient at the bedside or in the clinic. That clinician's duty to the patient must begin and end with the duty of advocacy. If the patient gives a detailed medical history and submits his or her body to be examined, it can only be with the expectation that the clinician will be acting solely in his or her interests. The clinician must not be looking to see whether there are other patients somewhere else who might need some scarce medical resources more than the patient does—or, even less, be looking to the size of the clinician's end-of-year bonus.

One problem is that although "bedside rationing" has a nice rhetorical ring, most critics using the term never define it carefully.[21] This lack of definition obscures the possibility that bedside rationing may actually be an inevitable

part of medical practice, whether one is engaged in fee-for-service practice or working within managed care.[22] Two examples help to illustrate this.

First, money is not the only scarce resource in medical care. The clinician's time is similarly scarce. Most clinicians have more than one patient and use some sort of appointment system (see Chap. 8). Some data suggest that patients could benefit much more if routine office visits were longer than average—for instance, up to 30 min per patient.[23] Family physicians, who now average perhaps 10 min for routine visits, could use 30 min as a scheduling minimum if they were willing to take substantial cuts in income and to reduce the size of their practices. How would the much-praised "pure patient advocates" respond in this situation? These clinicians, it would seem, must do whatever will benefit individual patients—regardless of how many other patients might be waiting in line for care (and regardless of the financial implications for clinicians themselves). But this is not how most clinicians act today. They engage in bedside rationing, treating time as a limited commodity with a lot of demand and trying to gauge as best as they can what portion of time each patient needs so that all get decent care. And whenever a patient has an unexpected, acute emergency, patient advocacy wins out and the clinician will spend more time with that patient even if others have to wait or be rescheduled. Is this unethical? Or is it the real world of limited resources and clinical judgment?

A second example may be drawn from an official statement of organized medicine condemning bedside rationing.[20] According to this statement, if a managed care plan or other organization imposes any sort of practice guideline on a clinician, the clinician has an ethical duty to determine whether any patient is an exception to the assumptions underlying the guideline; if so, the clinician should proceed to give that patient the special care needed, not what the guideline says to do. The authors of this statement seem to have assumed that one is rationing at the bedside when one says no to a patient but not when one says yes. But that is to miss the whole point of calling a decision *rationing*. The ethically vital point is not that one says yes or no to the individual but rather that the decision has the net effect of redistributing a scarce resource among a group of people who all want it. A decision to make this patient an exception to the standard guideline and to bestow care that will cost more is implicitly but inevitably a decision to deny care somewhere else in the system (assuming that resources are truly limited—a point to which we will return).[24] From this point of view, either a decision to follow the guideline when one is treating patient A or a decision to ignore the guideline when treating patient B, who has a serious chronic disease and so has special needs, is a bedside rationing decision. Since clinicians in practice must use their judgment on a case-by-case basis and either apply the guideline or not, bedside rationing is inevitable.

The deeper ethical problem with a "pure patient advocacy" ethical stance is that it urges clinicians to put on blinders and to see only the individual patients who happen to be in front of them at that moment. But when resources are scarce, it is essential to consider that clinicians' decisions affect not only one patient but the entire population of patients within the "pool" who must share the same resource base (such as all enrollees in a single managed care plan). Although individual advocacy remains the dominant duty (because the individual patient is especially needy and vulnerable in many cases), clinicians would seem reasonably also to owe *some* duty to the other patients who will be affected by the choice of resource allocation.[25]

If we are correct so far—that bedside rationing is inevitable and that primary care clinicians owe duties both to each individual patient and to the group sharing the same resource base—then what sorts of rules or

guidelines would give us ethical advice on how to balance those duties in practice? Sabin has proposed four such rules that we find especially fruitful, at least as a point of departure.[26] According to Sabin, primary care clinician/gate-keepers should:

1. View themselves as having a dual duty advocating for both the individual patient and for other patients in the group affected by the resource decision.
2. Always try to use the least expensive treatment unless there is substantial evidence that a more expensive treatment will be more effective for this patient.
3. Spend some portion of time reviewing and helping to formulate the rules and practices of the plan as a whole and assuring that these practices are fair.
4. If the guidelines developed by a fair plan call for the individual patient not to receive some treatment when the clinician thinks that treatment might offer substantial benefit, then *both* withhold the treatment (at least for now) *and* inform the patient of the clinician's judgment.

These suggested rules are counterintuitive. It is not uncommon for clinicians to think that their duty is to be an advocates for the individual patient, to do whatever will help the patient regardless of cost, to spend all their available time doing direct patient care and to assiduously avoid committees and administrative work, and always to side with the patient whenever it is a case of the patient versus the plan. So how can these rules be justified?

Let us focus especially on the second and fourth of Sabin's rules. Rule #2 might not be needed if American physicians had a long history of conservative practice; but, as above, the opposite is true. Many things are done commonly today not because there is good evidence that the patient will benefit but simply because that is the way it has always been done. We know, for instance, that many clinicians still prescribe antibiotics for viral illnesses even though they do not work and worsen the society-wide problem of bacterial resistance. In such a high-cost, low-evidence world, we cannot simply assume that having clinicians follow their own "clinical judgment" is doing what is really best for the patient. There is at least a substantial chance that the patient will not benefit and that the only result will be a resource depletion whose impact will be felt by other needy patients down the road.

Therefore, it makes sense to reverse the usual thought processes that privilege individual clinical judgment. Accordingly, the good clinician should perhaps first ask, "What is the lowest-cost, medically appropriate treatment for this condition?" and only then ask, "Is there good evidence that a more expensive treatment would provide this patient with substantially more benefit?" If such a sequence is followed with critical thinking and with a good grasp of the available medical evidence, then there is a greater likelihood that the clinician will achieve both goals at once—doing what is needed and desirable for the individual patient while at the same time assuring, for the good of the entire group of patients, that resources are not wasted. Note that "substantial evidence" of benefit need not necessarily be from a large-scale randomized controlled trial; in many cases the clinician's informed hunch will be good enough evidence, at least in the absence of any data to the contrary. However, in our case study, it is not quite clear what would make Dr. Wales's opinion about the inferiority of the local neurosurgeons "substantial" enough to require her to seek an out-of-area referral for Mr. Ireland.

Rule #4 brings up the ethics of a practice that has become commonplace in managed care: "gaming the system" (one of the temptations facing Dr. Wales).[27] *Gaming the system* refers to the common practice of redescribing the diagnosis or the clinical condition in a way that stretches the truth or is even frankly fraudulent in order to get the plan to pay for some test or treatment that is not strictly "covered" under the plan's criteria (see Chap. 2). The alternative, openly challenging the rules or trying to get an exception to the rules for a particular patient, is usually very time-consuming and might not work.

Rule #4, on inspection, turns out to be very complicated because it presumes that the clinician has accepted the duty of "being a good citizen" of the plan and has been actively involved in trying to make the plan work as fairly as possible for all patients (rule 3). This means, in turn, (1) that the rules are administered fairly, so that if one patient truly needs exceptional care, the appeals process to justifiably break the rule is reasonably streamlined, and (2) that the rules are based on good medical information, so that if patients really derive benefit from certain medical interventions, the plan covers those interventions. If the plan is that sort of fair plan, then the case where a treatment is really beneficial but the rules of the plan deny it anyway will arise very rarely; in such a rare case, the patient should still have a route of appeal that is likely to work quickly enough in light of the urgency of the clinical situation.

If the plan is fair, then what should the ethical clinician do? Merely to go around the rules and to find a way to get the treatment for the patient despite the initial denial (which would usually be a form of gaming) is to cease to be a good citizen within the plan and to give away resources which the plan has *fairly* decided really belong to other patients[27] But not to tell the patient that this other treatment, which is beneficial in the clinician's judgment, exists would be to fail as an individual patient advocate. The ideal outcome would be either that the patient, with the clinician's help, files an appeal and gets the treatment soon or else that the patient decides to spend personal funds to get the treatment if it truly cannot be covered by the plan.

We see that a good deal hinges upon the overall justice of the plan.[28] Whether gaming the system is ethically acceptable might be a different matter if we were to suppose that the plan

(1) excluded clinicians from membership on the key committees that define plan policies; (2) was a for-profit plan that last year spent only 75 percent of its funds on patient care, paying a good deal of the rest as dividends to stockholders[6]; and (3) as a result of its profitability, paid its chief executive a special bonus of several million dollars.

In discussing the pros and cons of gaming the system, we must add to the ethical concerns the question of whether gaming is a prudent long-term strategy. Suppose that clinicians routinely engaged in gaming. Then, plans could not take the clinicians' statements as to the patients' diagnoses and care needs at face value; they would know that clinicians routinely lied to get more services for their patients. In turn, that would predictably lead plans to try new techniques to monitor clinicians' decisions. The end result could be even more micromanagement, which would drives the clinicians crazy and in fact prompted them to try to game the system in the first place. Thus gaming the system turns out, in the long run, to be both unsustainable and counterproductive.[27]

What Sabin's list of rules suggests is that we can begin to sketch out a framework for balancing the two important duties owed by the primary care clinician as gatekeeper: the duty to be a strong advocate for the individual patient and the duty to conserve resources, so that all patients in the plan will receive adequate care to meet their current and future needs. Doing this, however, requires changing some of the attitudes and habits acquired in a fee-for-service environment. In particular, it demands active involvement in the management of the plan itself.

Gag Rules

Sabin's rule #4 requires that the clinician tell the patient about the possibly beneficial treatment even if it is not considered a covered benefit by the plan. That rule, in turn, requires that the plan place no restrictions upon the clinician's freedom to communicate such information to the patient.

In early 1997, national attention was focused upon "gag rules" in managed care contracts that restricted clinician-patient communications in one of two ways.[29] Clinicians might be prevented from disclosing to patients specific treatments or treatment options that were not covered by the plan. Or, more generally, clinicians might be prevented from disclosing to the patient the incentives under which the clinician operated, lest the patient learn that the incentives might interfere with the clinician's judgment of what was best for the patient.[30] In Dr. Wales's case, a gag rule might prohibit her from disclosing to Mr. Ireland her view than an "out of plan" surgeon was superior to one with whom the plan has an affiliation.

Where did these rules come from? In all likelihood they arose from a common business practice: the antidisparagement clause.[30] If you go to work as a salesperson for Ajax Corporation, your boss expects you to try to sell the customers Ajax products and especially not to tell them that some other company's product would actually meet their needs better, even if that is what you truly believe. So it is routine for business contracts to contain clauses preventing employees from saying anything to customers that would cause them to lose faith in the corporation or its products and services. At least some managed care gag rules seem to have been these standard antidisparagement clauses, transported into the medical setting without any consideration of the fact that the relationship between a clinician and a patient is ethically different from the relationship between a salesperson and a customer. However, at least some gag rules were quite specifically tailored for the medical setting, suggesting that these plans foresaw how clinicians might feel obligated to communicate some information to patients that was not in the plan's interests.

Once various sources blew the whistle on this practice, the response was swift. The American

Medical Association denounced gag rules and even offered its member physicians the services of its legal staff to determine whether a questionable phrase in a contract was a gag rule or not.[31] Several state legislatures immediately passed laws banning gag rules from managed care contracts.[30] Recognizing a burgeoning public relations disaster, the managed care industry first denied that its plans had any gag rules; then it removed them from clinicians' contracts.[30]

What are the ethical implications of this episode? First, gag rules illustrate one extreme end of a spectrum of business practices in medicine. At that end of the spectrum, something that might be acceptable in other business arrangements is simply flat-out wrong in medicine. The bedrock principle that underlies the clinician-patient relationship is the clinician's duty of disclosure of relevant information to the patient; without this principle, there could be no notion of informed consent (see Chaps. 11 and 19). If the clinician is being paid in a certain way that could affect the clinician's judgment about what treatment to offer the patient, then that information is arguably relevant and the patient has a right to know it. One could debate whether the plan or the clinician has the primary responsibility to communicate this information; at any rate, it is quite wrong to conceal the information if the patient asks for it. And certainly, if the clinician knows of some potentially beneficial treatment that the plan does not provide, the clinician is obligated to disclose that information as well. Perhaps the patient can find a way to secure that treatment, either inside the plan or outside it, or perhaps not. But in any event, assuring that the patient has at least the option of seeking the treatment is a far more critical ethical value than making sure that the patient does not think badly about the plan.

Another way to conceptualize the ethical problem with gag rules envisions the relationship between patient and clinician and patient and plan as built on trust and trustworthiness. The ethical relationship is one in which the patient feels entitled to trust the clinician or the plan and in which the clinician and plan act toward the patient in ways designed to build trust. But trust implies that critical information will be available when needed. It is precisely when trust has been called into question that the response "Just trust me" is totally inadequate. Therefore a plan that inserts a gag rule into a contract or a clinician who signs that contract is automatically acting in an untrustworthy manner.[14]

Hall and Berenson, suggesting practical rules for ethics in managed care, propose that managed care policies ought to pass what one might label a "red-faced test." If the general public knew that the plan was operating according to this policy, would the operators of the plan be embarrassed? If so, the policy is probably unethical.[32] Thus, gag rules fail this test in two different ways. When the public found out that such rules existed, the industry obviously had a very red face. And, by trying to prevent the disclosure of information that might cause embarrassment were patients to know it, plans were acknowledging in advance that they knew they could not pass the red-faced test but proposed to implement those unethical policies anyway.

A second major ethical implication of gag rules is the reminder that there are some situations in which it would be unethical for a clinician to sign a managed care contract. In most cases, the violations of ethical principles will not be so obvious or egregious; a clinician of integrity could still sign on with the plan, hoping to work within it to make it more fair and reasonable for the patients. But in the most extreme cases—represented by gag rules and by capitation budgets that are predictably too low to provide minimally decent services to the patients—the ethical clinician simply cannot sign a contract with the plan even if that plan dominates the local market and not signing threatens the clinician's livelihood. But it would be naive to suggest that such advice will not deeply threaten the financial interests of some primary care clinicians. Still, it is inescapably the case that clinicians who sign contracts with a plan while knowing of its ethical deficiencies cannot simply wash their hands and blame the plan if their patients later suffer harm as a result.

Closing Comments

Physicians like Dr. Wales are correct to worry about the impact that managed care will have on the ethics of practice. A few aspects of managed care, such as gag rules, turn out simply to be ethically indefensible. But many other managed care practices, on careful scrutiny, turn out to be justifiable or not depending upon a detailed analysis of the circumstances.[26,33]

How Dr. Wales advises Mr. Ireland will depend, therefore, upon a number of considerations. The basic ethical tension is between the duty of individual patient advocacy and the duty to conserve scarce resources to meet the predictable needs of other patients. If the plan is reasonably fair to all parties—and we would hope that if it were not, Dr. Wales would have refused to sign a contract—then money spent to provide more expensive care for Mr. Ireland is money that will not be available for some other patient. If Dr. Wales has good-quality data to show that Mr. Ireland is likely to have a substantially better outcome with the out-of-plan surgeons, she should advise this as a good patient advocate. If the data are less compelling or the difference in benefit is less substantial, Dr. Wales has a correspondingly greater obligation to adhere to the "rules" of the plan—as long as she answers all of Mr. Ireland's questions honestly and withholds no key information from him.

In assessing circumstances like these and drawing sound ethical conclusions, primary care clinicians will be challenged to put aside con-

cerns over personal autonomy, power, and income[34] in order to focus on the actual well-being and rights of patients.

References

1. Buchanan A: Managed care: rationing without justice, but not unjustly. *J Health Polit Policy Law* 23:617–634, 1998.
2. Hafner-Eaton C: Physician utilization disparities between the uninsured and insured: comparisons of the chronically ill, acutely ill, and well non-elderly populations. *JAMA* 269:787–792, 1993.
3. Smith BM: Trends in health care coverage and financing and their implications for policy. *N Engl J Med* 337:1000–1003, 1997.
4. Mariner WK: Business vs. medical ethics: conflicting standards for managed care. *J Law Med Ethics* 23:236–246, 1995.
5. Gray BH: Trust and trustworthy care in the managed care era. *Health Affairs* 16:34–49, 1997.
6. Kuttner R: Must good HMOs go bad? First of two parts: the commercialization of prepaid group health care. *N Engl J Med* 338:1558–1563, 1998.
7. Kuttner R: Must good HMOs go bad? Second of two parts: the search for checks and balances. *N Engl J Med* 338:1635–1639, 1998.
8. Hasan MM: Let's end the nonprofit charade. *N Engl J Med* 334:1055–1057, 1996.
9. Nudelman PM, Andrews LM: The "value added" of not-for-profit health plans. *N Engl J Med* 334:1057–1059, 1996.
10. Neff JM, Anderson G: Protecting children with chronic illness in a competitive marketplace. *JAMA* 274:1866–1869, 1995.
11. Sabin JE, Daniels N: Determining "medical necessity" in mental health practice: a study of clinical reasoning and a proposal for insurance policy. *Hastings Cent Rep* 24:5–13, 1994.
12. Daniels N, Sabin JE: Last chance therapies and managed care: pluralism, fair procedures, and legitimacy. *Hastings Cent Rep* 28:27–41, 1998.
13. Pellegrino ED: Rationing health care: the ethics of medical gatekeeping. *J Contemp Health Law Pol* 2:23–45, 1986.
14. Mechanic D, Schlesinger M: The impact of managed care on patients' trust in medical care and their physicians. *JAMA* 275:1693–1697, 1996.

15. Brody H: Common fallacies that stall discussions about ethical issues in managed care. *Fam Med* 28:657–660, 1996.

16. Franks P, Clancy CM, Nutting PA: Gatekeeping revisited—protecting patients from overtreatment. *N Engl J Med* 327:424–429, 1992.

17. Miles SH, Koepp R: Comments on the AMA report "Ethical Issues in Managed Care." *J Clin Ethics* 6:306–311, 1995.

18. Morreim EH: *Balancing Act: The New Medical Ethics of the New Medicine's Economics*. Boston, Kluwer, 1991.

19. Levinsky NG: The doctor's master. *N Engl J Med* 311:1573–1575, 1984.

20. Council on Ethical and Judicial Affairs AMA. Ethical issues in managed care. *JAMA* 273:330–335, 1995.

21. Ubel PA, Goold S: Recognizing bedside rationing: clear cases and tough calls. *Ann Intern Med* 126:74–80, 1997.

22. Ubel PA, Arnold RM: The unbearable rightness of bedside rationing: physician duties in a climate of cost containment. *Arch Intern Med* 155:1837–1842, 1995.

23. Kaplan SH, Gandek B, Greenfield S, et al: Patient and visit characteristics related to physicians' participatory decision-making style. *Med Care* 33:1176–1187, 1995.

24. Daniels N: Why saying no to patients in the United States is so hard. *N Engl J Med* 314:1380–1383, 1986.

25. La Puma J: Anticipated changes in the doctor-patient relationship in the managed care and managed competition of the Health Security Act of 1993. *Arch Fam Med* 3:665–671, 1994.

26. Sabin JE: A credo for ethical managed care in mental health practice. *Hosp Commun Psychiatry* 45:859–860, 1994.

27. Morreim EH: Gaming the system: dodging the rules, ruling the dodgers. *Arch Intern Med* 151:443–447, 1991.

28. Clancy CM, Brody H: Managed care: Jekyll or Hyde? *JAMA* 273:338–339, 1995.

29. Woolhandler S, Himmelstein DU: Extreme risk—the new corporate proposition for physicians. *N Engl J Med* 333:1706–1708, 1995.

30. Brody H, Bonham V: Gag rules and trade secrets in managed care contracts: ethical and legal concerns. *Arch Intern Med* 157:2037–2043, 1997.

31. Gianelli DM: Bound and gagged: AMA—unethical managed care rules stifle communication. *Am Med News* 39(5):1,26, 1996.

32. Hall MA, Berenson RA: Ethical practice in managed care: a dose of realism. *Ann Intern Med* 128:395–402, 1998.

33. Pearson SD, Sabin JE, Emanuel EJ: Ethical guidelines for physician compensation based on capitation. *N Engl J Med* 339:689–693, 1998.

34. Sobieraj J: Truth or consequences (letter). *N Engl J Med* 339:411, 1998.

Susan Dorr Goold

Conflicts of Interest and Obligation

Dr. Edwards is a second-year resident on an emergency room rotation. She is seeing a patient with atypical chest pain who has risk factors for coronary artery disease. Although she thinks the patient should probably be admitted to rule out a myocardial infarction, she is worried about the response she will get from the admitting team. Last time she admitted a patient to them the senior resident called it "soft," and she knows that they have already admitted many patients today.

Dr. Singh looks at his schedule and groans. Mr. Ehrlich is one of his first patients scheduled and routinely takes up so much time asking questions and raising concerns that Dr. Singh runs late for the rest of the day and has to rush through seeing some of his other patients.

Scope of the Problem

The very phrase "conflict of interest" conjures images of adversaries ready to fight for their own interests—an image that does not fit comfortably with the clinician-patient relationship. Yet the phrase, which has a legal origin, describes a fluctuating set of circumstances in which fiduciaries may be too strongly tempted to act in their own rather than in their clients' interests. This chapter reviews the concept of conflict of interest, the related concept of conflict of obligation, the aspects of these conflicts that are important for clinicians to recognize and consider, and the impact they can have on the trust-based clinician-patient relationship.[1,2]

Background Theory and Context

Types of Conflicts

Clinicians are fiduciaries or agents of their patients. They are required by law and professional ethics to pursue the patient's good in the same way as an attorney or financial broker is required to pursue a client's good. A *conflict of interest* can be narrowly defined as a set of circumstances in which the clinician's own interest conflicts with his or her patient's.*

Other conflicts need to be distinguished from conflicts of interest. *Conflicts of obligation* occur when a clinician, ethically or legally, must con-

---

*Conflict between clinicians' interests and patients' interests must be distinguished from *within patient* conflict of interest when a single patient has multiple goals or preferences. For example, a *patient* may have a conflict of interest when he or she considers delaying a surgery until after a vacation. This is not a conflict of interest between the clinician's interests and those of the patient.

sider the interests of two or more parties.[3] This occurs regularly in office practice, as clinicians must consider the needs of waiting patients when they choose to spend more or less time with a current patient. The medical researcher likewise considers the needs of future patients, perhaps to the detriment of current ones. Similarly, a clinician may have an obligation to attend an important family event, so that "family obligations" may conflict with the needs of patients.

A *conflict of value* occurs when actions directly or indirectly undermine professional values. Investment in tobacco firms, for instance, does not pose a conflict of interest, as the interests of the clinician's individual patients are not significantly affected, but it does pose a conflict between professional values (promoting health and preventing illness) and personal values (achieving return on investment). However, in some cases, conflicts of obligation and value overlap conflicts of interest. This chapter addresses conflicts of interest and conflicts of obligation, since both challenge the clinician's ethical duty to serve his or her patients' interests.

Examples of Conflicts

There are many examples of conflicts of interest for clinicians (Table 8-1). Clinician ownership of facilities providing ancillary services to which patients may be referred by an individual clinician can cause a conflict between the clinician's interest in a profitable investment and the patient's interest in getting the best-quality, most convenient service[4,5] (see Chap. 9). The way clinicians are paid for their services inevitably causes a conflict of interest. In any system of financial reimbursement, clinicians are paid better for some things (e.g., procedures) than others (e.g., advance care planning) (see Chaps. 7 and 20). Clinicians may have interests in career advancement (e.g., publication, recognition, reputation) that can influence clinical decisions

Table 8-1

Conflicts of Interest and Conflicts of Obligation—Examples

Conflicts of interest
Investment in medical facilities
Reimbursement for services
Gifts from industry (e.g., pharmaceutical companies)
Industry sponsorship of research
Pursuit of nonmonetary goods (e.g., reputation, power, personal fulfillment)
Peer pressure (e.g., to not admit a patient)

Conflicts of obligation
Clinical research
Educating clinicians in training
Needs of other patients for time
Family needs

or recommendations. A clinician who wishes to publish an unusual case study, for instance, may pursue a diagnostic workup that has little benefit for the patient. A specialist may feel pressure to please referring doctors in order to continue receiving referrals (see Chap. 9). For instance, a cardiologist may perform a catheterization for borderline indications in order to fulfill the (assumed) expectations of a referring clinician. Clinicians accept pens, meals, and other gifts (large and small) from pharmaceutical companies who hope to (and do) influence prescribing behavior that may or may not promote patients' interests.[6,7] Peer pressure and acceptance can be powerful incentives for medical decision making: residents in the emergency room cringe at the label "sieve" and are often loath to admit patients to their colleagues. All of these represent conflicts of interest.

There are numerous instances of conflicts of obligation as well. Since more than one patient may benefit from the clinician's limited time and effort, conflicts between patients' interests are inevitable. Medical educators may impose inconvenience, repeat examinations, a higher risk of complications, and unnecessary tests on patients for the good of future patients and current trainees.[8] Clinician-investigators consider the advancement of medical knowledge (and hence the good of future patients) in decisions and recommendations for patients as well as in the distribution of their time and talent.[9] The needs and demands of family, friends, church, and community pull at clinicians as much as (or more than) any individual patient. Some types of practice, such as occupational medicine and forensic medicine, inevitably serve two masters.[10] Serving two masters is morally problematic in part because it may undermine the trust-based clinician-patient relationship.

What Is Trust?

Trust is the foundation of relationships between clinicians and patients. These interpersonal trust relationships have moral content: fidelity to trust is morally praiseworthy while betrayal of trust is morally blameworthy.[14] The need to trust and the reliance on that trust are especially important in health care for several reasons. First, health is a primary good. It is necessary to achieve one's life goals and contributes to equality of opportunity.[15] Second, the sick are emotionally, physically, and spiritually vulnerable. Imbalances of knowledge and power, which contribute to this vulnerability, are present in interpersonal health care relationships to a greater extent than they are in other arenas.[16] Third, clinician-patient relationships occupy a central role during times when individuals confront physical weakness, suffering, death, and birth. These are life events with profound, even spiritual meaning.

To pursue his or her patients' good, the clinician must be trusted by them with private information, with their bodies (even to the extent of invading them with knives), and with their health and well-being.[17] Clinicians accept the trust of patients in a general way upon entry into the profession and add to and personalize

their moral obligation related to this trust when they enter into a relationship with a patient. Clinicians are morally required to justify or deserve trust (to be trustworthy).

Patients grant substantial power and discretion over health-related decisions to clinicians.[16] Patients expect that clinicians will act for their well-being and their interests. Along with these expectations of beneficence are expectations of advocacy, expecting the clinician to act on one's behalf in negotiations or dealings with third parties, such as insurance companies. Finally, patients expect competence and even good outcomes. All of these moral expectations—of beneficence, advocacy, and competence—are characteristic of trust-based clinician-patient relationships. These expectations can be influenced by real or perceived conflicts of interest or obligation.

What conditions predispose to stronger or weaker trust relationships? It is important to distinguish between actions that affect the strength of trust and those that affect its justification. Some behaviors, such as exhibiting compassion, both strengthen and justify trust. Some, like public relations, affect perceptions and thus trust but do not justify it. Other behaviors, for instance proper sterile technique or self-education, may not be perceived by patients but still justify the doctor as trustworthy. Finally, some actions, like deception, both weaken trust and justify distrust.

Toward Resolution

Evaluating Conflicts in Practice

As evidenced by the examples above, conflicts of interest and obligation are ubiquitous in primary care medicine. The ethical question is to what degree a particular conflict represents morally unacceptable behavior. To determine which conflicts are morally acceptable or morally blameworthy, we need to examine the characteristics of the conflict in a particular circumstance (Fig. 8-1). A conflict of interest may be *avoidable* or *unavoidable*, the result of *legitimate* or *illegitimate* interests, or *reasonable* or *unreasonable* interests, and it may have varying impact on patients' trust in physicians and the physician's willingness to serve a given patient's interest.

AVOIDABLE OR UNAVOIDABLE

First, to what extent is the conflict avoidable or unavoidable? A clinician's desire to leave work at a reasonable hour may conflict with the patient's desire or need for further education or explanations. This is an unavoidable conflict. The way clinicians are paid always generates a conflict of interest. Fee-for-service payment may

encourage more visits and procedures; salaries may discourage "adding on" urgent appointments; and prepayment may discourage the provision of needed services.[11] Conversely, investments in medical care facilities or the acceptance of gifts from pharmaceutical companies are avoidable, conflicts of interest. *Unavoidable conflicts*, which cannot be eliminated, cannot be considered morally blameworthy. Rather, efforts can and should be made to minimize their impact. On the other hand, *avoidable conflicts* of interest, because of effects (perceived or real) on the clinician's duty to promote the patient's interests, should be avoided. Conflicts of obligation, of course, are inherently unavoidable, since they represent competing duties to two or more parties. Nevertheless, again, efforts to minimize the impact of such conflicts should be made.

Figure 8-1   Proposed algorithm for evaluating conflicts of interest or obligation in clinical practice.

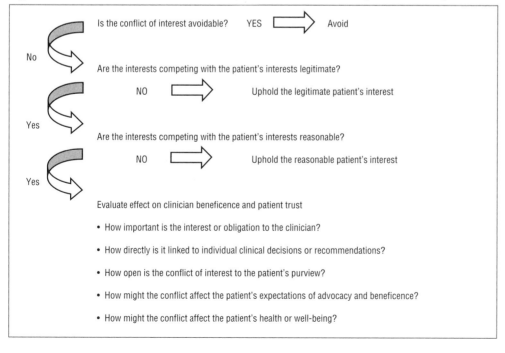

Legitimate or Illegitimate, Reasonable or Unreasonable

Once a conflict is known to be unavoidable, one must ask to what extent the clinician's interest is legitimate or reasonable. *Illegitimate* interests on the part of the clinician may be morally blameworthy to begin with, as in desires to harm others, or may be morally indifferent until they conflict with patients' interests or become manifest in the clinician's role as a clinician. For example, although the desire for sexual gratification is legitimate in some contexts, it becomes illegitimate when pursued in the context of the clinician-patient relationship.[12] Even *legitimate* interests may become unreasonable if pursued too vigorously. Time for oneself and one's family and the right to a "fair wage" are legitimate, reasonable expectations. The desire for a grandiose home or to avoid being available to patients after hours are, arguably, legitimate but perhaps unreasonable.

Reasonable and legitimate clinician interests that unavoidably conflict with patient interests must be further evaluated for their impact on patients' trust of clinicians. Reasonable and legitimate conflicting obligations to others (e.g., waiting patients) should be similarly examined for their impact on this trust.[13]

Effects on Clinician Beneficence and Patient Trust

Conflicts of interest (even or perhaps especially when disclosed) may affect patients' expectations for clinicians' beneficence and their trust in clinicians. The *intrusiveness* of this interest of the clinician's into individual treatment decisions and recommendations is a key concern. How likely is it that this interest will influence a recommendation for a particular patient?

The intrusiveness of conflicting clinician interests affects expectations of advocacy and beneficence and has two main components. First, the *strength* of the interest—that is, the amount of benefit or harm that could potentially accrue to the clinician—affects the likelihood that the interest will, consciously or subconsciously, influence patient care decisions and thus weaken and undermine trust. Second, the *linkage* of a clinician's self-interest to an individual patient care decision affects its intrusiveness. For instance, suppose a clinician wants to attend his or her son's school play. The importance attached to attendance at that event and the anticipated enjoyment of doing so are measures of the strength of the clinician's obligation and interest. The conflict of interest (and obligation, in this case) will have an indirect linkage to decisions made throughout the day, including the amount of time spent with individual patients. The indirect linkage for most of the patients that day makes the conflict minimally intrusive. However, in the case of the last patient of the day who—because of complexity, medical need, or demands—threatens to take a substantial period of time and directly contribute to the clinician's tardiness to the school play, the linkage is direct; every minute with this patient makes the clinician a minute later for the play. Thus the conflict, although of similar strength for all patients throughout the day, is most evident and salient in the case of the last patient and has the greatest potential to influence the clinician's judgment as to the amount of time necessary for that patient; it has the most potential to affect beneficence, advocacy, and even competence.

A similar example could be derived for a clinician's investment in a medical care facility. The strength of the conflict of interest is proportional to the financial gain or loss the clinician can sustain and the importance the clinician attaches to it. The linkage is most direct in the (usually illegal) "kickback" form of compensation, where clinicians receive a specific dollar amount per referred patient.[5] It is least direct where the clinician, as one of many investors, has a small interest in the overall profitability of the center. Small gifts from drug company detailers—personal notepads and pens, for instance—are moderately linked to individual patient care decisions because they are often present during or near encounters with patients and have been documented to influence decisions.[6,7] However, they are relatively weak, because their presence or absence is not usually of great importance to clinicians. Of course, increasing the value of the gifts (expensive dinners, travel, research money, honoraria) increases the strength and hence the intrusiveness of this type of conflict of interest.

Disclosure of and *openness* about conflicts has several *potential effects on patients' trust* in clinicians. For patients previously unaware of such conflicts, "opening their eyes" to them may weaken trust. Honest communication about financial incentives to limit prescription drug costs, for instance, may lead patients to wonder if, when given a prescription, economics or effectiveness is driving the choice. On the other hand, conflicts that are hidden from patients can, if discovered, lead to an even greater sense of betrayal. Patients who find out about the same financial incentives for drug costs from someone other than the clinician are likely to be additionally distrustful because of the perceived deception. Patients who hear via a newspaper that their esteemed clinician was paid a great deal to promote a particular health care product are likely to feel profound betrayal and distrust.

Finally, conflicts of interest and obligation need to be considered for their *potential impact* on the patient's health and well-being—on the patient's expectations for a good outcome. For example, when the last patient of the day is having crushing, substernal chest pain, the consequences for the patient of rushing the visit are potentially devastating. On the other hand, explaining one more time the content of a low-fat diet or how to quit smoking has both less urgency and less overall impact on individual patient's health and well-being. In the first example, the clinician's interest must be subjugated, at least until the patient is stabilized and transferred to an appropriate site of care. In the second example, postponement of the beneficial service of counseling can be done with little or no immediate harm.

One can evaluate the investment in a medical testing facility in a similar fashion. Although in some communities such investment may be essential in order to have the facility available at all, usually the clinician's investment is not necessary. Even where the strength of the incentive is low (e.g., the clinician has a 1 percent interest in the testing facility) and the linkage indirect, one must not underestimate the impact over time on the population of patients of potentially unnecessary tests because of the availability of and financial interest in testing facilities.

Similarly, pharmaceutical companies' influence on prescribing affects the public health through antibiotic resistance and excess cost. Patients, third-party payers, and society bear the costs and risks of less appropriate or more expensive drugs as a result of the influence of pharmaceutical company gifts, events, and advertising.

Resolving the Representative Vignettes

In the first hypothetical case described at the beginning of this chapter, Dr. Edwards, a resident confronts a conflict between the patient's well-being and her own reputation (that is, a conflicting obligation to her patient and her colleagues). Absent complete apathy on her part for her reputation or for her colleagues, this conflict is unavoidable; she has a legitimate interest in her professional reputation. Concern for being labeled "soft on admissions" might be considered unreasonable, although one could argue that peer regard is an important mechanism of social control and thus a reasonable concern. The admitting team may or may not have legitimate, reasonable interests in avoiding another admission; absent more details about the workload and training program, we are unable to tell. Thus, we have moved (in Fig. 8-1) to evaluating this conflict's impact on the clinician and the patient's trust. How much importance does this clinician place on her reputation? The more important it is to her, the more influence this conflict could have on her willingness to act to achieve the patient's well-being. In this case, she also perceives a very direct linkage between her decision for the patient and her reputation; if she admits a "soft" case, she faces ridicule. The conflict is, generally, not open to the patient's purview; it would be a rare patient indeed who realized that house officers are loath to admit patients to their colleagues. She could disclose the conflict by telling the patient, "The admitting team is extremely busy today and is likely to balk at another admission, so I'm reluctant to admit you." In this case, the conflict certainly affects the clinician's willingness to advocate for her patient and pursue the patient's good. It might even, should reputation "win" over beneficence, result in a deleterious outcome for the patient. Accordingly, in honoring the trust inherent to the clinician-patient relationship, the resident ought to advocate for her patient and have her admitted. Perhaps explaining this decision-making process to her colleagues might mitigate the presumption that she has regarding the impact on her reputation.

We can pursue a similar analysis for the second case, involving a conflict of obligation, since it is the later patients who will suffer for the time afforded Mr. Ehrlich. Like all conflicts of obligation, this one is unavoidable. All patients take some time, and this, in turn, affects the time available for later patients. The obligation to spend time with patients is legitimate, although the expectation for huge amounts of time is, in this case, unreasonable. Following the algorithm, it is important for clinicians to "uphold the reasonable patient interest." In other words, Mr. Ehrlich should be constrained from taking extreme amounts of time per visit, perhaps by having him come back frequently for shorter visits.

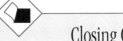

Closing Comments

Trust in clinicians is strongly influenced by public perceptions of clinicians generally, as well as by patients' perceptions of their individual clinicians. Reports of the medical profession's financial investment in medical facilities, pharmaceutical companies, or other ventures can undermine the trust that individual patients have in individual clinicians. On the flip side, individual clinicians, members of a medical and professional community, can influence the relationships that *other* clinicians will have with their patients in the present and the future by strengthening and deserving the trust placed in them by their patients. Conflicts of interest that are avoidable or represent illegitimate or unreasonable interests should be avoided in order to strengthen and justify the trust of individual patients and, generally, in the medical profession. Those conflicts that are unavoidable must be recognized and then evaluated for their impact on patients' trust, health, and well-being. Those unavoidable conflicts that undermine trust in the medical profession or individual clinicians through concealment, strength, linkage to patient care decisions, or their impact on patient well-being should be "reengineered" to minimize their effect.

References

1. Khushf G: A radical rupture in the paradigm of modern medicine: conflicts of interest, fiduciary obligations, and the scientific ideal. *J. Med Philos* 23:98–122, 1998.
2. Rodwin MA: The organized American medical profession's response to financial conflicts of interest: 1890–1992. *Milbank Q* 70:703–741, 1992.

3. Toulmin S: Divided loyalties and ambiguous relationships. *Soc Sci Med* 23:783–787, 1986.

4. American Medical Association, Council on Ethical and Judicial Affairs: Conflicts of interest: physician ownership of medical facilities. *JAMA* 267:2366–2369, 1992.

5. Relman AS: "Self-referral"—what's at stake? *N Engl J Med* 327:1522–1524, 1992.

6. Lurie N, Rich EC, Simpson DE, Meyer J, et al: Pharmaceutical representatives in academic medical centers: interaction with faculty and housestaff. *J Gen Intern Med* 5:240–243, 1990.

7. Chren MM, Landefeld CS: Physicians' behavior and their interactions with drug companies: a controlled study of physicians who requested additions to a hospital drug formulary. *JAMA* 271:684–689, 1994.

8. Shooner C: The ethics of learning from patients. *Can Med Assoc J* 156:535–538, 1997.

9. Batchelor JA, Briggs CM: Subject, project or self? Thoughts on ethical dilemmas for social and medical researchers. *Soc Sci Med* 39:949–954, 1994.

10. Kelly K, Moon G, Savage SP, Bradshaw Y: Ethics and the police surgeon: compromise or conflict? *Soc Sci Med* 42:1569–1575, 1996.

11. Pearson SD, Sabin JE, Emanuel EJ: Ethical guidelines for physician compensation based on capitation. *N Engl J Med* 339:689–693, 1998.

12. Yarborough M: The reluctant retained witness: alleged sexual misconduct in the doctor/patient relationship. *J Med Philos* 22:345–364, 1997.

13. Gray BH: Trust and trustworthy care in the managed care era. *Health Affairs* 16:34–49, 1997.

14. Pellegrino ED, Thomasma DC: *The Virtues in Medical Practice.* New York and Oxford, Oxford University Press, 1993.

15. Rawls J: *A Theory of Justice.* Cambridge, MA: Belknap Press, 1971.

16. Brody, H: *The Healer's Power.* New Haven, CT, Yale University Press, 1992.

17. Rhodes R, Strain JJ: "Trust and transforming medical institutions," unpublished manuscript, 1998.

Blaire S. Osgood
Alex J. Krasny
Linda L. Emanuel

Consultation and Referral

Ms. Cates asked Dr. Brown, her oncologist, to refer her to another oncologist so she could receive a second opinion on her diagnosis. After reviewing Ms. Cates' test results, the second oncologist, Dr. Klein, felt that Dr. Brown sorely underestimated the seriousness of her condition. Furthermore, after visiting with Dr. Klein, Ms. Cates asked if he would replace Dr. Brown as her primary clinician. Typically, Dr. Klein does not take on patients who have been referred to him solely for second opinions. However, he feels uncomfortable sending Ms. Cates back to a physician whom he suspects has seriously misjudged her condition.

Dr. Kolton has been Mr. Johnson's primary care physician ever since he signed up for the Wellness Health Plan HMO. When Dr. Kolton discovers that Mr. Johnson has prostatic hypertrophy and an elevated prostate-specific antigen (PSA), he decides that this patient should be referred to a urologist for a biopsy. He could refer Mr. Johnson to a urologist located in the same rural area, which would be covered by Wellness Health Plan HMO. However, Dr. Kolton thinks that even though it would not be covered by the health plan, a large academic medical center 100 miles away might be better equipped to diagnose and possibly treat Mr. Johnson's condition.

Dr. Harris, an internist, owns a private practice in a small community. Dr. Smith, a nephrologist who has a financial interest in the local dialysis clinic, approaches Dr. Harris with a business proposition. Dr. Smith suggests that for every patient Dr. Harris refers to her clinic for kidney dialysis, Dr. Smith will pay her a percentage of the fees collected from the patient. The financial incentive is appealing to Dr. Harris, yet the nature of the arrangement disturbs her.

Scope of the Problem

In great part, medical ethics now focuses on issues that arise during clinicians' interactions with patients. However, ethical considerations regarding referrals and consultations mark the nexus where patient care ethics intersect with *interprofessional ethics:* the ethics of interactions between professionals. It is an important premise in traditional medical ethics that clinicians have ethical obligations to other health care professionals as well as to patients. This is explicit in the Hippocratic Oath, where physicians are advised to "give a share of precepts and . . . all other learning . . . to pupils who have signed the covenant and have taken an oath according to the medical law."[1] More recently, the *Principles of Medical Ethics* of the American Medical Association specifically state that physicians have responsibilities to patients and health care professionals.[2] The obligations to patients and to other health professionals are guided by the physician's essential purpose—namely, to provide competent medical service with compassion and respect for dignity.

This chapter focuses on the obligations of the primary physician and the consultant to one another as well as their obligations to nonphysician health care professionals within the context of referrals and consultations. We then offer guidance in some specific circumstances: how primary clinicians should respond to patients' requests for referrals and consultations; how primary physicians should address concerns arising from referrals or consultations with incompetent or unethical colleagues; and whether primary clinicians should use referral as a means to terminate an unsatisfactory patient-clinician relationship. We conclude with a discussion of the obligations of primary clinicians in situations where policy restrictions on consultation and referral exist as well as the ethical issues related to fee-splitting and self-referral.

Consultations and Referrals and Who Makes Them

Referrals and consultations can be thought of as occupying different points on a continuum measuring the degree to which the primary clinician involves another clinician in patient care. On one end of the continuum, the primary clinician simply seeks information from another clinician, which he or she then uses in caring for the patient. Arrangements of this sort include informal "curbside consultations." No transfer of care occurs with a curbside consultation, and there is no transfer of responsibility. For instance, one study illustrated that general internists working in an HMO often sought informal consultations with gastroenterologists.[3] Although the safety and efficacy of curbside consultations are uncertain, since the consulting clinician has not evaluated the patient face to face, they can provide continuous need-driven education. These collegial discussions often allow primary clinicians to spend less time sorting their way through the medical literature in order to access information or advice in a timely manner.

At the other end of the continuum, the primary clinician refers a large portion of a patient's care to another clinician. At this extreme, responsibility for the overall care of a patient may be assumed by the clinician to whom the primary clinician has referred the patient, at least until the patient is cured, stabilized, or dies. This might be the case when a primary clinician, for example, refers a patient with cancer to an oncologist. Referrals of this nature begin to overlap with transfer of the patient. The majority of referrals and consultations involve shared care that falls between these two extremes.

Although both referrals and consultations have the same general aim of providing the patient with a health benefit, the responsibilities held in either case differ. *Consultations* occur when a clinician other than the primary clinician performs a specific diagnostic or therapeutic task. Consultants are responsible for their own actions, but overall responsibility for the patient's care is not assumed.[4] In contrast, in *referrals*, another clinician assumes a greater degree of responsibility for the patient's care from the primary clinician.[4] With both referrals and consultations, the implicit assumption is that the primary clinician will continue to coordinate the patient's care unless transfer arrangements have been made.

In this chapter, the term *primary clinician* is understood to mean the clinician with principal responsibility for the overall care of the patient. Depending on the nature of the situation, the primary clinician can be either a generalist or a specialist. A *generalist* is typically a physician such as a family physician or an internist without formal medical specialty training. A *specialist* is defined here as a physician with expertise in a particular field. The term *consultant* denotes a physician, either a generalist or a specialist, who is asked by the primary clinician to assist in the care of a patient.

Background Theory and Context

The Purpose of Referral and Consultation

The underlying purpose in providing patients with referrals and consultations is to serve their interest by providing comprehensive, quality health care. Those reasons include but are not limited to the following: to assist in making a diagnosis or determining an optimal treatment plan, to obtain expert advice, to reassure the patient or family or offer alternative perspectives with a second opinion, as a legal precaution, as a teaching or learning tool, or to obtain a procedure that requires specialized training. Perhaps the most common reason for referring patients to another clinician is to provide specialty care.

When caring for patients, primary clinicians have a responsibility to seek the input of other clinicians when they cannot alone address the problem at hand. This responsibility stems from the ethical principle that individuals should not inflict harm on others, also known as the *principle of nonmaleficence*.[5] In accordance with this principle, clinicians must acknowledge the limits of their own expertise and, when indicated, use the talents of other health professionals. Collegial interactions such as these help avoid harm and enhance patient care.

Some referrals are clearly indicated, such as referring a patient to an oncologist for chemotherapy or a gastroenterologist for endoscopic retrograde cholangiopancreatography. Other situations are more nebulous and can illustrate how the moral obligation that gives impetus to referrals and consultations can be weighed and balanced in different ways. What, for instance, are the responsibilities of primary clinicians when they have some experience in treating a particular disorder, but a specialist might have more experience doing so? For example, a primary clinician might diagnose a skin disorder and be able to treat it even though a dermatologist has more experience with the condition.

The precedent set forth by case law offers one type of standard for evaluating appropriate actions regarding referral and consultation. In cases such as these, the courts have held that clinicians have an obligation to inform the patient fully about the problem and then to describe their expertise in that area compared to that of a specialist.[6] If the patient elects to have the primary physician treat the disorder, the physician could be held liable for wrongdoing only if the patient had been led to believe that the primary clinician would provide care of equal or greater quality than that of a specialist. That is, case law indicates that the obligations to provide information and choice are sufficient. This standard, though legal in origin, begins to describe the clinician's professional obligations. It also has relevance to situations where referral options are constrained by prior contract or policy—a matter considered later in this chapter.

Although the primary clinician's duties in making a referral or requesting a consultation encompass these legal considerations, they also go further. Besides objectively evaluating the skin disorder and disclosing potential treatment options, the primary clinician has an obligation to act in the patient's best interest. In that capacity, the obligations of primary clinicians are obligated not only to disclose information and make options available but also to be the patient's advocate. If the goal of providing comprehensive quality care is furthered by consultation or referral, the primary clinician should recommend it. Only if this goal is not furthered might a greater goal outweigh this obligation. This could occur if a referral paid for out of pocket would prevent a patient from being able to afford essential medications (although the danger here lies in setting different standards of care for those who can afford to pay for referrals and those who cannot). Determining the best interest of patients in light of factors such as these can prove difficult for clinicians, especially when they are working within the constraints of certain health care systems (see Chap. 7).

Obligations of the Primary Clinician and Consultants to One Another

The primary clinician and the consultant are bound by the obligation to support each other's activities in the patient's best interest. This obligation is aimed at improving patient care. Ensuring that referrals or consultations are beneficial requires the primary clinician and the consultant to uphold their obligations to each other.

Whether the degree of involvement of the consultant or consultants is large or small, good care requires that one clinician maintain the role of care coordinator. That is, one physician assumes the role of primary clinician. This approach emphasizes the concept of accountability.[7] Coordinating care among clinicians, and thereby appropriately placing accountability, involves communicating the terms of the interprofessional relationship effectively. For clinicians to work in concert, the roles of the primary clinician and consultant must be appropriately delineated. Failure of communication about responsibilities can lead to discordant expectations, inadequate or duplicative care, and increased costs. This uncoordinated care has been termed *split care*, being dispersed among specialists without mutual acknowledgment of the need for communication with a primary clinician.[8] It is perhaps especially common in academic tertiary care centers, but can occur in any patient care setting.

Without an explicit understanding of roles and expectations, confusion about authority and responsibility may arise. Primary clinicians may dominate the relationship because they, by definition, are the patient's primary provider of health care, and the consultant is dependent on them for referrals. On the other hand, consultants could assume a more controlling role, since they might dictate the therapeutic action within their areas of expertise. The consultant could also interfere with the primary clinician's relationship with the patient by undermining the primary clinician's credibility.[8] Some boundary and jurisdictional conflicts such as these can be avoided by opening appropriate channels of communication.

MODELS OF COMMUNICATION

There are several models of communication.[9] Ideally, there is the chance for multilateral deliberation in shared decisionmaking to include all relevant parties. The circumstances will dictate what is realistic. In some instances, the primary clinician may be responsible for transmitting the consultant's opinion to the patient. In other instances, as in a hospital setting, direct three-way communication may be expected between the primary clinician, the consultant, and the patient.

Although there is no single best model of communication, there are definite pitfalls if communication is not coordinated. Without coordinated communication, the patient ends up orchestrating the clinicians, which may result in poor care and strained relationships with the physicians.[8] Lack of communication may result in the failure to provide the full and necessary information for quality decisionmaking and for the patient's informed consent. Communication breakdowns may also lead to the inappropriate disclosure of confidential information.

The primary clinician who asks for a consultation must define the purpose of the consultant's involvement. Assumptions by all parties may simply not be correct. An appropriate written request provides relevant clinical information and poses specific questions. The motivation behind the primary clinician's request is also typically exposed by such requests. For example, if the consultant is being called on primarily to respond to the concerns of a worried spouse, to assist in a diagnosis, or to provide an obviously needed procedure, the consultant generally should be informed of this.[8]

The goal of consultants is to support primary clinicians and their relationships with patients. Consultants are mainly responsible for addressing primary clinicians' requests and responding to those requests appropriately. Appropriate responses include providing the requested specialized care and communicating back to the primary clinician regarding the service provided. It is also appropriate for the consultant to offer additional indicated care and make suggestions that assist patient care. However, the consultant should proceed with such services or suggestions only with the primary clinician's concurrence. Even if such services and suggestions are not used, the information may contribute to the primary clinician's continuing education.

The job of defining and communicating roles and expectations is often a continuing process. Ideally, the patient and the consultant as well as the primary clinician should participate. When the patient understands the reasons for the consultation, the chance that the patient will follow the plan of care and, subsequently, be more satisfied with the outcomes may increase.[10] The consultant may have an evaluation suggesting an adjustment in the physicians' respective roles, in which case direct communication and appropriate adjustment should be made.

Obligations of Primary Clinicians to Nonphysician Health Professionals

Primary care is practiced among a network of interprofessional relationships. In the current medical environment, physicians work with pharmacists, nurses, social workers, physical and occupational therapists, technicians, pastors, and other allied health professionals. Sometimes these professionals make up a team, so that formal referrals and consultations are unnecessary. In other settings, referrals and consultations are made, whether in the form of a requisition for an imaging study, referral for physical therapy, or assessment and intervention by a social worker.

The primary clinician has an obligation to the nonphysician professional that is the same as the obligation to a physician. The scope of the job requested by the primary clinician, appropriate background information about the patient, and the nature of the possible intervention should be clear. The nonphysician professional who is providing referred care has the counterpart obligation to relay back to the primary clinician pertinent information such as the

assessment of the patient's condition, the treatment goals, plans or recommendations, and family concerns.[8]

Each nonphysician health care professional plays a unique role and has corresponding bilateral obligations. Without detailing each, one relationship may be worthy of specific mention—namely, that of the pharmacist with the primary clinician. This professional relationship is noted in particular, partly as an illustration and partly because it may not typically be thought of as a consultative or referral relationship. However, there is much similarity in the obligations of pharmacists and other consultants. The pharmacist reviews the clinician's orders or prescriptions, watches for potentially conflicting medications, and offers suggestions to the clinician. The pharmacist's obligation to communicate to the primary clinician important information regarding contraindicated drugs that have been prescribed is a central part of error reduction in a patient's care and treatment. Pharmacists can extend the scope and quality of care effectively, as do more commonly defined consultations and referrals.

Toward Resolution

Responding to Patients' Requests for Referrals, Consultations, or Second Opinions

When a patient requests a referral that concurs with the primary clinician's judgment, there is no dilemma. Responding to patients' requests for referrals to, for instance, dubious providers of alternative medicine requires the primary clinician to balance conflicting considerations (see Chap. 3). Similarly, there is a need to balance competing considerations when the patient wishes to avoid referral or consultation that is contrary to the clinician's judgment of the patient's best interests. Note that meeting patients' demands and acting in their best interest are not necessarily equivalent obligations. Clinicians are first required to consider objectively medical indications that would call for a consulting or referring health professional even if this is contrary to the desires of the patient. Indeed, patients may be honestly persuaded when their primary clinician frankly discloses his or her medical opinion. Primary clinicians must act as advocates for patients' health needs, not necessarily for their misguided preferences (see Chap. 1). The primary clinician should try to persuade the patient toward needed consultation or referral and against misguided specialty attention.[11] However, a primary clinician should take seriously patients' views for or against services and recall always that patients have appropriate final authority over health decisions as long as they are competent.[12]

Consultants may also be faced with requests from patients. Although consultants are free to offer independent advice, they should be mindful of their interprofessional relationships and support the efforts of the primary clinician.[8] Most requests, such as requests for referrals to other specialists, should be transmitted back to the primary clinician so that continuity of care is maintained. Either the original primary clinician can handle the request or there can be an agreed-on adjustment to the roles, so that the consultant assumes this responsibility.

Requests for a second opinion may come from a referring clinician, whether at that clinician's initiative or at the patient's request. In order to respect the ability of patients to receive care from clinicians of their choice, consultants must decide independently of their colleagues whether to treat patients who ask for a second opinion.[13]

Responding to the Involvement of Incompetent or Unethical Colleagues

Situations in which the primary clinician or consultant has doubts about the other's ability to provide the patient with quality medical care may occur. These doubts could concern the clinician's lack of technical expertise, limited experience with a particular problem, or problems with his or her bedside manner or ethical conduct.

One type of situation might involve primary clinicians who feel forced to refer a patient to a clinician that they suspect to be lacking some necessary skill. For example, clinicians who practice in a rural environment in which there are few specialists may experience this sort of dilemma. Or the primary clinician may practice in a managed care arrangement that limits the number of available specialists to a preapproved panel (see Chap. 7).

In those situations when primary clinicians do have referring options, patients should be provided with the best reasonable referral. If realistic choices among equally talented clinicians are possible, then patients should be informed about a clinician's qualifications, experience, professional style, and any other relevant information so that they can make an informed decision. As set forth by both ethical and legal precedents, the primary clinician should be forthcoming with relevant information rather than waiting for the patient to ask questions.[14] Ultimately, primary clinicians should not refer patients unless they are confident that the services provided on referral will be performed competently and in accordance with accepted medical standards.[15] Clinicians' collegial obligations to one another go only as far as promoting the best interests of the patient.

Conflicts between the primary clinician and the consultant may not be discovered until after the services of the consultant have been employed. If the primary clinician and the consultant disagree on certain aspects of the patient's care, this is not necessarily incompetence or unethical behavior on either party's part. In these situations, the clinicians should resolve their conflict in a way that serves the best interest of the patient. Although the clinicians may wish to disclose the disagreement to the patient and acknowledge that they have different opinions, it would be inappropriate to make derogatory comments to the patient about the other clinician's abilities or recommendations.[8] Such comments impede care and erode the patient's trust in and respect for the clinicians.

Primary clinicians and consultants should help each other avoid errors by communicating between themselves. Feedback that is supportive and neutral is also a good way to resolve disagreements. If the disagreement between the primary clinician and consultant is not simply a case of differing opinions but is more obviously malpractice or a breach of ethical standards on behalf of one of the clinicians, then the suspect clinician should be confronted or, when appropriate, reported to the in-house peer review body or state licensing board. Physicians are responsible for upholding the profession's integrity, and to do so may sometimes require reporting a colleague's behavior.[16] In cases where the disagreement or perceived error has relevance to the patient's future medical decisions, the disagreement or perceived error should certainly be fully disclosed to the patient. Preferably the clinician responsible for the disagreement or error should be the one to disclose all the facts necessary to ensure understanding of what has occurred and allow for informed decisions regarding future medical care.[17]

Referring as a Means to Terminate the Patient-Clinician Relationship

Disagreements may arise not only between the primary clinician and the consultant but also between the primary clinician and the patient. Although a primary clinician certainly has duties to his or her patients, these duties have limits. Clinicians may need to terminate the patient-clinician relationship under some circumstances. This, however, is a step that should not be taken without serious consideration. Occasion-

ally, a patient might make a request that would call upon the clinician to do something incompatible with his or her personal or professional belief, such as performing an abortion or providing a seemingly futile intervention. In these cases, it would be permissible to refer the patient to another clinician who may not hold the same ethical values. In other circumstances, the appropriateness of referring a patient as a means to terminating the patient-clinician relationship is less clear.

Concerns about appropriateness are raised in cases that involve, for example, a patient who does not cooperate with an agreed-upon treatment plan, a patient with a borderline personality, or one with whom the clinician has a major personality clash. Such situations have been characterized as care of the "difficult" or "hateful" patient.[18] Although these cases are certainly difficult to handle, withdrawing from the case may not be the appropriate resolution, as doing so may simply shift the encumbrance of the case to another clinician. A second and perhaps more important reason to question the use of referral in these situations is related to the notion that clinicians are bound by their calling to serve patients of all types. This is articulated in the Daily Prayer of a Physician (Prayer of Moses Maimonides) which says, "Preserve the strength of my body and of my soul that they ever be ready to cheerfully help and support rich and poor, good and bad, enemy as well as friend. In the sufferer let me see only the human being."[19]

Nonetheless, under the right circumstances, a clinician can withdraw from a patient's care and refer that patient to another as long as the proper steps are taken. A major concern in referring a patient as a means of terminating the patient-clinician relationship is to avoid abandoning the patient. *Abandonment* has been defined as "the unilateral termination by the physician of the patient-physician relationship without adequate notice to afford the patient the opportunity to obtain equally qualified replacement care and at a time when medical care is needed."[20] Once a patient-clinician relationship has been established, the clinician is obligated to provide treatment or arrange for treatment to be provided elsewhere. Clinicians risk being accused of *patient dumping* if they fail to uphold these responsibilities, because once a clinician assumes the care of a patient, the clinician cannot neglect that patient.[21]

To avoid claims of abandonment, the primary clinician ought to take certain steps. For example, the clinician should make sure that any limitations on the patient-clinician relationship are communicated to the patient early and are documented in the medical record.[22] Also, in some cases, it may be necessary to ensure that the clinician to whom the patient is being referred is willing to accept the patient. It would defeat the fundamental purpose of referring the patient to a new clinician if the new clinician were unwilling to assume care for the patient. Last, most state medical societies as well as the American Medical Association have developed guidelines for physicians as to how to appropriately terminate the patient-clinician relationship.[23] Clinicians should be familiar with such guidelines.

Restrictions on Consultations and Referrals

GATEKEEPERS

In the delivery of fee-for-service care, there are few limits on referrals and consultations as long as the patient or his or her insurance will pay for these services. However, other types of service arrangements limit consultation and referral. For example, to work within the constraints of managed care, primary clinicians must justify their decisions to seek referrals and consultations and may face an uphill battle in accessing these services for patients.

Arrangements that employ policy restrictions on available services have essentially reproportioned the functions of primary care by expanding the primary clinician's role into one of a "gatekeeper." Gatekeeping policies and procedures have been implemented in response to health care expenditures and the need to contain costs. As a *gatekeeper*, it is the responsibility of the primary clinician to decide which medical services patients should be allowed to access and which medical services are not necessary or appropriate. In addition to reducing costs, gatekeeping is expected to improve the quality of care by increasing coordination, assisting communication, and promoting continuity of care.[24]

The role of the gatekeeper may be well intended. However, gatekeeping also makes explicit the ethical problems associated with financial incentives, which can affect the quality of care a patient receives. On the one hand, the primary clinician, as the gatekeeper, must determine to what services the patient needs access, including referrals to specialists. On the other hand, the primary clinician is often encouraged by financial incentives to be conscious of the overall constraints of the managed care entity of which he or she is a part. Under these circumstances, the clinician may be inclined to weigh the quality of a patient's treatment less than the organization's need to serve all patients and control costs. Although gatekeeping for referrals and consultations may decrease costs and improve coordination of care, it may do so at the expense of increased administrative work, diminished freedom in clinical practice and decision making, and strained patient-clinician and interprofessional relationships.[24]

The deepest and most immediate obligation of a clinician is to be an advocate for the patient. If financial incentives or policy restrictions limit meaningful treatment options, disclosure is appropriate. Further, primary clinicians are professionally obligated to recommend treatments, including referral, when they believe that the treatment would materially benefit the patient. Clinicians should not withhold treatment options or stretch their services beyond their expertise merely as a means to enhance their own or the plan's profitability.[25]

Upholding ethical requirements such as these while working within policy restrictions potentially places clinicians in uncomfortable "gray zones." For example, what if the patient would receive a higher quality of care from a specialist but the primary clinician is restricted from referring the patient to the specialist owing to the terms of the plan? The plan may include restrictions such as denying coverage for certain services (e.g., pelvic exams) when performed by a specialist (e.g., a gynecologist) because, according to the terms of the plan, such services should be provided by the primary clinician. Primary clinicians in this scenario may be unsure as to the limits of their obligation to function as patient advocates. For instance, if the primary clinician embellishes the patient's medical history so as to secure the specialist's care, this may be considered *upcoding* (i.e., falsely claiming that a condition is more serious for purposes of access to services or reimbursement[26]) rather than patient advocacy.

In general, clinicians should avoid actions that could be construed as deceitful, even when done in the patient's best interest. Even the patients in question may feel that, if their clinician is willing to tell "white lies" in these scenarios, the clinician may also be acting fraudulently in other contexts. When primary clinicians are faced with the dilemmas created by the interface of ethical obligations and policy restrictions, they must work within the constraints of honesty. As a patient advocate, primary clinicians charged with gatekeeping must remain committed to lobbying on the behalf of patients against policies that force inappropriate denials, such as denying access to needed specialists.[25] This responsibility entails not only challenging denials of treatment but also advocating—at the health plan's or governmental policymaking level—elimination or modification of inappropriate regulations. Nonetheless, although clinicians are expected to do everything possible to secure the best care available for their patients, they remain obligated not to lie or commit fraud. Patient advocacy does not justify this.

FEE SPLITTING

Medical care should be patient-centered and in the name of service, not clinician self-centered. Selfish motives, whether intentional or unintentional, are manifest in situations where clinicians inappropriately tie their personal financial concerns to patient services, resulting in a conflict of interest (see Chap. 8). Legislation on the practice of fee splitting addresses situations in which clinicians might be tempted to make decisions about health care utilization that could directly benefit themselves financially.

Fee splitting involves a payment by or to a clinician solely for the referral of a patient. It is considered to be unethical. According to the ethics policy of the American Medical Association, "[a] physician may not accept payment of any kind, in any form, from any source . . . for prescribing or referring a patient to said source. The payment violates the requirement to deal honestly with patients and colleagues."[27] Moreover, fee splitting is illegal. Medicare and Medicaid statutes prohibit willful solicitation, receipt, offer, or payment of any kickback, bribe, or rebate as compensation for the furnishing of referrals.[28]

The reasoning behind these strict prohibitions is that patients depend on their clinicians for unbiased advice and medical care. A patient should be referred to a specialist based on the specialist's skill and his or her ability to meet the patient's needs. When clinicians receive a financial benefit from patient referrals, personal financial gain threatens to bias decision making.

SELF-REFERRAL

Self-referral guidelines aim to prevent clinicians from referring patients to facilities in which they have a financial interest but where they do not provide services. A comprehensive set of federal regulations known as *Stark I*[29] and *Stark II*[30] prohibit self-referral of Medicare and Medicaid patients. The Stark Acts prohibit clinicians from referring patients to an entity within which they or an immediate family member have an ownership interest or compensation arrangements for specified services covered by Medicare or Medicaid.

In general, self-referral prohibitions are not intended to deter clinicians from investing in health care facilities. Rather, the prohibitions are aimed at preventing clinicians from profiting solely from their ability to refer patients. If a clinician has a financial interest in a facility but does not provide care there, his or her decision to refer a patient to the facility could seem profit-motivated. Even if clinicians disclose their financial interest and wholeheartedly believe that the patient would receive quality care at the facility, the appearance of impropriety is cause for concern. Nevertheless, the prohibitions are not intended to prevent patients from getting the care they need when no other alternatives are available. Self-referral may be acceptable in the absence of adequate alternative facilities and alternative financing and when a medical need can be demonstrated.

Self-referral guidelines aim to curb referrals motivated by the financial gain clinicians would receive in return. Like the reasoning behind the fee splitting prohibitions, self-referral prohibitions ensure that referral decisions are made exclusively with patients' best interests in mind. Within the medical profession, self-referral, as well as other issues that fall within the framework of fraud and abuse, is particularly egregious because of the potential for inappropriately influencing clinicians' medical judgment.[31] Self-interested arrangements are out of place in the medical profession because they interfere with what should be clinicians' primary goal: to serve the best interests of patients.

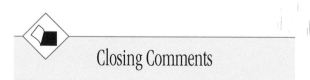

Closing Comments

The hypothetical cases at the beginning of this chapter illustrate that referral and consultation arrangements can introduce many dilemmas both for primary clinicians and their colleagues. Although Dr. Klein is wary of undermining his colleague, he also has obligations to ensure that Ms. Cates's condition is diagnosed and treated correctly and that her right to choose a physician is respected. Dr. Klein should communicate openly both with Dr. Brown, to evaluate whether he can treat her condition properly, and with Ms. Cates, to explore her motivations for requesting him as a physician, before deciding whether to undertake her care.

In the case of Dr. Kolton, who thinks that Mr. Johnson might receive better care outside of his health plan, he clearly has an obligation to disclose his opinion to his patient. Although the ultimate decision will depend on Mr. Johnson's preferences and resources (such as his willingness to travel and ability to pay) Dr. Kolton has an immediate obligation to recommend the best available options for Mr. Johnson's care and a long-term responsibility to be an advocate for improved care within the health plan.

Dr. Harris's intuition that the profit-sharing arrangement proposed by Dr. Smith creates a conflict of interest is correct. She has an obligation to be aware of state and federal law regarding fee splitting and related practices as well as a professional responsibility to ensure that her referrals are motivated by what is best for her patients, not her pocketbook.

Clinicians in all of the situations discussed above have a primary responsibility to act in the best interest of patients. Nevertheless, these vignettes underscore the complex balancing act clinicians must perform, in which the best interests of patients, collegial obligations, principles of professionalism, and other factors come into play. This is especially true for the primary clinician, who has the duty to serve as a general health care provider and as a coordinator for the patient so as to ensure that the patient has no gaps or overlaps in medical care. Although the specific services provided by the primary clinician may vary, the responsibility to act as a case manager and patient advocate remains the same.

As medicine becomes more advanced and specialized, more individuals and resources are required to provide patients with the highest possible quality of care. This forms the basis for a collegial, and collaborative health care system. As a result of burgeoning knowledge, clinicians have come to rely upon interprofessional assistance. Effectively managing patients' access to needed medical resources has become a job in itself. As this job becomes increasingly difficult in the years to come, the responsibility to manage and coordinate care will fall squarely on the shoulders of primary clinicians and present yet a new set of challenges.

Referrals and consultations exemplify the dual obligations that clinicians have to collegiality and to patient care. Despite this duality, the two rarely need be mutually exclusive since the notion of collegiality is grounded in the belief that patient care must always be of primary importance. This notion also recognizes the need to rely on teamwork, coordinate the provision of care, communicate effectively, assure quality among colleagues' standards, and ensure access to specialty services without profiting inappropriately from referrals and consultations. Patient care motivated collegiality can guide most judgments about when referrals and consultations are appropriate.

References

1. Edelstein L: The Hippocratic Oath: text, translation and interpretation. *Bull Hist Med Suppl.* Baltimore, Johns Hopkins Press, 1943.
2. American Medical Association Council on Ethical and Judicial Affairs: Principles of Medical Ethics, in American Medical Association Council on Ethical and Judicial Affairs (ed): *Code of Medical Ethics: Current Opinions with Annotations, 1998–1999.* Chicago, American Medical Association, 1998, p xiv.
3. Pearson SD, Moreno R, Trnka Y: Informal consultations provided to general internists by the gastroenterology department of an HMO. *J Gen Intern Med* 13:435–438, 1998.
4. Nutting PA: Referral and consultation in primary care: do we understand what we're doing? *J Fam Pract* 35:21–23, 1992.
5. Beauchamp TL, Childress JF: *Principles of Medical Ethics,* 4th ed. New York, Oxford University Press, 1994, p 28.
6. *Morgan* v. *Engles,* 372 Mich 514, 127 NW2d 382.
7. Pearson SD: Principles of generalist-specialist relationships. *J Gen Intern Med* 14:S13–S20, 1999.
8. Stoeckle JD, Ronan L, Emanuel LL, et al: A manual on manners and courtesies for the shared care of patients. *J Clin Ethics* 8:22–23, 1997.
9. Emanuel LL, Richter J: The consultation and the patient-physician relationship. *Arch Intern Med* 154:1785–1790, 1994.
10. Eyers K, Brodaty H, Parker G, et al: If the referral fits: bridging the gap between patient and referrer requirements in a tertiary referral unit. *Aust NZ J Psychiatry* 30:332–336, 1996.
11. Gallagher TH, Lo B, Chesney M, et al: How do physicians respond to patients requests for costly, unindicated services. *J Gen Intern Med* 12:663–668, 1997.
12. Baergen R, Baergen C: Paternalism, risk and patient choice. *J Am Dental Assoc* 128:481–484, 1997.
13. American Medical Association Council on Ethical and Judicial Affairs: Opinion 8.041, "Second opinions," in American Medical Association Council on Ethical and Judicial Affairs (ed): *Code of Medical Ethics: Current Opinions with Annotations, 1998–1999.* Chicago, American Medical Association, 1998, p 127.
14. Morreim EH: Am I my brother's warden? Responding to the unethical or incompetent colleague. *Hastings Cent Rep* 23:19–27, 1993.
15. American Medical Association Council on Ethical and Judicial Affairs: Opinion 3.04, "Referral of patients," in American Medical Association Council on Ethical and Judicial Affairs (ed): *Code of Medical Ethics: Current Opinions with Annotations, 1998–1999.* Chicago, American Medical Association, 1998, p 76.
16. American Medical Association Council on Ethical and Judicial Affairs: Opinion 9.031, "Reporting impaired, incompetent, or unethical colleagues," in American Medical Association Council on Ethical and Judicial Affairs (ed): *Code of Medical*

Ethics: Current Opinions with Annotations, 1998–1999. Chicago, American Medical Association, 1998, p 161.

17. American Medical Association Council on Ethical and Judicial Affairs: Opinion 8.12, "Patient information," in American Medical Association Council on Ethical and Judicial Affairs (ed): *Code of Medical Ethics: Current Opinions with Annotations, 1998–1999*. Chicago, American Medical Association, 1998, p. 142.

18. Groves JE: Taking care of the hateful patient. *N Engl J Med* 298:883–887, 1978.

19. Friedenwald H: Daily prayer of a physician: translation. *Bull Johns Hopkins Hosp* 28:260–261, 1917.

20. Thieman S: Avoiding the claim of patient abandonment. *Missouri Med* 93:634–635, 1996.

21. American Medical Association Council on Ethical and Judicial Affairs: Opinion 8.11, "Neglect of patient," in American Medical Association Council on Ethical and Judicial Affairs (ed): *Code of Medical Ethics: Current Opinions with Annotations, 1998–1999*. Chicago, American Medical Association, 1998, p 139.

22. Torres A, Wagner R, Proper S: Terminating the physician-patient relationship. *J Dematol Surg Oncol* 20:144–147, 1994.

23. American Medical Association Council on Ethical and Judicial Affairs: Opinion 8.115, "Termination of the patient-physician relationship," in American Medical Association Council on Ethical and Judicial Affairs (ed): *Code of Medical Ethics: Current Opinions with Annotations, 1998–1999*. Chicago, American Medical Association, 1998, p 141.

24. Halm EA, Causino N, Blumenthal D: Is gatekeeping better than traditional care? A survey of physicians' attitudes. *JAMA* 278:1677–1681, 1997.

25. American Medical Association Council on Ethical and Judicial Affairs: Ethical issues in managed care. *JAMA* 273:330–335, 1995.

26. Kongstvedt PR: *Essentials of Managed Care*. 2d ed. Gaithersburg, MD, Aspen Publications, 1997, p 135.

27. American Medical Association Council on Ethical and Judicial Affairs: Opinion 6.02, "Fee splitting," in American Medical Association Council on Ethical and Judicial Affairs (ed): *Code of Medical Ethics: Current Opinions with Annotations, 1998–1999*. Chicago, American Medical Association, 1998, p 108.

28. Weber RD: Practice management contracts/illegal fee-splitting. *Michigan Med* 97:8–10, 1998.

29. 42 USC Section 1395nn (January 1, 1992).

30. 63 Fed Reg 1659 (January 9, 1998).

31. A Hearing on Physician Ownership/Referral Arrangements. Friday, August 16, 1991. Press Release #19, Subcommittee on Health, Committee on Ways and Means, United States House of Representatives.

Robert M. Arnold
Maryanne Fello

Chapter 10

Hospice and Home Care

Mr. Smith, 62 years old, was admitted to home hospice with progressive lung cancer, metastatic to his left femur and right shoulder. During the initial hospice visit, the nurse found that the family was close-knit but had difficulty talking about Mr. Smith's diagnosis or prognosis. The patient was stoic, in charge, and denying the import of his illness. Following his last chemotherapy session, Mr. Smith's clinician informed him that further treatments would be ineffective. However, Mr. Smith told his hospice nurse that he was getting better and responding well to treatment. Although the family and staff believe the patient to be in extreme pain, he refused aggressive pain management. When questioned about his pain, he responded "You just live with it." Without adequate pain control, he had difficulty ambulating or even moving in bed. The family begged for something that would relieve Mr. Smith's horrible back pain.

Mrs. Jeanai, 85 years old, has severe chronic obstructive pulmonary disease (COPD) and was admitted to hospice in Pittsburgh. Some 3 months later her COPD had progressed to the point that she was usually bed- and chair-bound. Her family consisted of her 96-year-old husband, who had severe heart failure and mild dementia, and two adult children. Her son lived in Houston and had not seen his mother in 2 years. Her daughter lived in Pittsburgh and was the primary caregiver for both parents. She had a full-time job, was a single parent with three teenage children, and had her own health problems. She was overwhelmed and told the social worker that she had to go to the emergency room because her diabetes was so poorly controlled, that she had nearly passed out. Acknowledging her limitations, she asked the social worker about nursing home placement for her parents. Her mother, on the other hand, refused to think about going anywhere. "We were married, we raised the kids in this house, and we are going to die here," she yelled.

Mr. Yuns, 45 years old, has AIDS. Over the previous 2 months he had become increasingly debilitated and anorectic. He was often confused and had trouble making decisions. A week ago he stopped eating solids altogether and could take only liquids. His partner has called Mr. Yuns' physician, inquiring about what could be done to feed him.

Mr. Knoweld, 72 years old, has widespread colon cancer and was therefore admitted to hospice 6 weeks ago. He lived with his wife in a modest home, had a loving family, and worried about what would happen to him as he got sicker. Many discussions with him over time led the family to know that he wanted to "die in his own home." He was reluctant to allow his family to help, insisting that his wife and he could manage. However, he became increasingly debilitated and, during the previous 2 weeks, fell three times getting out of bed to go to the bathroom. Moreover, he was quite stubborn, refusing to stay in bed or use a bedside commode. Initially, his 70-year-old wife was able to take care of him, but she was not strong enough to help him transfer. Mr. Knoweld had limited financial resources other than his house, which he was proud of having fully paid off. The hospice nurses wondered whether he would be better off in a nursing home. One of the hospice nurses volunteered to go over a couple of extra times each day to help Mr. Knoweld's wife.

Danny Silverstein, 8 years old, has a terminal brain tumor. The hospice team met Danny's mother, the day she returned home from Tijuana, Mexico, where Danny had just undergone a course of alternative therapy, including "bovine thymus" and colonics. Even though Danny's neurosurgeon did not support the decision to obtain this treatment, he continued to support Mrs. Silverstein and to care for Danny. At home, Mrs. Silverstein asked the hospice nurses for guidance on how to provide this alternative therapy, needing to know how to give an injection and to administer colonics.

Scope of the Problem

The five hypothetical cases presented above illustrate some of the common ethical issues that arise in home hospice. The purpose of this chapter is to describe the types of ethical issues that hospice professionals confront, describe how ethical principles can play a role in understanding these issues, and present a framework one can use to help resolve these issues as they arise in practice.

Characteristics of Hospice Programs

In 1996, about 20,000 health care providers worked in roughly 3000 hospices in the United States.[1] Most hospices are nonprofit, although an increasing number of for-profit hospices exists. By regulation, hospices are multidisciplinary. Clinicians must certify that patients have less than 6 months to live, advise nurses regarding difficult cases, and sometimes make house calls. Nurses make frequent home visits and teach family caregivers how to manage the bulk of the day-to-day care. Aides and volunteers also provide home care, including basic activities of daily living, helping with chores, and providing respite for family caregivers. Social workers and psychologists help patients and families deal with the stresses of the illness, the dying process, and bereavement. Chaplains help patients with spiritual and existential issues. Physical, speech, and occupational therapists are also available.

Hospices serve nearly 450,000 patients or roughly 15 percent of patients who die in America every year. Over 80 percent of the patients have cancer, although the number with diseases of the heart, liver, kidneys, and lungs as well as those with dementia is increasing. Roughly 70 percent of patients are over 65 years of age, 80 percent are white, and 50 percent are married. Over 80 percent of these patients' care is provided in the home, with short periods in nursing homes or hospitals for family respite or the management of acute symptoms.[1] The median length of survival after hospice admission is 36 days. Some 15 percent of patients die within a week of admission and 25 percent die within 2 weeks.[2]

Ethical Issues That Arise in Hospice

Many of the ethical issues that arise in hospice (e.g., forgoing life support, questions of capacity, respecting advance directives, etc.) also arise in other settings (see Chaps. 17, 18, and 20). There is a difference, however, when these issues arise in hospice care, among patients who have chosen a palliative mode of care rather than life-prolonging therapies. Moreover, these issues arise in the patient's home, where the patient's family, however defined, rather than paid professionals, provides the majority of care. Questions regarding how to balance the desire to remain at home and the effect on the family caring for the dying patient are specific to home care.

These problems are magnified because of hospices' commitment to the family. Hospice treats both the ill individual and the caregivers.[3] This dual focus on patients and their families can cause conflicts. For example, most patients say they would rather die at home. At home, patients have more freedom to engage in the activities of their choosing. The benefit of dying at home, however, may impose costs on the caregivers, typically, in the U.S., women.[4] Caregivers often suffer financially, emotionally, and socially in their efforts to tend a dying patient. Caregivers must take time off from work, use savings to pay for private-duty nurses, or remodel the house to accommodate the patient. In addition, there are physical and emotional costs. Caregivers stay up at night giving medicine and attending to the patient. They must often give up social activities and neglect their own health. Balancing these conflicts is a central component of hospice practice.

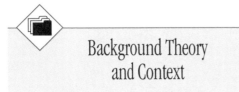

Background Theory and Context

Historical Development of Hospice Care

Before World War II, much of health care was delivered by physicians making house calls. A good part of available diagnostics and therapeutics could be easily transported in the physician's black bag. It was expected that family members would convalesce or deteriorate at home. However, advances in medical technology shifted medical practice from home to hospital.[5] For the dying patient, this meant that the terminal phases of the illness were often managed by hospital staff, directed by the physician. Converging forces met in the decade of the 1960s, spurred on by the initiation of Medicare (1966) and the burgeoning advances in medical technology. Richard Nixon signed into law the National Cancer Act (1971), enabling the creation of the National Cancer Institute (NCI) and beginning the "War on Cancer." Concomitant advances in critical care made it possible for doctors to keep patients alive with dialysis, ventilators, and cardiopulmonary bypass machines. For the first time physicians had to decide when to use or not use these technologies in patients with incurable, progressive illnesses. Moreover, these new technologies markedly increased the cost of medical care and led to debates over the proper role of hospitals and medical technologies, especially in end-of-life care.

The modern hospice program developed in part as a reaction to the overtreatment of dying patients. Hospice emphasizes palliative care, rather than treatment, for patients with incurable, progressive illness. The goal is to achieve an optimal quality of life through relief of suffering, control of symptoms, and maintenance of functional capacity while remaining sensitive to the patient's and family's values.[3] Hospice views dying as a natural process that is profoundly personal.

In the mid-1960s, the work of Elizabeth Kübler-Ross and Dame Cicely Saunders led individuals in the United States to put their concepts of death, dying, and palliative care to work. These new programs were home-based. Most significant in creating uniformity among hospice programs was the Federal Medicare program in 1982. It provided a mechanism for making hospice—which requires extra services such as spiritual care, counseling, and bereavement and volunteer care—financially viable.

Ethical Principles in Hospice Care

As an outsider invited into the patient's domain, the hospice worker must consider carefully the ethical principles of autonomy, beneficence, justice, and dignity in attending to the hospice patient and his or her family. Although all but the last principle are the same as those used to analyze cases in the hospital or ambulatory setting, there are differences in how these principles are conceptualized in the context of home care and hospice.

AUTONOMY

Promoting autonomy is justified both *consequentially* (i.e., on the action's consequences) and *deontologically* (i.e., on the process or duty).[6] First, respecting an autonomous decision typically maximizes patients' *best interests*. What is in someone's best interest is not objectively determined but can be seen only in the context of the particular patient's values and goals. Given the subjective nature of "best interest," persons whose interests are at stake are best qualified to determine the proper goals of medical therapy. Second, it is felt to be intrinsically good to allow individuals to direct their own lives, regardless of whether the decision optimizes their well-being. We wish to define our own values and decide how to act to achieve our goals even if these decisions are sometimes incorrect in the eyes of others. This value is deeply ingrained in cultural ideals throughout the Western world.

While there is a clear consensus regarding the importance of respecting autonomy, what it means to promote autonomy is less clear.[7] Autonomy has a variety of different meanings, which can lead to different and sometimes conflicting actions. For example, should one be respectful of a patient's current decision to refuse physical therapy even if it will decrease her ability to be self-sufficient in the future? What we do to honor an individual's autonomy depends on what we mean by it.

Common conceptions of autonomy include autonomy as free action, autonomy as effective deliberation, and autonomy as consistency.[8]

AUTONOMY AS FREE ACTION   This notion of autonomy centers on promoting intentional and voluntary activities. According to this view, most of our daily actions are autonomous, such as getting out of bed in the morning and wearing a particular shirt.[8,9] Autonomy as free action is met by simply having the ability to form preferences and having a sense of self involving the belief that one's actions can influence the environment in predictable ways. This notion of autonomy incorporates "negative" and "positive" conceptions. The law of battery, which precludes health care providers from nonconsensual touching, exemplifies a negative aspect of autonomy as free action (that is, a right to be left alone). In hospice, the attempt to limit restraints, even for demented patients, may be seen as an effort to promote free action. In contrast, attempts to increase patients' ability to function can be seen as positive efforts to promote free action.

AUTONOMY AS EFFECTIVE DELIBERATION   This is a richer notion of autonomy than autonomy as free action. Effective deliberation consists of making a decision based on an adequate understanding of the situation and the possible alternative courses of action.[8,10] Autonomy as effective deliberation requires an understanding of the situation and the action as well as its consequences and possible alternatives. To act autonomously requires the ability to understand options, to weigh options in a rational way, and to make a decision.

This notion of autonomy, typified in the doctrine of informed consent, is the most prevalent in the bioethics literature.[10,11] In hospice, this notion is most important when a patient faces a significant decision with clearly identifiable options, typically in choosing therapeutic goals and deciding whether to forgo treatment. Three questions are typically asked: Is the patient competent to make the decisions? Has the patient been given enough information about the various options, including the risks and benefits, to make an informed decision? Has the patient been coerced into making a decision or, alternatively, is his or her decision voluntary?

AUTONOMY AS CONSISTENCY   Autonomy as consistency emphasizes that the autonomous activity is consistent with an individual's commitments, values, and life plans.[8,12] Autonomy as consistency places special emphasis on the coherence between the activity in question and the patterns of activity and commitment with which one has been or is involved or foresees oneself involved in the future. Thus, autonomy as consistency is unlike the other conceptions of autonomy discussed above, which focus on isolated, discrete acts.

This model of autonomy has particular relevance for hospice. Autonomy in hospice care must not focus exclusively on discrete actions.[8,12] Hospice has to do with helping patients make sense of their lives and thus of their dying. Hospice consists of trying to maximize functions and allow dying patients to live their lives as fully as possible. As such, hospice, deals more with promoting meaning and quality of life than with specific, discrete choices.[13]

Promoting autonomy as consistency means seeing how the dying person's daily experiences cohere with his or her larger life story. It means viewing the last part of one's life as a time for active growth and meaning—for living as fully as possible in this phase of life. Autonomy as consistency requires hospice to provide the resources needed for people to achieve their goals. For instance, hospice will offer physical therapy to help a patient achieve the goal of being as independent as possible while ensuring that another patient has the spiritual support needed to achieve peace before death occurs.

These three notions of autonomy place different obligations on the hospice provider. Free action requires noninterference, effective deliberation requires giving help in making informed decisions, and consistency requires offering the support and options needed to help terminally ill patients fulfill their values. Moreover, in some cases these different notions may seem to conflict, requiring the hospice staff to decide which conception of autonomy is most important.[13,14] Hospice staff need to be aware of autonomy's many facets as they struggle with promoting their patients' self-determination.

BENEFICENCE AND NONMALEFICENCE

These are important concepts in hospice care, as they are in health care generally.[15] Given hospice's focus on terminally ill patients, however, long-term risks and benefits are rarely part of the equation. Instead, benefits and burdens focus more on quality-of-life issues, such as relief of pain and shortness of breath. Recent studies have demonstrated the distress that dying patients experience in the last weeks of life. For example, the Study to Understand Prognoses and Preferences for Outcomes and Risks

of Treatment (SUPPORT) showed that over half of conscious patients suffered moderate or severe pain in their last week of life.[16] Therefore, the hospice teams' obligation to promote beneficence requires them to aggressively seek to identify such symptoms and to treat them emergently.

Promoting beneficence also requires hospice staff to attend to patients' psychosocial well-being. Studies have shown that psychological symptoms are prevalent and bothersome.[17] Good hospice care thus requires screening for anxiety and depression. In addition, Hospice staff need to know how to elicit dying patients' existential and spiritual concerns. Finally, quite frequently, dying patients' major concerns involve their loved ones' well-being. Thus, the notion of beneficence needs to be expanded to include the terminally ill patient's loved ones.

In hospice care, difficulties sometimes result from a conflict or perceived conflict between the obligation to promote autonomy and that to promote beneficence. Traditionally, the objection to allowing patients to forgo life-sustaining treatment was based on health care providers' belief that their obligation to promote life overrode all other values. In hospice, the relevant question is whether, from the patient's point of view, the therapy's benefits outweigh the burdens.[18] This determination is made by asking a series of more specific questions: Do the current benefits of being alive outweigh its burdens? For some patients, continued existence itself is a burden. What are the therapy's benefits and burdens? This question can be broken down into a series of more specific questions. First, will the therapy be likely to result in a life worth living? Second, even if successful, are the therapy's side effects "worth" the chance of a positive outcome? Does it make sense to try a therapy for a short time to see if it will work, discontinuing the treatment if it is not achieving the patient's goals?

JUSTICE

Justice requires that differences in treatment reflect ethically relevant differences in individuals. Although most agree that promoting justice is important, what this means is controversial. Does justice require allocation resources according to need or desert or random allocation?

Issues of justice arise in hospice care in a variety of forms that can be categorized as issues of *macroallocation* and *microallocation* of resources. The former are related to the funding of different types of health care. In the past, palliative care received little funding compared to curative or preventive medicine. Given the dismal state of end-of-life care,[16] one might argue that justice demands that more money be allocated to palliative care.

In contrast, microallocation of resources involves the distribution of resources among specific individuals.[19] Two issues often come up in hospice care: how to distribute financial resources and how to distribute the energy of staff. For example, imagine a patient in a hospice who might benefit from elevated blood counts if she received expensive injections. The government and insurers pay hospices a fixed amount per day per patient, so spending a great deal of money on this patient's medicine may mean the hospice has less money to use to help other patients. Most hospices try to deal with this issue, at least partially, by developing policies to ensure that similar individuals are treated similarly. Typically the policies take into account factors such as the severity of symptoms, probability of benefit, the amount of benefit, and the availability of less expensive alternatives.

Similarly, staff time and energy are limited and must be allocated among the many patients and families. A family may want the nurses present 8 hours a day or may continually ask for volunteers to help with household chores. Meeting these needs may limit a hospice's ability to serve its other patients. Thus, on a day-to-day basis, hospice administrators must try to allocate fairly the staff's services to meet all of their patients' needs.

DIGNITY

Although it is not typically considered a "principle" of medical ethics, respecting a dying patient's dignity is clearly a moral goal of hospice care. The dictionary defines *dignity* as "the quality of being worthy, honored or esteemed," but this does not tell us what makes a dying person worthy of honor or esteem. Some say what counts as dignity is subjective and that each individual should be free to define a dignified death however he or she sees fit. Others argue that human dignity has an objective basis, depending on social worth, freedom, or pleasure and pain. Sulmasy argues that "human dignity has its basis in the moral proposition that every human life has intrinsic meaning and value."[20] Death with dignity therefore means respecting the intrinsic meaning and value of the dying process. However, determining how to operationalize this principle in practice is difficult and may result in disagreement.

Toward Resolution

Rules of Thumb

How can one arrive at a justified decision when different values seem to compete? A few rules of thumb can help[21] (Table 10-1).

MAKE SURE OF THE FACTS

Good decisions require accurate data in both clinical ethics and clinical care. For example, in

Table 10-1

Rules of Thumb for Resolving Cases

1. Makes sure of the facts.
2. Clarify the values at stake.
3. Think creatively about possible solutions.
4. Clarify the value conflict
5. Determine who is the appropriate decision maker.

the hypothetical case described at the opening of this chapter of Mr. Yuns who is anorectic and has AIDS, it is important to know the answers to factual questions such as the following:

• Does artificial nutrition increase the quality or length of life in patients with terminal illnesses? (At least for patients with metastatic cancer and advanced dementia it does not prolong life, but there are few data on quality of life. Moreover, these technologies have side effects.)[22,23]

• Is death without artificial hydration and nutrition painful? (The preponderance of evidence suggests that if the patient receives good oral hygiene, it is not.)

• What are the patient's religious beliefs? (Some religions, in particular Orthodox Judaism, hold that artificial hydration and nutrition are morally required.)

• What does the law say about forgoing artificial hydration and nutrition? (The law is quite clear that this medical technology, like all others, can be forgone.)[18]

• Had the patient expressed any preferences regarding artificial hydration and nutrition?

CLARIFY THE VALUES AT STAKE

Once the values at stake are made explicit, it is possible to develop solutions to optimize them or to determine how they should be weighed in an individual case. Returning to the vignettes at the opening of this chapter, when

Mr. Smith refused pain medications, the relevant values include autonomy as effective deliberation, autonomy as consistency, and beneficence toward the patient. For Mrs. Jeanai, whose daughter can no longer provide adequate care, the values at stake include the patient's autonomy, beneficence toward the patient, beneficence toward the daughter and justice. For Mr. Knoweld, who wants to be at home despite having inadequate support, the values include autonomy, beneficence toward the patient, beneficence toward the surrogate, and justice. Finally, for Danny Silverstein, the boy with a brain tumor whose mother wants help with alternative medicine, the primary value at stake is beneficence toward the patient.

THINK CREATIVELY ABOUT POSSIBLE SOLUTIONS

In many cases this is the most important step. The best choice is to find a solution that promotes the values of all involved parties. For example, in the case of Mrs. Jeanai, a solution that both respects Mrs. Jeanai's desire to stay at home while also ensuring her daughter's well-being is better than a solution that forces a choice between the two values.

Educating caregivers regarding how to care for their loved ones is an essential task of hospice, and may promote both the patient's and caregiver's well-being. Family members often have little experience tending to the terminally ill. This can cause unnecessary grief and anguish.[4] Families need to know that they can access a health care provider when they have questions or need help. Certification of hospices requires a hospice nurse to be on call and available for home visits 24 hours a day, 7 days a week. Providing adequate volunteers and respite care to weary family members is another hallmark of hospice. For example, a volunteer once a week allows the caregiver time to attend to business outside of home or to her own needs. This opportunity can mean the difference between a sustained effort at home care and a "bailout." In addition, when families are overwhelmed, hospice allows the patient to be trans-ferred to an inpatient hospice or nursing home for a short period of time.

CLARIFY THE VALUE CONFLICT

Disagreements over values can be of three different sorts. First are disagreements about what values should be considered. In the case of Mr. Smith, individuals may disagree about what conception of autonomy is at play. Adherence to his current refusal of pain medicine may decrease his ability to engage in other activities that he enjoys. On the other hand, one might question whether his refusal of pain medicine is consistent with his values and beliefs regarding suffering and redemption.

Second, sometimes there is disagreement about how to weigh different values. For example, in the case of Mr. Knoweld, the disagreement may be over whether his well-being is more important than respecting his desire to stay at home.

Third, there may be disagreement about how the different proposed solutions will promote various values. Even when individuals agree on the most important values, they may disagree about the best way to promote these values. Reasonable people can disagree, for instance, about the efficacy of artificial nutrition and hydration in promoting Mr. Yuns's comfort.

DETERMINE WHO IS THE APPROPRIATE DECISION MAKER

In many cases, disagreement over values can be resolved by determining who should make decisions. Appeals to patient autonomy and the doctrine of informed consent are used to determine, in cases of conflict, who should make the decision. Unfortunately, in hospice care, this often does not resolve the problem. First, as described above, in hospice there is a responsibility to care for the patient and the family, not just the patient. Thus, when patients' and fami-

lies' best interests conflict, the right answers are not always clear. Second, it is often unclear what to do when family members disagree. For example, two sons may both feel they are representing the patient's best interest, but they may disagree about what should be done. Finally, in hospice care, decisional autonomy is an insufficient action guide. For example, a patient who says she wants to go home but whose family is unwilling to support her at home will typically not be able to go home. Being able to make a decision is not worth much if one cannot execute it. Sadly, dying patients often lack the physical, emotional, and financial resources to execute their preferred choices. Hospice staff must both determine who has decisional authority and seek to fulfill this person's wishes.

Revisiting the Hypothetical Cases

Let us return again to the vignettes described at the beginning of the chapter and examine two of them in depth.

MRS. JEANAI

The case of Mrs. Jeanai and her family poses a relatively common challenge for the hospice team. Family caregivers have a legitimate moral stake in the decisions to give care at home, particularly when their time and energy are needed for the plan to be possible. Gathering the facts is crucial to the resolution of this case. Medical facts, such as prognosis and what symptoms to expect as death approaches, are needed. If the prognosis is a few weeks of continued life, the situation may be manageable; a prognosis of several months may be impossible for the caregivers to endure and may require a totally different approach. If the patient's expected outlook includes increasing somnolence and becoming "bed-bound," the family may plan differently than if shortness of breath and restlessness are likely to increase during the dying process.

Another important fact to be clarified is Mr. Jeanai's potential contributions to caretaking. Even if he is totally incapable of physical caregiving, can he be counted on to provide an "anchor" in the home, attending to simple needs of the patient and being able to call the hospice when a problem arises?

Finally, financial facts must also be explored. Both the patient's ability to cover out-of-pocket expenses and the daughter's loss of income must be determined.

Now let us examine the values at stake. The sense of duty to care for other family members is often (but not always) operative. Promises are sometimes made about future caregiving. Couples often guess about being "the first to go" and plan accordingly. Children are given caregiving messages as well. Exploring which messages are operative may serve to mitigate a bereavement complicated by guilt or unfinished business. Another obvious value in this case is the couple's (or at least the patient's) value of independence as evidenced by her wish to die in her home. Competing with these values is the daughter's well-being as well as possible harm that may befall Mrs. Jeanai should her care be suboptimal.

With these facts and values in mind, thinking about creative solutions becomes possible. With an aggressive symptom management plan, the family can be reasonably assured that the patient's sensation of shortness of breath will be minimized. Support for Mr. Jeanai can include home health aides, volunteers, and a simplified alert system. If paid help is a requirement and the couple's only asset is their home, a reverse mortgage may provide necessary cash. A family leave may free the daughter to participate without jeopardizing her own health. Finally, one may find that support from the patient's or daughter's church, or other friends may help to alleviate the family's stress.

If there is still a conflict about the setting (home or nursing home) in which the care will be given, the hospice must clarify the most appropriate decision maker(s). If the patient still has the capacity to participate in the decision-making process, her desires should be respected. One should not forcibly remove her from her home. However, this respect for the patient's negative autonomy does not require that others harm themselves to care for her. The daughter's responsibility to her mother is not endless and must be balanced against her own and her family's needs. One of the most important roles the hospice can play in this case is helping the daughter establish the boundaries of her ability to contribute both physically and financially.

Mr. Knoweld

The hypothetical case of Mr. Knoweld and his family raises another issue common in hospice. We begin, once again, by establishing the facts of the case. Mr. Knoweld, although debilitated, is a competent and stubborn man. His prognosis is measured in months, so the caregiving issues need to be considered on a long-term basis by hospice standards. His family is local, and despite his attempts to keep them away, remains supportive. Mr. Knoweld's wife is in reasonably good health but cannot support Mr. Knoweld's much desired periods out of bed. Funds with which to cover out-of-pocket caregiving costs are again limited. This case, however, also requires factual information about the hospice. What are the likely effects of allowing this nurse to volunteer? How big is the hospice? How many persons do they have on staff and how many patients do they cover?

The values at play in this case are not only the patient's but also those of the hospice staff. Certainly Mr. Knoweld's value of maintaining his independence in his own home seems paramount. The hospice nurse who has also volunteered extra visits sees her role as that of a caring professional and friend. She is clearly trying to do the right thing. The question is whether these efforts for one patient will detract from the hospice's ability to care for other patients. This case therefore raises questions of justice as well as autonomy and beneficence.

The interdisciplinary team meeting is often the milieu for creative problem solving on the part of the hospice staff. Upon presentation to the full team, the occupational therapist may offer an evaluation visit and suggest ways to preserve Mr. Knoweld's mobility. For example, a slide board or the installation of extra rails might be employed at minimal expense and without jeopardizing Mrs. Knoweld's health. The staff may also know of other volunteers who live near the patient who might be able to help.

Sometimes there are competing values and a need to negotiate, even with a dying patient. For instance, does Mr. Knoweld value staying at home or getting up more? If he can articulate his priority, then pointing out a compromise such as letting his relatives pitch in or not getting up unless someone other than his wife is there might be a way to stay at home longer. If his priority is being up and about, then the possibility of nursing home placement or private-duty help should be considered. Finally, team members can be instrumental in helping each other see their professional boundaries. Trusting other members of the team, including on-call staff, to monitor the needs of "favorite patients" serves not only to preserve time and energy for other patients, but also establishes a relationship between the family and the hospice team rather than with a sole staff member.

Closing Comments

Hospice care emphasizes care rather than treatment for patients with incurable, progressive illness and their families. Staff involved in this care regularly confront ethical issues regarding end-of-life care and attempt to reconcile them based on competing values of autonomy, beneficence, justice, and dignity. By recognizing several rules of thumb, one may be able to resolve most of these issues in practice, ultimately to the benefit of patients and their families.

References

1. Harrold JK, Lynn J (eds): *A Good Dying: Shaping Health Care for the Last Months of Life.* New York, Haworth, 1998.
2. Christakis N: Timing of referral of terminally ill patients to an outpatient hospice. *J Gen Intern Med* 9:314–320, 1994.
3. Task Force on Palliative Care, Last Acts, Robert Wood Johnson Foundation: Precepts of palliative care. *J Palliat Med* 1:109–112, 1998.
4. Pearson C, Stubbs ML: *Parting Company: Understanding the Loss of a Loved One: The Caregiver's Journey.* Seattle, WA: Seal Press, 1999.
5. Keenan JM, Hepburn K: The role of physicians in home health care *Clin Geriatr Med* 7:665–674, 1991.
6. Buchanan AE, Brock DW: *Deciding For Others.* Cambridge, UK, Cambridge University Press, 1989.
7. Dworkin G: *The Theory and Practice of Autonomy.* Cambridge, UK, Cambridge University Press, 1988.
8. Lidz CW Fischer L, Arnold RM: *The Erosion of Autonomy in Long Term Care.* New York, Oxford University Press, 1992.
9. Miller B: Autonomy and the refusal of life saving treatment. *Hastings Cent Rep* 11:22–28, 1981.
10. Appelbaum P, Lidz CW, Meisel A: *Informed Consent: Legal Theory and Clinical Practice.* New York, Oxford University Press, 1987.
11. President's Commission for the Study of Ethical Problems in Medicine and Biomedical and Behavioral Research: *Making Health Care Decisions.* Washington DC, U.S. Government Printing Office, 1982.
12. Dworkin R: Philosophical issues in presenile dementia. Washington DC: Office of Technology Assessment, 1986.
13. Lidz CW, Arnold RM: *Rethinking Autonomy in Long-Term Care.* U Miami Law Rev 407:603–623, 1993.

14. Collopy BJ: Autonomy in long term care: some crucial distinctions. *Gerontologist* 28(suppl):10–17, 1988.
15. Beauchamp T, Childress J: *Principles of Biomedical Ethics.* New York, Oxford University Press, 1997.
16. The SUPPORT Principal Investigators: A controlled trial to improve care for seriously ill hospitalized patients: the study to understand prognoses and preferences for outcomes and risks of treatments. *JAMA* 274:1591–1598, 1995.
17. Doyle D, Hanks GW, MacDonald N (eds): *Oxford Textbook of Palliative Medicine.* New York, Oxford University Press, 1998.
18. Meisel A: Legal myths about terminating life support. *Arch Intern Med* 151:1497–1502, 1991.
19. Jennings B (ed): Ethics in Hospice Care: challenges to hospice values in a changing health care environment. *Hospice J* 12(spec vol) 1997.
20. Sulmasy DP: Death and human dignity. *Linacre Q* 61:27–36, 1994.
21. Forrow L, Baden L: *Clinical Ethics for the Medical House Officer: General Principles and Cases.* Boston, Beth Israel Deaconess Medical Center, 1997.
22. Ripamonti C, Genta BT, Bezzetti F, et al: Role of enteral nutrition in advanced cancer patients: indications and contraindications of the different techniques employed. *Tumori* 82:302–308, 1996.
23. Bezzetti F, Amadori D, Breura E, et al: Guidelines on artificial nutrition versus hydration in terminal cancer patients: European Association for Palliative Care. *Nutrition* 12:163–167, 1996.

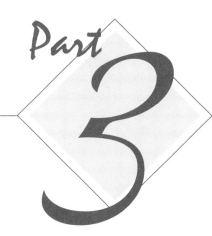

Part 3

Problems Related
to the Process
of Care

Jeffrey H. Burack

Truth Telling

Ms. Abbott, 21-years-old, seeks routine primary care from a new clinician in her college town. She has been in good health except for a history of depression. When the new physician request prior records, her pediatrician responds by telephone and reveals that the patient is a genotypic male (XY) with androgen-insensitivity syndrome. (In this condition, also called testicular feminization, a defect in the testosterone receptor protein results in the development of a female appearance. However, secondary sexual maturation is limited, the vagina ends in a blind pouch, and the undescended intraabdominal testes pose a high risk of malignant transformation.) Her parents and previous physicians had decided not to tell Ms. Abbott about her condition for fear of the psychological trauma that might result. The home-town pediatrician believes now, when she is away from the prying eyes of her small town, would be an excellent time to have the surgery necessary to remove her intraabdominal testes. He urges the new physician to arrange for the operation, telling the patient that the purpose is to remove her "diseased ovaries" or "diseased reproductive organs" and to continue to conceal her condition, the divulgence of which he fears would "shatter her." The new physician wonders about how to obtain informed consent for such a procedure.

Ms. Bennett, 73 years old, is brought for medical attention by her son because he finds her often lethargic and confused, and she has fallen twice in the previous month. Since being widowed 2 years earlier, she has suffered from insomnia and anxiety, for which benzodiazepine sedatives have been prescribed. She is drowsy, inattentive, and slow-moving but has an otherwise normal mental status and neurologic exam. Concerned that her symptoms may be the result of excessive use of sedative medications, the physician recommends tapering Ms. Bennett off the drugs, but she absolutely refuses to try this. The physician believes that she is addicted to benzodiazepines and fears that continued use might result in a devastating fall or other injury. He contemplates withdrawing her gradually and unwittingly from benzodiazepines using placebo pills.

Mr. Carver, an anxious but otherwise-healthy 43-year-old, undergoes unilateral nephrectomy for chronic pyelonephritis. At laparotomy, the surgeon discovers and resects a small mass in the tail of the pancreas. Pathology reveals adenocarcinoma with clean surgical margins. The overall 5-year survival for pancreatic cancer is percent 2 to 5 percent, and most patients die within a year. But the consulting oncologist believes that this patient's prognosis is probably much better than average, given the limited extent of his tumor and the lack of symptoms. She recommends a course of experimental chemotherapy. The primary care physician is prepared to tell the patient that he has pancreatic cancer but is reluctant to reveal the dismal overall prognosis, both for fear that the patient will refuse treatment and to prevent him from losing hope.

Ms. Dickens, 57 years old, has severe hypertension and chronic obstructive pulmonary disease (COPD). She has been hospitalized and intubated several times in the past for her COPD but over the past 2 years has done so well on inhaled steroids that her lung disease has required little attention from her long-time primary care physician. Her blood pressure, on the other hand, has become increasingly difficult to control and remains dangerously high despite a combination of three medications. In frustration, the physician adds a long-acting beta blocker to her regimen, not thinking about its potential to exacerbate her bronchospasm. Three days later, Ms. Dickens experiences severe shortness of breath that does not respond to her usual inhalers. She is brought by ambulance to the emergency department and is precipitously intubated for respiratory failure. Her son asks: "Doc, what brought this on?" The physician feels terrible for having prescribed the beta blocker but sees little to be gained from revealing the error.

Mr. Eng, 82 years old, complains to his primary care physician of weight loss, early satiety, and epigastric pain. The physician refers Mr. Eng for esophagogastroduodenoscopy, at which a large tumor is seen at the gastroesophageal junction; thereafter, abdominal ultrasound reveals innumerable hepatic metastases. Biopsies of the mass show poorly differentiated adenocarcinoma. Before the patient's scheduled visit, his eldest son, a 58-year-old executive, telephones the physician to express his and the family's concern that the physician not "say anything that will upset Dad." Further discussion reveals that the patient's children have suspected for some time that their father is seriously ill and specifically have thought it likely that he has cancer. The son fears that knowledge of a cancer diagnosis would frighten and perhaps kill his father. In any case, he reports, "in our Chinese culture, old people are not told such things," and he makes it clear that as the eldest son, responsibility for receiving information and making treatment decisions should be his. The physician wonders what to say to the son and what to tell the patient.

Scope of the Problem

Clinicians should generally tell the truth to their patients. There can be little argument with this broad prescription. But questions about whether the truth can or should sometimes be concealed or modified are surprisingly common. In this chapter, I discuss the sorts of situations in which questions about truth telling arise, and their relationship to the general issue of medical paternalism. I discuss arguments for and against being truthful in medical practice and suggest a taxonomy of different types of deception and concealment. Although such behavior should almost always be avoided, unsettling questions remain as to whether offering the unvarnished truth is always desirable in the practice of primary care medicine.

History

Some problems in biomedical ethics are new; others have been around as long as the practice of medicine itself. The authors of the Hippocratic works were well aware of the range of clinical situations in which a physician might be tempted to lie to or hide the truth from a patient. In the Hippocratic volume *Decorum*, physicians are cautioned to conceal most things from patients and to appear always cheerful and serene, so as to distract the patient's attention from what is happening.[1] Throughout medieval and early modern times, the physician's role as authoritarian healer was emphasized, with little evident concern for truthful disclosure of information. Thomas Percival, the first codifier of modern medical ethics, concluded in 1803 that any right patients may have to true information about their own conditions would be "suspended, and even annihilated" if the consequences of having that information were deemed likely to prove harmful.[2] This position was formalized in the American Medical Association's founding Code of Medical Ethics in 1846.[3] Although there were always dissenting voices, this approach was espoused by most influential medical authorities until very recently. In a much-cited study conducted in 1960, Oken reported that 88 percent of physicians had a usual policy of not explicitly telling cancer patients their diagnosis.[4]

By 1977, this attitude had undergone an abrupt and dramatic reversal. Using a survey similar to Oken's, Novack et al. found that 98 percent of physicians now reported preferring to disclose a cancer diagnosis.[5] Many factors may have contributed to this striking turnabout.

Certainly, recent advances in cancer treatment had by that time made a diagnosis of cancer seem less an irrevocable death sentence. More subtle social forces were also at work during the intervening years, including the greater recognition of personal dignity and autonomy fostered by the civil rights and women's movements and the increased hostility toward authority wrought by the Vietnam War and the Watergate scandal. These social factors have undoubtedly accounted for much of the shift toward a general policy of honest disclosure in medicine. Moreover, the present consumerist climate in medicine, the emphasis in medical ethics on individual autonomy, and the astronomic rise in the general public's access to medical information have combined to make routine deception appear so unwise and impractical that questions about its rightness or wrongness might not even appear relevant. One is tempted to ask, then: Why ever do anything short of telling the whole truth?

Background Theory and Context

Basic Arguments for and against Truth Telling

WHY NOT JUST TELL THE TRUTH?

As illustrated by the case of the college student with androgen-insensitivity syndrome, Ms. Abbott, the motive that most often conflicts with the desire to tell the truth is the desire to help and certainly to avoid harming the patient. Clinicians have a duty not to lie but also another duty to act beneficently toward patients. A dilemma arises when it appears that one cannot simultaneously satisfy both obligations: one must either lie or hurt the patient emotionally. That is, clinicians may be tempted to hide,

shade, or lie about clinical information because of the fear that it will upset the patient and be to his or her overall detriment.

This fear takes many forms: that patients will misunderstand or exaggerate the importance of the information; that they will worry unnecessarily about something for which there is nothing to be done; or that the information will cause psychological distress, depression, or even suicide. Ms. Abbott has lived a "normal" life as a woman, and it is incontestably appropriate and humane to worry that disclosure of her genetic and anatomic peculiarities might shake the deepest foundations of her self-regard and life plans. The well-intentioned clinician, thinking only of the patient's welfare, might reasonably believe that she would be much better off never knowing about her disturbing diagnosis.

It was in light of such concerns that classical medical authorities considered that the physician stood in the best position from which to judge the overall likely impact of the information. This assertion exemplifies medical *paternalism*, the position that physicians could and indeed ought always to do what they judged to be in patients' best interests, regardless of those patients' own preferences. It was the physician's privilege, even a responsibility, to make this judgment and consequently to reveal only that information which would be beneficial. The reasons to avoid the truth in such circumstances seem clear: the physician's goals are to minimize harm and maximize benefit to the patient. Why, then, worry so much about being truthful in the first place? Why not simply make a carefully considered judgment of the overall best course of action, weighing the benefits and burdens as clinicians do in virtually every area of clinical decision making?

WHY BOTHER TELLING THE TRUTH?

CONSEQUENTIALIST REASONS *Consequentialist* arguments involve the likely consequences or outcomes of taking a particular course of action.

The classical argument for nondisclosure must be understood as a purely consequentialist one: the decision about whether and what to tell ought to be made solely on the basis of how things will subsequently go for the patient.

Yet a variety of negative consequences might be expected to flow from a policy of lying or concealing the truth suggesting many reasons for clinicians to be truthful (Table 11-1). For example, patients who are lied to might feel angry or humiliated if they learned the truth. These negative feelings are themselves bad outcomes. Similarly, patients who discover that they have been deceived may be less inclined to pursue future appropriate medical care, and their health may suffer as a result.

Apart from the immediate consequences to the patient at hand, there are longer-term consequentialist reasons for clinicians to endorse a policy of telling the truth. Mounting evidence indicates that litigation against clinicians results at least as much from patients' and families' sense of having not been dealt with honestly as

from bad outcomes.[6] Furthermore, there is evidence that patients who are told the details of their condition and who participate in health care decision making generally are more satisfied with their care and have better health outcomes.[7,8]

More directly, research indicates that the vast majority of patients desire clear, concrete, detailed diagnostic and prognostic information.[8] The picture is perhaps clouded in that, once given such information, many patients prefer that a trusted clinician advise or decide upon a course of action.[9] However, a preference for a direct recommendation as to what to do should not be construed to imply endorsement of not being told what is wrong.

Perhaps most difficult to assess may be the effects of deception on the clinician's integrity, character, and self-perception. Clinicians practice and live by an integrated set of core personal and professional beliefs, the preservation of which is itself an ethical imperative. Routinely deceiving patients might inure clinicians to

Table 11-1

Fifteen Reasons to Be Truthful

Consequentialist reasons	Avoiding anger and humiliation
	Encouraging patients to pursue future care
	Improving health outcomes
	Emphasizing good communication
	Enhancing clinician-patient relationships
	Reducing liability risk
	Giving patients what they want
	Preserving social trust
	Preserving clinician integrity
Deontologic reasons	Upholding the general moral prohibition against deception
	Honoring the professional obligation of veracity
	Respecting patient autonomy
	Preserving patient dignity
	Preserving clinician dignity
	Enhancing social equality

minimize concerns about truthfulness and respect and thus undermine professional integrity. Trainees who are taught that deception is acceptable may not come to incorporate veracity into their sense of professional virtue. Clinicians who conceal or modify information may also be burdened by the unforeseeable and cumulative strains and risks of the further deceptions required to support an initial one.[10] Finally, clinicians must recognize that any efforts at concealment or deceit, and especially any systematic policy that condones them, will further erode public trust in medicine. Any one of these consequential considerations may seem to be minimally affected by any particular clinical choice, but the weight of them all taken together supports a strong presumption in favor of truth-telling.

DEONTOLOGIC REASONS There are also compelling deontologic reasons for such a strong presumption (Table 11-1). *Deontologic* moral rules are ones meant to stand on their own, without reference to the possible consequences of contemplated actions. Most deontologic moral systems include a general prohibition against lying. These everyday prohibitions may not forbid milder forms of deception (see below, "What Is the Truth?") and generally do not require specific forms of disclosure—that is, although they proscribe lying, they do not generate obligations to reveal information that is not directly asked for.

Since clinicians are subject to the same rules as others, they would be forbidden to lie. However, particular relationships between people create additional obligations and prohibitions, so that there are extra rules by which clinicians have to abide in their roles as clinicians. The clinician-patient relationship is a *fiduciary* one: the patient surrenders power to the clinician in the expectation that the clinician will use that power for the patient's good.[11] Medicine encourages and relies upon this extension of trust and surrender of control and in return promises assistance, support, fidelity, and truthfulness. Deception is inimical to such a relationship. In practice, clinicians are thus subject to rules about truth telling that are more stringent than those governing relations between strangers.

One of the most compelling arguments in favor of a policy of full disclosure is that giving patients relevant information about their own situation maximally respects and enhances their *autonomy*: their ability to control, make decisions about, and determine the course of their own lives. In order to make autonomous decisions, we need to be fully informed. Before making their own personal health-related decisions, clinicians generally want all information that might be even remotely relevant. Respect for autonomy demands that clinicians extend the same degree of control to patients, even to those who might make decisions that are short-sighted or otherwise not in their own best interests. The clinician's task then becomes one not of limiting the information given to patients but of adequately preparing the ground on which those patients will make important choices, by checking understanding, discussing options, and helping to clarify values and priorities.

Autonomy is closely related to *dignity*, which at a minimum involves some measure of self-awareness, self-control, and honest self-representation. Our dignity is undermined when we are *manipulated* or *coerced*—that is, when someone else circumvents our free will and causes us to act in certain ways. Deception and nondisclosure are manipulative, since their goal is to produce or prevent specific sorts of behaviors by others who would be expected to act differently if given full information. Lack of truthfulness therefore undermines patients' dignity.

What Is the Truth?

If falsehood, like truth, had only one face, we would be in better shape. For we would take as certain the opposite of what the liar said. But the reverse of truth has a hundred thousand shapes and a limitless field.

—Michel de Montaigne[12]

Arguments about whether or not to engage in some form of telling less than the full truth often devolve into definitional conflicts about whether that behavior actually constitutes lying or deception. It is therefore worthwhile to be precise about what these terms mean. Table 11-2 presents a taxonomy of forms of not telling the truth. It is organized from the most direct, most obvious, and typically most egregious (lying), at the top, to the more subtle and less evidently problematic at the bottom (selective disclosure). However, there can be no rigid hierarchy of "worse" versus "better" or less bad types of not telling the truth. The evil, harm, and justifiability of any episode of not telling the truth will depend, among other factors, on its intent, its consequences, and the availability of alternatives.

We must first distinguish deception from concealment (Table 11-2). *Deception* may be defined as actively and intentionally causing another person to adopt a false belief or to fail to reject a false belief. Three elements are implicit in this definition: (1) the result must be the production or reinforcement of a false belief, (2) one's actions must be causally related to that production or reinforcement, and (3) it must be one's deliberate intent in acting to so cause a false belief. Deception involves a misinforming act and therefore stands in contrast both to truthfully informing another and to doing nothing at all. *Concealment* is a broader phenomenon that consists of intentionally avoiding the communication to another person of all the relevant information one has as one understands it. While deception aims at creating or reinforcing a particular false belief, concealment typically aims to avoid the production of particular true beliefs. Though it may occur in the context of action, concealment in its essence is passive and stands in contrast to full disclosure of information.

DECEPTION

The most direct and easily grasped form of deception is *lying*, which is the direct communication of a statement which one knows or believes to be false with the intention of thereby causing a false belief. Lying is per se a linguistic act, whereby one uses language to deceive. It need not, however, be a verbal act, since one can surely lie using sign language, writing, or electronic media. It is lying specifically that is the object of most categorical moral and religious prohibitions concerning deception.

Outright lying may be quite infrequent in medical practice, but other more common clinical practices come under the heading of *misleading*, which might be taken to include all nonlying forms of active deception (Table 11-2). The use of therapeutic placebos, as are being considered for Ms. Bennett in the hypothetical case above to facilitate withdrawal of benzodiazepines, provides an example. As the physician hands the patient the bottle of inert tablets, the statement, "Take this pill, it will help you" may not, strictly speaking, be a lie, particularly given the surprising effectiveness of placebos in many clinical contexts.[13] Nothing said is technically false, and the pills may indeed help the patient

Table 11-2

Forms of Not Telling the Truth

CATEGORY	FORM	EXAMPLES
Deception	Lying	Falsehood
	Misleading	Placebo, euphemism, nonverbal response
Concealment	Withholding	Nondisclosure, timing
	Selective disclosure	Omission, emphasis

to feel better. Yet the very point of giving the placebo is to ameliorate symptoms and to do so by creating in the patient the (false) belief that she is receiving a physiologically active agent. Since the production of the false belief is intended, the practice is unarguably deceptive.

Similarly, one can actively mislead by using euphemisms. This is exemplified by the once common practice of not disclosing that cancer had been discovered at biopsy but instead using either common terms such as "growth," or medical jargon such as "neoplasm." Again, such statements are not lies, since the tissue biopsied indeed is both a growth and a neoplasm; but to the extent that one intends the patient to believe that she has a benign lesion, the act is deceptive.[14] Finally, though more difficult to identify, episodes in which nonverbal behavior is aimed at producing or reinforcing false beliefs may represent an even more prevalent form of deception. These might include physical examination maneuvers intended not to discover or to exclude signs of disease but simply to reassure an anxious patient.

CONCEALMENT

Withholding and *selective disclosure* are forms of concealment of information (Table 11-2). The goal of withholding information by deliberate nondisclosure is not that the patient form a false belief. Instead, the formation of a specific true belief is thereby avoided. Thus, in the hypothetical case of Ms. Abbott, should her physician decide not to disclose the diagnosis of androgen-insensitivity syndrome, information would be withheld from the patient in order to prevent her from coming to hold the true belief that she is genetically male. Many of the same issues raised by deception are relevant in such cases of nondisclosure, including especially the ways in which it may compromise the patient's autonomy. Because the physician is not actively deceiving the patient, it could be argued that his

or her action in such instances would be less blameworthy. Nevertheless, from a consequentialist standpoint, the outcomes for the patient and for trust may be comparably deleterious.

Information can also be temporarily withheld to affect the timing of the delivery of bad news. One often cited example goes as follows: A clinician is seeing a very anxious man whose recent biopsy of a colonic polyp shows cancer. The patient is scheduled to leave the next day for a week-long vacation. The clinician must decide whether to give the patient his results today or to wait until his return. The clinician's concern is that the results will so upset him as to ruin this much-needed vacation for both the patient and his wife. There would in any case be no intervention recommended within the week, and a week's hiatus seems extremely unlikely to affect the course of his disease. In the end, the clinician intends to fully disclose the diagnosis—just not today. Would waiting in this case be deceptive?

That depends on how the conversation goes. The patient may ask, "Do you have results?" In that case, answering "no" would be a lie. Answering "yes" and informing the patient that he has a "neoplasm" that will need further follow-up on his return would be a euphemistic deception. If the patient does not ask at all, not telling him at this time that the results are available would not constitute deception but would be a type of concealment. To determine whether any of these actions would be justified, one would have to appeal to many of the same features of the case: the likely consequences to the patient of being told his diagnosis, the compromise to his autonomy of not being given important information about himself, the effect on his relationship with his clinician, and so on.

In everyday practice, probably the most common form of not telling the entire truth is selective disclosure. This may occur by omitting elements of the truth—telling "the truth" but not "the whole truth"—or, more subtly, by emphasizing and focusing the patient's attention on certain elements of what is being disclosed. Clinicians may believe that by selectively disclosing information, they can influence patients in the direction of choices they believe to be in those patients' best interests. The hypothetical case vignette involving Mr. Carver illustrates the subtleties of selective disclosure. Telling Mr. Carver that he has pancreatic cancer but not mentioning prognostic statistics may aim at preventing him from concluding that treatment is futile—that is, the goal again is to avoid the formation of a particular belief. But in the *Arato* case, from which this case is adapted, a California court ruled that clinicians must give statistical life-expectancy data to patients with life-threatening diseases, on the grounds that such information is necessary to making informed choices about whether to undergo treatment.[15]

In one, almost trivial sense, virtually every medical conversation involves selective disclosure, as it would not be possible, let alone desirable, for a clinician to disclose every potentially relevant medical fact. For example, in recommending a particular antihypertensive drug to patients, it is improbable that clinicians would have at their command all medical knowledge pertinent to that drug's efficacy, toxicity, and interactions. Even if they did, it would be absurdly time-consuming to mention every last rare side effect and risk, confusing or overwhelming patients, who would be left unable to see the forest (the therapeutic rationale) for the trees (myriad medical details).

However, the practical impossibility of such full disclosure should not be taken to justify all instances of selective disclosure. One can distinguish between different sorts of selective disclosure according to the reasons and intentions behind them. For example, if sexual dysfunction is so rare a side effect of an antihypertensive that it has only been described in isolated case reports, it is reasonable not to mention such dysfunction in discussing the pros and cons of the medication. If, on the other hand, sexual dysfunction is actually a very common side

effect but one of which the clinician is not aware, the failure to disclose it may be blameworthy, but not because the clinician has concealed it. Rather, the fault would then be attributable in not keeping adequately up to date with pertinent medical literature—surely a moral obligation to one's patients, but not one having to do directly with truth telling.

Finally, imagine that the clinician indeed knows that sexual dysfunction is a common side effect but chooses to omit it from the potential toxicities discussed with the patient because of a belief that the patient is inordinately concerned about his sexual functioning and is therefore likely to refuse the drug if impotence is mentioned. The clinician believes that this would be an irrational choice, which would very likely deprive the patient of significant clinical benefit. Therefore, the clinician is motivated by the beneficent desire to bring about improved health for the patient. Nevertheless, the temptation to so act is fundamentally paternalistic. The patient's autonomy is violated in that he is not given the opportunity to choose for himself, however wrong-headed one may believe that choice to be.

Nonpaternalistic Deception

The foregoing discussion applies to situations in which the truth is disguised or withheld because of the belief that doing so will in some way benefit the patient who is so deceived—that is, to *paternalistic* deceptions.[16] As difficult as these instances may be to justify, *nonpaternalistic* deceptions, in which the patient is misled or uninformed in order to serve *someone else's* ends, are even more highly suspect. There are a variety of circumstances under which clinicians may be tempted to withhold or modify the truth for nonpaternalistic reasons. These include situations in which obligations to the patient appear to conflict with perceived obligations to others. Clinicians may collude, for example, to keep a colleague's impairment by substance abuse a secret from mutual patients for fear of humiliating the colleague or destroying his or her livelihood. Such concealment cannot be justified, particularly as it may put those very patients at risk (see Chap. 9).

Other forms of nondisclosure may be motivated by clinician self-interest. Questions of whether and how medical errors should be disclosed to patients may present clinicians with particularly difficult dilemmas. Revealing an error in medical judgment would appear to offer little benefit to Ms. Dickens who was prescribed a beta blocker that precipated a flare of COPD in the hypothetical case described above, while potentially causing harm to the clinician and to the patient-clinician relationship. There are, however, powerful reasons for judicious disclosure in such cases. The patient may be confused and discouraged by what she takes to be a sudden and unexplained worsening in a condition she had thought had stabilized. She may blame herself for the exacerbation. Informing her of the precipitant and emphasizing the need to avoid beta blockers may help prevent such episodes in the future. Such disclosure surely cannot reasonably be imagined to harm the patient.

The fear that patients like Ms. Dickens will lose confidence in their clinicians and may go elsewhere for care provides no justification for withholding information from them. Revealing the information might actually increase her confidence in the clinician. As discussed in Chaps. 7, 8, and 9, clinicians may hesitate for similar reasons to reveal to patients their financial arrangements with various health care organizations. But withholding or disguising the truth to prevent a patient from making certain choices is a form of manipulation and hence a violation of autonomy, particularly when the clinician believes that the patient would likely act differently with the information in hand.

◆ Toward Resolution

Recognizing the Problem

Some clinical situations share features—of the patient, the information at issue, and the anticipated consequences—which ought to serve as "red flags" that a significant issue of truth telling has arisen or is likely to and which should thus prompt careful deliberation (Table 11-3). Patients who may be at increased risk for not having the truth told to them are those with whom clinicians have the most difficulty identifying and whose values might be expected to diverge most from the clinicians'; such patients would include the elderly, the poor, members of other cultures, and disenfranchised minorities. Clinicians may be likely to stereotype these patients and to assume that they either do not

Table 11-3

Red Flags for Truth Telling Issues

Patient characteristics	Disenfranchised
	Adverse health behaviors
	Unlikable
	Intellectual or emotional limitations
Type of information	Potentially upsetting
	Serious diagnosis or prognosis
	Already known to others
Potential consequences	Strong emotional reaction
	Likely to affect decision making
	Effects on others

want to know the truth or cannot handle it. Likewise at risk are patients whose behavior clinicians might be inclined to try to manipulate, such as those who use tobacco, alcohol, or other recreational drugs; who do not adhere to prescribed therapies; or who otherwise engage in health-threatening behavior. These patients, and others who are simply unlikable, may evoke anger or other negative emotions in clinicians. Clinicians may also be inclined to adjust the truth for patients whose intellectual capacity they believe to be limited or whose emotional balance may be precarious, such as those with affective disorders.

Information that is frightening, discouraging, bizarre, or potentially stigmatizing may be especially likely to be withheld or disguised. This will, of course, be true for virtually all new diagnoses of serious, life-threatening, or potentially disabling conditions, for much data about prognosis and risk, and for bad news about relapses or failure to respond to therapy. The other situation that must always raise concern is when information already known to others is being kept from or modified for the patient or other persons it affects.

Finally, the potential consequences one considers in deciding whether and how to deliver information can be illuminating. Fear of a strong emotional reaction on the part of the patient—perhaps of the loss of hope, depression, or even suicide—is one flag indicating the need for careful scrutiny. Concern about the decisions the patient will subsequently make, and particularly the fear that he or she will make the "wrong" ones, is another. In these situations, clinicians generally find themselves wondering whether the patient is "better off not knowing." In others, clinicians contemplate the possibility that "it wouldn't make a difference to the patient anyway." This often marks circumstances, as in Ms. Dickens' case described above, in which the clinician is concerned about the possible effects of the disclosure on others, including the clinician, rather than on the patient.

Special Circumstances

SENSITIVE DISCLOSURE

The deleterious impact of bad medical news can often be mitigated by the way in which such news is communicated. Clinicians, dedicated to the welfare of their patients, understandably balk at being "brutally honest" and giving information in such a way as to cause pain. In the case of a distressing diagnosis or prognosis, however, brutality may be based in the facts, over which the physician has had no control; life is manifestly cruel to some patients. The clinician's task is therefore not to change or hide those facts but to deliver them in a way that embodies concern and empathy for the patient. "The truth may be 'brutal,' but the telling of it should not be."[17]

There is a well-developed literature on the sensitive delivery of bad news.[18] Breaking bad news can be thought of in three stages: preparation, discussion, and follow-up (Table 11-4). For example, knowing that there is difficult news to deliver, the clinician must set aside adequate time for discussion. The stress of a routine 10- or 15-min office visit may be inimical to sensitive discussion and may frequently result in unintended "brutal" honesty. Furthermore, patients are apt to feel abandoned or isolated after receiving calamitous medical news, particularly since friends and loved ones may sometimes withdraw in fear or confusion. This feeling of abandonment may be the ultimate "brutality" that accompanies bad news. With forethought, the clinician can encourage the patient to express fears and worries about what has been

Table 11-4

Twelve Tips for Clinicians Breaking Bad News to Patients

Preparation	Set aside adequate time for discussion
	Provide privacy and a comfortable setting
	Come prepared with information and a plan
	Sit and, if appropriate, touch the patient
	Warn the patient that you have something difficult to discuss
Discussion	Speak straightforwardly and get right to the point
	Keep terms simple and check for understanding
	Watch for nonverbal cues and be aware of your own
	Acknowledge and address strong emotional reactions
	Allow the patient time to express fears and worries
Follow-up	Schedule follow-up with yourself and consultants
	Be available

disclosed, ask questions, and depart feeling supported and cared for rather than abandoned.

EXCEPTIONS TO THE DUTY TO DISCLOSE

There are clinical situations in which it is commonly supposed that the usual duty to disclose information may be abridged. In each, however, the circumstances under which disclosure can rightly be avoided are much narrower than would at first appear, and the physician contemplating nondisclosure takes on significant responsibilities to probe, understand, and be candid about the reasons justifying it. Five clinical situations are discussed below: patient's waiver, patient's incapacity, medical emergency, therapeutic privilege, and cultural difference.

PATIENT'S WAIVER   Patients may explicitly waive their claims to full information about their own conditions or prognoses. A patient may, for example, agree to undergo a biopsy but state: "Doctor, I don't want to know the results." In such a case, it would seem at first blush that most of the arguments typically supporting full disclosure—respecting patient autonomy and

promoting trust, for example—would support honoring the request not to disclose.

Yet when the full implications of such nondisclosure are explored, it will most often turn out to be either untenable or contrary to the patient's overall wishes. For example, not disclosing the findings of cancer on a biopsy would seem to preclude the possibility of obtaining informed consent for appropriate therapy. The patient's request may be motivated by inordinate fear of bad news, by concern about being unable to cope with such news, or by anxiety about being abandoned to do so alone. When a patient asks not to know, the clinician must explore the reasons for the request, must offer reassurance and support, and must play out various implications and hypothetical scenarios that the patient might not foresee.

Alternatively, patients may sometimes state that they simply do not want to know "if it's bad news." This sort of conditional waiver is almost always impossible to honor: since the patient appears to want to hear good news, silence will likely be interpreted as bad news. This may, in effect, be tantamount to disclosure and may possibly be worse, since fear will often make patients project onto that silence a grimmer diagnostic or prognostic situation than actually obtains. Such conditional waivers should never be accepted at face value. They should be viewed as marking fear and ambivalence and should serve to prompt more in-depth exploration and discussion.

PATIENT'S INCAPACITY   It would seem self-evident that patients should not be told more than they are capable of understanding. Informing a small child, for example, about the harsh details of her condition and the intricacies of the therapeutic options would appear to cause terror without countervailing benefit, and delivering a lengthy litany of medical details to a severely demented adult would be a cruel farce. The rationale and criteria for assessing decision-making capacity are described in Chap. 18 and apply here in the consideration of how that capacity ought to affect disclosure. Yet clinicians must scrupulously avoid using a patient's limitations as an excuse to avoid difficult discussions or the revelation of information that might result in decisions with which they would disagree. And, as with issues of informed consent (Chap. 19), when decisions are made to limit disclosure because of diminished capacity, the clinician must assiduously seek an appropriate surrogate to whom fuller disclosure can be made. That is, the same sorts of arguments that support truth telling to fully competent patients support equally truthful disclosure to those close to and responsible for patients who lack decision-making capacity.

MEDICAL EMERGENCY   The duty of beneficence occasionally demands, under emergency conditions, that the usual processes of disclosure, discussion, and informed consent be abridged. The paradigmatic example is the trauma victim, rushed bleeding but still conscious toward a hospital operating room, for whom fully describing the diagnostic possibilities, planned interventions, and potential outcomes might cause a fatal delay. To invoke the emergency

exception to disclosure, like imposing unconsented treatment, the following may generally be required: (1) that significant harm is highly likely to occur in short order to the patient or to others; (2) that limiting or avoiding disclosure directly makes such harm considerably less likely to occur; and (3) that there is no alternative approach which is likely to accomplish the same ends but avoids deception or concealment. The fact that the word "likely" appears in each of the three criteria serves as a reminder that no hard and fast formulae can be devised that will process clinical factors into an ethically appropriate response. Rather, a good-faith assessment of probabilities and alternatives, grounded in the individual patient's actual circumstances and the best available evidence, is essential.

THERAPEUTIC PRIVILEGE   A commonly invoked reason for avoiding full disclosure is to extend the "therapeutic privilege" to nonemergency situations, claiming that fully informing a capable patient of relevant information might harm that patient. Most cases of nondisclosure, like those above, appeal to some version of therapeutic privilege to justify the concealment or alteration of information. However, clinicians must recognize that, in so doing, they are essentially arguing on the basis of medical emergency and must therefore be prepared to defend their decisions on the grounds of averting grave harm, direct causality, and the absence of alternatives. When these criteria are considered, exceedingly few cases satisfying this standard will arise in primary care. If the emergency justification is eschewed in favor of a broader and weaker one, therapeutic privilege as applied to nonemergencies becomes simply a restatement of paternalism: the clinician is entitled to decide what, of all possible behaviors and interventions, is most likely to benefit and least likely to harm the patient, and to choose that course of action. As we have seen, this position is generally unacceptable, particularly where it regards control of information about the patient.

CULTURAL DIFFERENCE Since many clinicians in the United States see a population of increasingly multinational and multicultural origins, the argument is frequently made that the American emphasis on autonomy and subsequent insistence on full disclosure are conceits peculiar to the individualistic, litigious, mainstream American culture of the late twentieth century. A rigid practice of detailed disclosure, the argument continues, may be not only optional in other cultural contexts but even inappropriate or harmful to persons immersed in those cultures. Mr. Eng's case vignette illustrates these concerns.

Family and community concerns should never be dismissed as irrelevant or disparaged as being against the patient's interests: the presumption should generally be that these individuals have the patient's welfare at heart. On the other hand, in Mr. Eng's case, his son's fears about the detrimental power of "bad news" are not supported by evidence and may be amenable to change. He may hold incorrect beliefs about the diagnoses or prognoses under consideration, which should be explored. Furthermore, as with patients' waivers, nondisclosure may complicate subsequent decision making about treatment options, advance care planning, and, in this case, the sort of end-of-life reconciliations and arranging of affairs in which many persons would choose to engage (see Chap. 20).

Withholding information from this patient because "in our Chinese culture, old people are not told such things" unacceptably pigeonholes the patient by age and ethnicity. Just as one cannot presume, without asking, what a young person in "our" culture might choose, one equally cannot reduce the individual from a different culture to a stereotypic caricature. The clinician must gently explain that, from within the perspective of American medicine, respect for persons dictates that clinicians understand and honor individual preferences and, furthermore, that while this no doubt is a culturally biased perspective, it is one that cannot easily be abandoned.

Most importantly, however, much of this conflict might have been anticipated and averted by discussions, while the patient was still well, about what sorts of things he does and does not want to be told. It is above all with the patients about whom clinicians are most likely to hold stereotypes, and for whom they might therefore be most inclined to invoke the cultural difference exception, that they most need to seek clarity in advance. That is, these patients should be asked about their preferences regarding disclosure, consent, advance directives, and the like. A waiver that one is convinced legitimately reflects the patient's own previously expressed preferences is on surer moral ground than the objection to disclosure, however well-intentioned, of a third party. In some communities, however, simply discussing the hypothetical possibility of a bad outcome would be considered inappropriate or even harmful.[19] The clinician's pursuit of such clarity must therefore be moderated by genuine sensitivity to cultural concerns.

Finally, in any such situation of conflict, whether explicitly cultural or not, the clinician is not obliged to act alone and ought not do so. Taking care to safeguard patients' confidentiality, the clinician should seek assistance from other clinicians, from community groups or leaders, and from hospital or organizational ethics committees and consultants.

IMPLICIT MODULATION OF DISCLOSURE

The foregoing exceptions to truth telling all refer to explicit characteristics of a clinical situation that might militate against full disclosure. But the implicit, partial "waiver" that probably governs most clinician-patient relationships is much more difficult to characterize. People rely on trusted professionals to filter the technical information they provide.[20] Most patients do not want to hear every detail of their differential diagnosis, therapeutic options, risks and complications, and possible outcomes. Clinicians, in turn, make constant and perhaps often accurate judgments about what individual patients want to hear and are able to bear, and they adjust the manner and content of their disclosures accordingly.

But herein lies one of the most subtle, perilous, and underexamined challenges of day-to-day clinical medicine. For although such judgments may often reflect precisely the sort of individualized understanding and nuanced practice that professionals are expected to bring to their work, they also point to the glaring possibilities of stereotyping and discrimination, whether conscious or not. It would be unrealistic and probably contrary to the fiduciary responsibility to individual patients to expect clinicians to behave identically with everyone and thus never to make such judgments.[21] But the risks inherent in doing so strongly recommend that, rather than operate from presumptions and prejudice, clinicians base their determination of the level of discussion appropriate to each patient on an exploration, with that patient, of the patient's own priorities and preferences. Such determinations are most appropriately made in the context of a significant relationship with the patient over time and in no way should be taken to justify snap paternalistic assessments of what information patients can and cannot handle. And since clinicians tend to underestimate their patients' desire for information, the "default" condition ought always to be a strong presumption in favor of full disclosure.

When Considering Not Telling the Truth

It would be naive to suggest that special circumstances will never arise in which a reasonable course of action—or even the best course—involves concealment or deception. But because of the special prohibition against deception in a fiduciary relationship and its generally damaging consequences, the burden falls heavily on clinicians to convince themselves and others that such special circumstance exist. The cases discussed in this chapter demonstrate that the range of clinical situations in which such behavior is permissible is far narrower than is often imagined. To state this most clearly: in primary care practice, concealment and deception may be appropriate only in exceedingly rare situations. Typically, when clinicians think that they have to deceive, they either are wrong about the facts of the situation or its likely outcomes or have not adequately thought through nondeceptive alternatives. What steps should the clinician who is considering hiding or disguising the truth take before doing so? (Table 11-5)

First, before acting on the impulse to deceive, the clinician must step back and take time to consider the situation, the patient, the clinician's own motives, and the likely outcomes. Deception or concealment should never be undertaken as a reflexive response to the exigencies of the moment. The impetus to deception often springs from the unarticulated belief that the information in question is something the

Table 11-5

Steps for Clinicians to Take When Considering Deception or Concealment

Step back and take time before acting
Try to find out what the patient really wants
Consider the patient's special needs and background
Be explicit about goals and benefits sought
Imagine yourself in the patient's place
Seek out and consider nondeceptive alternatives
Seek advice
Imagine and prepare for revelation of the deception
Take responsibility

patient would "really" rather not know. One of the first steps should therefore always be to probe more deeply—to find out what the patient's actual values and preferences are regarding the disclosure of medical information. Clinicians should not, for example, project their own distress about giving bad news and assume that patients are equally loath to receive it. The clinician must consider the patient's special circumstances, including his or her cultural and ethnic background and medical and psychosocial history, but must not substitute stereotypes for individualized exploration of values and wishes.

In considering any action that intentionally falls short of offering the complete truth, clinicians must carefully examine their own motives and consider the goals of the proposed action and the benefits sought through it. Making a sincere effort to be explicit about what one really hopes to gain is perhaps the most difficult step in deciding whether to deceive or conceal. Concealment is typically undertaken for precisely the wrong reason: the clinician fears that the information will unduly influence the patient's choices. Information that is potentially influential must be revealed. The clinician's task is to explain and situate that information in ways that express any reservations about how the patient might use it.

One powerful technique for clinicians to clarify their own intentions is to project themselves into the patient's place, asking: If I were in this patient's shoes, what would I hope my clinician would do for me? How would I feel, for example, if the deception were successful but I later found out about it? This sort of empathic projection can be a powerful antidote to the tendency to assume stereotypic values on the patient's part and can also bring to life the very real potential consequences of deception.

The clinician must also actively seek out and consider nondeceptive alternatives. At a minimum, deception should always be considered *prima facie* prohibited, so that it may only be considered as a last resort. No such morally charged action can be considered justified in isolation from its alternatives. Deception should never be entertained unless one can say, in good conscience and after critical review, that there are no nondeceptive ways to achieve the same important clinical goals.

At this stage, if not before, it is important to seek advice from colleagues, including ethics consultants or committees. It is neither appropriate nor prudent for a clinician alone to bear the burden of having made a decision to deceive. If one is justified in hiding the truth, the compelling facts of the case ought to hold up under scrutiny by uninvolved peers. Others can often point out flaws in assumptions or expectations and can help to generate workable, nondeceptive alternative courses of action that may not have been apparent to the clinician closely involved in the case. In the exceptional situation in which a clinician has had to act on the spot, consultation and review after the fact will help determine how to proceed subsequently. Should the deception be revealed, for example, and if so, how? Consultation may also help the clinician recognize how the situation could have been prevented or otherwise addressed in the first place, so that future deceptions can be avoided.

If, after such thorough consideration and consultation, the clinician still believes that not telling the truth is the best course of action, the next step involves imagining and preparing for exposure of the deception at some later time. This serves several purposes. First, however foolproof one imagines one's deception to be, revelation is always a realistic possibility, and must therefore be factored in as a potential consequence. Second, speculation on how things may go will help determine the shape of the action that one does choose to take. Third, the unpleasantness and possible professional and legal repercussions of being found out serve as potent stimuli for a final round of frank scrutiny of goals and motives and for an all-out search for alternatives. And finally, such moral imagination is an essential element in accepting responsibility for the action one is about to take. Clinicians should feel comfortable in imagining having to justify their behavior to themselves, their colleagues, the patient, and the community.

Truthful disclosure about medical errors is undeniably further complicated by the litigious environment in which American medicine is practiced. The clinician's chief concern may be the fear of being sued. But mounting evidence suggests that honest disclosure and acceptance of responsibility for understandable errors may prevent rather than promote lawsuits.[8] It would certainly mark a salutary change in social expectations of clinicians were errors to be openly discussed. Nevertheless, it would be disingenuous to urge full disclosure in such circumstances without consultation with hospital risk managers or other legal counsel. Clinicians may fear that if they disclose errors, patients will lose confidence in their care and seek other clinicians. But it is precisely the possibility that the informed patient will behave differently that *demands* disclosure. For while an error may be understandable, it may nevertheless seem to patients to be a legitimate reason to seek care elsewhere, in which case they ought to be enabled to do so.

Postscript: Telling the Truth to Ms. Abbott

The new physician must talk honestly to Ms. Abbott about her diagnosis of androgen-insensitivity syndrome. The patient is at a point in her life at which many make choices about sexuality, marriage or other commitment, and reproduction. Her autonomy in making such choices is severely impaired without clear information about her anatomy and genetics; it is an affront to her dignity that so many others have this information while she does not. The sort of paternalistic protection the pediatrician recommends may have been appropriate when she was a child, but must give way before her status as an autonomous adult and her new physi-

cian's fiduciary obligation to her can be realized. The consequences of disclosure are likely to be far less severe than the new physician imagines, for several reasons: patients in such circumstances typically already suspect or know that something is unusual about their sexuality (she has not had menses, for example, by age 21); many have unexpressed questions about their gender identity, for which they are often in fact relieved to have an explanation; and the sort of despair or self-destruction the physician fears is decidedly unusual and probably reflects projection of the physician's own distress and discomfort. There are no compelling reasons to continue to hide the truth, and many to come forward with it. The physician should follow guidelines for sensitively breaking difficult news (Table 11-4), and should be readily available for follow-up during what will likely prove a challenging time for Ms. Abbott.

Closing Comments

Not telling the truth in medicine is typically motivated by beneficent concern for patients. Nevertheless, there are compelling consequentialist and deontologic reasons for clinicians to try always to offer them the truth. Although there is a spectrum of not telling the truth, from lying to selective emphasis, little ethical work is done by categorization alone. The relative good or evil of any such behavior is a function less of its type than of the intentions, consequences, and alternatives associated with it.

The risks of the truth being altered or hidden are heightened in dealing with disenfranchised populations, threatening information, and the possibility that patients might make decisions deleterious to their health. In such circumstances, careful preparation and sensitive disclosure will often obviate the perceived need to deceive or conceal. Clinicians can practice preventive ethics by making it a priority to learn their patients' preferences regarding disclosure.

Clinicians must therefore always make a sincere effort to be explicit about what they really hope to gain by any deception or concealment. Other steps to take before considering such action include actively seeking nondeceptive alternatives, soliciting advice from colleagues and consultants, and ultimately taking responsibility for the proposed action and its potential consequences.

References

1. Hippocrates: Decorum, in *Hippocrates*. Vol 2. Jones WHS (trans). Cambridge, MA, Harvard University Press, 1923.
2. Percival T: *Medical Ethics*, 3d ed. Oxford, England, John Henry Parker, 1849.
3. American Medical Association: First code of medical ethics, in *Proceedings of the National Medical Convention 1846–1847*. Chicago, American Medical Association, 1847.
4. Oken D: What to tell cancer patients: a study of medical attitudes. *JAMA* 175:1120–1128, 1961.
5. Novack DH, Freireich EJ, Vaisrub S: Changes in physician attitudes toward telling cancer patients. *JAMA* 241:897–900, 1979.
6. Levinson W, Roter DL, Mullooly JP, et al: Physician-patient communication: the relationship with malpractice claims among primary care physicians and surgeons. *JAMA* 277:553–559, 1997.
7. Stewart M: Effective physician-patient communication and health outcomes: a review. *Can Med Assoc J* 152:1428–1431, 1995.
8. Hébert PC: *Doing Right: A Practical Guide to Ethics for Physicians and Medical Trainees*. Toronto, Oxford University Press, 1996.
9. Kelly WD, Friesen SR: Do cancer patients want to be told? *Surgery* 27:822–826, 1950.
10. Bok S: *Lying: Moral Choice in Public and Private Life*. New York, Pantheon Books, 1978.
11. Pellegrino ED: Toward a reconstruction of medical morality: the primacy of the act of profession and the fact of illness. *J Med Philos* 4:32–56, 1979.
12. Montaigne M de: Of liars, in *The Complete Works of Montaigne*. Frame DM (trans). Stanford, CA, Stanford University Press, 1957.
13. Brody H: *Placebos and the Philosophy of Medicine: Clinical, Conceptual and Ethical Issues*. Chicago, University of Chicago Press, 1980.
14. Veatch RM: The dying cancer patient, in Veatch RM (ed): *Case Studies in Medical Ethics*. Cambridge, MA, Harvard University Press, 1977.
15. Annas G: Informed consent, cancer, and truth in prognosis. *N Engl J Med* 330:223–225, 1994.
16. Dworkin G. Paternalism. *Monist* 56:64–84, 1972.
17. Jonsen AR, Siegler M, Winslade WJ: *Clinical Ethics*, 3d ed. New York, McGraw-Hill, 1992.
18. Buckman R: *How to Break Bad News : A Guide for Health Care Professionals*. Baltimore, Johns Hopkins University Press, 1992.
19. Carrese JA, Rhodes LA: Western bioethics on the Navajo reservation: benefit or harm? *JAMA* 274:826–829, 1995.
20. Nyberg: *The Varnished Truth*. Chicago, University of Chicago Press, 1993.
21. Thomasma, David C: Telling the truth to patients: a clinical ethics exploration. *Cambridge Q Health Ethics* 3:375–382, 1994.

Amir Halevy

Confidentiality

Beth Williams, who is being treated for depression, expresses anger and hostility toward her husband during a clinic visit. She states repeatedly that her husband is constantly nagging her and that she is so tired of his complaints that she wants to kill him. She reveals that she has fantasized about stabbing him to death while he sleeps. The clinician, who feels that Ms. Williams poses a risk to her husband, but is uncertain if she would actually follow through on her threat, is uncertain about what to do with the information. Choices include preserving confidentiality and counseling only Ms. Williams, violating confidentiality by informing the police or other authorities, and finally, violating confidentiality by informing both the police and Ms. Williams's husband.

Brad Lyons, a married man in his early thirties, is concerned that he might have acquired HIV infection during unprotected sexual intercourse with a prostitute on a recent business trip. After pretest counseling, his primary care clinician orders an HIV antibody test. The test returns positive and the diagnosis is confirmed by Western blot. During posttest counseling, the patient states that he will not inform his wife and he demands that the clinician not inform her of either his extramarital affairs or of his HIV status. Should the clinician maintain confidentiality and not inform the wife of his HIV positivity? Or should the clinician tell Mr. Lyons that she will inform his wife of his status and the need for her to be tested and protected?

Dr. Santini has a thriving primary care practice. More than half of Dr. Santini's patient's work for a large, locally based factory. The head of human resources for the company contacts the physician to report that their workers' compensation and overall health insurance premiums have skyrocketed. An internal analysis reveals that a significantly disproportionate share of the costs are attributable to pregnancy-related events. The company asks Dr. Santini to inform them of all pregnancies as soon as they are diagnosed. Furthermore, they ask Dr. Santini to tell the company which workers are using contraceptives and which are actively trying to conceive. The human resource director also mentions that they are considering looking at another insurance plan that would force her patients to find a new primary care physician. Should Dr. Santini comply with the request and violate confidentiality or refuse the company's request and potentially lose a significant percentage of the practice?

Scope of the Problem

Confidentiality, or the promise not to share personal information inappropriately, is fundamental to the clinician-patient relationship. In legal circles, it is grounded in an individual's right to *privacy*—a relatively new concept in the law that includes the right to be left alone, the right to bodily integrity, and the right to control information of a personal nature. Without a guarantee of confidentiality, in most circumstances patients would be unlikely to reveal potentially embarrassing but relevant information or even to go to a clinician for evaluation and treatment.

Although absolute confidentiality is neither practical nor desirable, questions about when confidentiality may or should be violated can pose important clinical and ethical challenges.

Range of Issues

Confidentiality affects nearly all aspects of a clinical practice. The basic rule, discussed more fully below (see "Background Theory and Context"), is that the clinician must preserve confidentiality in all matters regarding the patient. However, there are some exceptions.

For instance, the practicing clinician must occasionally deal with the patient who poses a risk to others. Such risks range from an overt threat to harm an individual or group of people to an unwillingness to change potentially threatening behavior. Consider the patient infected with a communicable disease, like Brad Lyons, in the hypothetical case above, who does not wish to disclose his infection, or patients with either seizures or syncope who insist on continuing to drive. The clinician must be aware of ethical duties as well as required reporting laws that may pose competing obligations upon him or her regarding confidentiality. For example, depending on the jurisdiction, there may be laws requiring the reporting of certain diseases and suspicions regarding violence or abuse. Such laws create a legal duty on the part of clinicians to violate confidentiality in certain circumstances.

Confidentiality is also challenged in dealing with interested third parties. These include, but are not limited to, concerned family and friends, neighbors, employers, lawyers, and, in some cases, the media. In addition, if the clinician desires compensation for his or her services, he or she must understand what information may be disclosed to third-party payers and under what circumstances. Finally, the changing technological environment and the increased emphasis on electronic means to both store and transmit information, threatens confidentiality if appropriate safeguards for protecting it are not instituted.

Background Theory and Context

Reasons for the Rule

Two basic requirements of a successful health care encounter are that the patient actually visit the clinician and that the patient disclose to the clinician all relevant information. Confidentiality is important for both. Patients must trust their clinicians not to reveal private and privileged information. For example, in the scenario involving Dr. Santini, how many patients would go to see a clinician—especially for such conditions as depression and other potentially disabling disorders—if they believed the clinician would report anything of interest to their employers? And how many patients who are HIV-positive or who suspect that they are would go to a clinician for either testing or treatment if they were not assured of confidentiality?[1]

The promise of confidentiality also encourages the full disclosure of information needed to make an appropriate diagnosis. A complete history includes questions not usually asked at parties! Most people do not reveal a detailed sexual history or recount exactly what illicit drugs they have used, or how much they drink, or other private matters to anyone who asks. However, such data are often important if the clinician is to diagnose and appropriately treat the patient. If patients were not assured of confidentiality, they might be much less likely to reveal their entire stories, if they were even to go to the clinician in the first place.

History and Codes of Ethics

The commitment to respecting patients' confidentiality is not new. The Hippocratic oath includes this promise:

> "What I may see or hear in the course of the treatment or even outside of the treatment in regard to the life of men, which on no account one must spread abroad, I will keep to myself, holding such things shameful to be spoken about."

Modern codes follow this tradition. The World Medical Association's code of medical ethics, first adopted in 1949, states that "a physician shall preserve absolute confidentiality on all he knows about his patient even after the patient has died."[2] These codes view confidentiality as absolute and inviolate, even after the death of the patient.

In the United States, various bodies of organized medicine, the courts, and legislatures have viewed confidentiality as a fundamental but not absolute right. The American Medical Association, through its Council on Ethical and Judicial Affairs, holds:

> "The physician should not reveal confidential communications or information without the express consent of the patient, unless required to do so by law. The obligation to safeguard patient confidences is subject to certain exceptions which are ethically and legally justified because of overriding social considerations. Where a patient threatens to inflict serious bodily harm to another person or to himself or herself and there is a reasonable probability that the patient may carry out the threat, the physician should take reasonable precautions for the protection of the intended victim, including notification of law enforcement authorities."[3]

The American College of Physicians states:

> "The physician must not release information without the patient's consent. However, confidentiality, like other ethical duties, is not absolute. It may have to be overridden to protect individual per-

sons or the public—for example, to warn sexual partners that a patient has syphilis or is infected with HIV—or to disclose information when the law requires."[4]

Various other specialty bodies have issued similar statements.[5]

Legal Precedents

Although, in an ideal world, ethical principles and pronouncements of organized bodies of medicine would be sufficiently powerful to cause all clinicians to conform to an accepted code of practice, legal reinforcement is often still required. The legal repercussions of violating confidentiality can take two forms. The first is potential sanction by the state medical licensing board for violating state specific professional standards. The second is civil tort law, where clinicians can be liable for monetary damages for breach of confidentiality.

Since the first successful civil action in 1917 finding a physician liable for breach of confidentiality,[6] there have been numerous cases in many jurisdictions that have established liability for inappropriate breach of confidentiality. The legal theories have varied from case to case but include defamation, invasion of privacy, and breach of an implied contract.[7] Regardless of the specific legal theory, clinicians clearly have a legal duty to protect confidentiality within accepted social constraints. This legal duty to guard confidentiality has also been shaped in recent years by cases such as *Tarasoff*, discussed more fully below, arguing that the clinician also has a balancing duty to breach confidentiality when vital third-party interests are at stake.

Exceptions to the Rule

As noted above, the basic rule that clinicians must preserve the confidentiality of patients' personal and medical information is not absolute. Aside from a patient's waiver of confidentiality, the exceptions to the rule are rooted in the protection of third parties and the public health. The exceptions require a balancing between the patient's right to privacy and the rights and interests of others. Specifically, when does the potential harm to others reach enough significance to warrant limiting the patient's rights? Two main types of exceptions are relevant: statutory reporting requirements, and case law generated duties to third parties.

STATUTORY EXCEPTIONS

All states have mandatory reporting laws of some type that require a clinician or other health care professional to notify either the state or appropriate authorities of certain diseases or conditions. The theoretical justification is that in certain cases, the public good outweighs the individual's right to privacy and confidentiality. Although the details vary from state to state, three major exceptions exist. One set of exceptions revolves around violence and violent crime. Most states have reporting requirements that mandate immediate reporting of knife wounds and gunshot wounds to the local police department.

As described in Chap. 13, a second set of exceptions encompasses abuse and neglect of vulnerable persons. All states have mandatory reporting laws for suspected child abuse and neglect and some states have laws requiring reporting of suspected abuse of dependent persons regardless of age. Additionally, clinicians have an ethical obligation to report such suspected abuse.

The final set of statutory exceptions is required reporting of certain contagious diseases, including tuberculosis, hepatitis, certain types of encephalitis, and various sexually transmitted diseases including syphilis and gonorrhea. Historically, the combination of required reporting and contact tracing (that is, notifying

individuals who may have had contact with the infected person so they may receive diagnostic testing and treatment as needed) have been effectively used to control the spread of communicable diseases. Again, the argument made for the breach of confidentiality through required reporting is that maintaining public health is more important than an individual's privacy concerns. Of note, many states have intentionally excluded HIV infection and AIDS from this public health model because of fears of discrimination against HIV-positive individuals. This HIV exceptionalism has created difficulty for many practicing clinicians regarding the appropriate limits to confidentiality.[8] Note that this tension between maintaining confidentiality and protecting third parties at risk for infection is discussed more fully below.

CASE-LAW DUTIES TO THIRD PARTIES: THE TARASOFF CASE

Case law also provides exceptions to the rule of confidentiality by creating a duty on the part of clinicians to warn or to protect innocent third parties. The case that initially established this new duty to violate confidentiality in certain instances was *Tarasoff* v. *Regents of the University of California.*[9] In 1969, Prosenjit Poddar, a graduate student at the University of California, sought counseling at a university clinic. While being seen by a psychologist, he confided that he intended to kill an unnamed woman, readily identifiable as Tatiana Tarasoff. The psychologist was sufficiently concerned to notify the campus police in order to detain Poddar and have him involuntarily committed. The campus police released Poddar after a brief detention when they concluded that he was rational and did not pose a threat. Neither Ms. Tarasoff nor her family was informed. After Poddar was released by the campus police, the psychologist's supervisor ordered the records destroyed and that "no further action be taken to deter Poddar." Two months later, Poddar stabbed Tarasoff to death.

Ms. Tarasoff's parents brought suit against the university and the psychologist, alleging negligence in the death of their daughter. The case was heard by the California Supreme Court in 1974, which ruled that the Tarasoffs had a cause of action against the therapist for breaching a duty to warn. The court concluded that a therapist has a duty to warn the identified victim, thereby violating patient confidentiality, when the therapist "determines, or should determine, that a warning is essential to avert danger arising from the medical or psychological condition of the patient." The original *Tarasoff* decision was vacated by the California Supreme Court in 1976. In an unusual rehearing, the court broadened the duty on the part of therapists to include a duty to protect.[10] The Court held that

> "when a therapist determines, or pursuant to the standards of his profession should determine, that his patient presents a serious danger of violence to another, he incurs an obligation to use reasonable care to protect the intended victim against such danger."

The Court also noted that notifying the potential victim, notifying the police, or taking "steps reasonably necessary under the circumstances" could discharge this duty. The Court specifically addressed the issue of patients' confidentiality by noting that it was limited by public health concerns; the Court concluded that the "protective privilege ends where the public peril begins."

Since the original *Tarasoff* decision and *Tarasoff II*, other courts and jurisdictions have used *Tarasoff* as precedent to broaden the duty to protect and warn.[11] Some have argued that the *Tarasoff* precedent extends to all clinicians and can be applied to those situations where the clinician should reasonably foresee that a patient's action could cause harm to third parties. Examples include school bus drivers—or any motor vehicle operators for that matter—with seizure disorders or syncope. The implications of extending the precedent in *Tarasoff* for

cases such as the representative vignettes provided at the beginning of this chapter are further discussed below.

Toward Resolution

This section is devoted to evaluating specific problems commonly faced in primary care. Four major areas are considered. First are practical points for clinicians dealing with patients' friends and family as well as the media. The second involves issues related to releasing records to others, including third-party payers. The third is an evaluation of obligations regarding confidentiality in situations involving risks to others, such as infectious diseases and driving. The fourth reviews the problems posed by new computer-based technologies.

Practical Points

The clinician-patient relationship does not exist in a vacuum. In most cases there are third parties, either family or friends, who are interested in the health of the patient. Clinicians practice in consultation with many health care professionals and are in contact with many individuals. The primary care clinician must be aware of potential problems in maintaining confidentiality on a day-to-day basis.

FAMILY AND FRIENDS

Most patients have family and friends who are interested in their care. Spouses, children, curious cousins, nosy neighbors, and multiple "best friends" all want to know how a particular patient is doing and about the plan of care. To whom should the clinician disclose information? A standard policy—that the clinician will reveal no information to anyone other than the patient—although potentially laudable from the perspective of confidentiality, is problematic. In most cases, disclosure of general information is appropriate, while sensitive or potentially embarrassing information should be withheld. Moreover, providing no information may be misinterpreted by concerned others as indicating that the patient's condition is much worse than it actually is. Clearly, the clinician must exercise discretion and judgment in determining what should be disclosed and to whom. Ideally, the clinician should ask the patient about his or her wishes regarding the disclosure of information to family and friends. The wishes of a competent patient should be followed. When patients lack decision-making capacity, the clinician should turn to surrogate decision makers for guidance.

Determining what constitutes appropriate disclosure to friends and family can be complicated by patients and families whose cultural background is different from that of the treating clinician. In the United States, the medical decision-making model is rooted in the concept of informed consent, which places the patient in the central role of key decision maker and thus allows the patient to determine with whom to share information. Some cultures have traditionally centered medical decision making around family members to "protect" patients from having to make difficult choices. When faced with a patient from such a culture, the clinician should not necessarily impose an "American" view of the centrality of the patient in decision making. However, the clinician should not automatically accept the family's insistence on making the decision for the patient. Rather, the clinician should ask patients about their wishes regarding both decision making and disclosure of information to family and friends. (see Chap. 11)

ADOLESCENT PATIENTS

Adolescent patients may pose particular dilemmas for the clinician regarding confiden-

tiality. Adolescents are not typically adults, in either the legal or the financial sense, but they can act independently in many matters and some require medical treatment for sensitive issues such as sexuality, substance abuse, and mental health (see Chap. 14). It is especially important to address these sensitive issues if the clinician is to have a reasonable impact on major causes of adolescent morbidity and mortality. Adolescents may not want their parents to know about problems involving matters such as sexuality, abuse, or use of drugs and alcohol. Or, they may be estranged from their parents. Regardless of the reasons for the adolescent's concern, adolescents are much more likely to seek medical attention and confide in their clinicians if they are assured of at least some degree of privacy and confidentiality.[12] The practicing clinician must deal with two separate but interrelated issues, informed consent (discussed in detail in Chap. 19) and confidentiality. Adolescents may provide legally valid informed consent to their own treatment in a number of situations. These exceptions vary somewhat from state to state but usually include provisions regarding treatment for sexually transmitted diseases, pregnancy, contraception, drug abuse, and obtaining abortions.

In some cases, the clinician may believe that parental involvement is in the patient's best interest. Here, the clinician should encourage the adolescent to allow the participation of the parents—but, as the American Medical Association (AMA) notes in its *Ethics Manual*, "Physicians should encourage parental involvement in these situations. However, if the minor continues to object, his or her wishes ordinarily should be respected."[3] The AMA allows for violating confidentiality over the objections of adolescents in those cases where the clinician is concerned about serious harm.

In cases when the physician believes that without parental involvement and guidance, the minor will face a serious health threat, and there is reason to believe that the parents will be helpful and understanding, disclosing the problem to the parents is ethically justified. When the physician does breach confidentiality to the parents, he or she must discuss the reasons for the breach with the minor prior to the disclosure.

The standard exceptions to confidentiality—namely, potential harm to self and/or others—also apply to adolescent patients.

Confidentiality for adolescents, however, is made somewhat more problematic by financial issues. Even in those cases where the patient's privacy concerns outweigh any arguments favoring disclosure to parents, the financial reality of most clinical encounters is such that most care is paid for either directly or indirectly by the parents. Insurance companies are unlikely to send blank checks to clinicians; they are also unlikely to deny a parent access to a dependent's records. Ideally, the clinician who treats adolescent patients should make a discussion regarding confidentiality part of the initial visit with both the patient and the parents. The discussion should focus on what can and will be kept confidential and what must be disclosed to the parents. In addition, it is important to discuss payment options and mechanisms that may increase the adolescent patient's likelihood of obtaining needed medical services.

HOSPITAL TALK AND GOSSIP

Clinicians sometimes have especially interesting cases. The case of a particular patient might be interesting because of the underlying medical condition or because the patient is famous. In either case, the clinician must guard against inappropriate disclosure of confidential information to uninvolved third parties. A fine line can exist between consulting colleagues for second opinions and gossiping in the doctors' lounge. In addition, the clinician must be careful not to make inappropriate disclosures in public set-

tings, ranging from social gatherings to hospital elevators. A study by Ubel and colleagues of elevator conversations revealed a not infrequent rate of disclosure of confidential patient information during a series of monitored elevator trips.[13] One can never know who—in the elevator, hospital corridor, or hospital lobby—may be connected in some fashion to the patient being discussed.

THE MEDIA

Some patients generate media attention either because of who they are or because of some unique or interesting aspect of their medical condition. Examples range from local politicians and socialites to celebrities and patients with multiple births. It is important to note that the media attention associated with caring for such patients may be flattering and potentially practice-enhancing for the clinician. How should the primary care clinician deal with media requests for information? The clinician owes no less an obligation to the celebrity patient than to the obscure patient. According to the American College of Physicians, "Physicians of patients who are well known to the public should remember that they are not free to discuss or disclose information about a patient's health without the explicit consent of the patient."[4] Ideally, the clinician should discuss with the patient his or her wishes regarding media disclosure. Some patients may want a complete information embargo, others might invite the tabloid reporters and photographers into their rooms. Either way, the clinician is ethically obligated to abide by the patient's wishes.

Releasing Records to Third Parties

Medical records occasionally need to be shared with third parties. While unauthorized release of medical records is a violation of confidentiality, the patient always has a right to authorize release to specified parties. The most common reason for a release of records is to obtain payment from a third-party payer, either an insurance company or the government. Of course, there are many other legitimate reasons for a release. Unfortunately, medical records can also have value for persons and organizations that should not have access to the records. Some might desire the records out of curiosity. Others might want to use the records to identify people at higher risk for certain diseases, in an attempt to sell insurance only to "healthy" people or to employ only those individuals who are unlikely to generate significant health care costs. Prior to releasing any records, the clinician should have authorization from the patient or the responsible surrogate decision maker. Ideally, the authorization should be in writing and be signed by the patient. Additionally, it should identify which data should be disclosed and to whom. The duration of validity of such a release varies from state to state. Although the Uniform Health Care Information Act recommends that the release be valid for no more than 30 months, some states have set a limit of only 90 days.[14]

The prohibition on unauthorized release of medical records also applies to any marketing company or organization, even if it promises to guard patient privacy. As noted by the AMA:

"Patients divulge information to their physician only for purposes of diagnosis and treatment. If other uses are to be made of the information, patients must give their permission after being fully informed about the purpose of such disclosures. If permission is not obtained, physicians violate patient confidentiality by sharing specific and intimate information from patients' records with commercial interests."[3]

Clinicians are occasionally faced with telephone requests for information. As a general rule, the clinician should be wary of such requests and not provide information over the phone without conclusively establishing the identity of the caller and the legitimacy of

the request. The same warning also applies to requests via facsimile machines and electronic mail.

Is There a Duty to Warn?

The *Tarasoff* decisions,[5,6] as discussed above, created a duty on the part of clinicians to warn and protect identifiable third parties of potential harm from patients. The *Tarasoff* case involved a patient who threatened to kill and subsequently did kill a former girlfriend; it would clearly apply to the first scenario depicted at the beginning of this chapter, involving Beth Williams. However, what is the clinician's obligation if there is no intent to cause harm but the patient's action or lack of action might still cause serious harm? In recent years, two areas of clinical practice have attracted considerable discussion concerning whether the *Tarasoff* precedent should be extended. One is the potential transmission of HIV; the other concerns the driver of a motor vehicle who has a medical condition that increases the likelihood of an accident. Both are discussed below.

HIV INFECTION

Infection with HIV has become a major problem throughout the world. As is well known, transmission of the usually fatal virus occurs mostly through sexual contact, injection drug use, and vertical transmission. As noted above, nearly all other communicable diseases, including sexually transmitted diseases such as syphilis and gonorrhea, are subject to state-mandated reporting rules that often include contact tracing and partner notification. However, HIV infection has been treated differently because of concerns regarding discrimination against patients infected with the virus or perceived to be infected with the virus. As a result, the standard public health model of reporting and contact tracing, which places public health above individual concerns of confidentiality, has not been used.

Moreover, some states prohibit disclosure of a person's HIV status to any third parties; some states make exceptions that allow informing a spouse.

Given the tension between maintaining patient confidentiality and preventing harm to third parties, the practicing clinician faces a dilemma such as that presented in the hypothetical case of Brad Lyons, described at the beginning of the chapter. As discussed previously, the *Tarasoff* decision argued that when there was a direct threat to an identifiable other, the clinician had a duty to warn or protect the third party and to violate confidentiality. In cases where the sexual partner of an HIV-infected individual is readily known, a strong argument can be made that the clinician is required to violate confidentiality and notify the partner. However, no such cases have yet been litigated, and although many, including the above-referenced American College of Physicians *Ethics Manual*[4] and the American Psychiatric Association's AIDS policy[15] argue that it is permissible for a clinician to violate the patient's confidentiality and inform a sexual partner, others have disagreed. Thus, at this time, much is now left to the judgment of the individual clinician. However, as advances are made in the management of HIV infection, especially those advances that require early detection to be effective, the argument in favor of disclosure will become more compelling.

IMPAIRED DRIVERS

What is a clinician supposed to do with a patient diagnosed with a medical condition that could impair the operations of a motor vehicle? There is little conflict when this occurs in airplane pilots, because of requirements for periodic health clearances. However, no similarly stringent requirements exist for an individual to renew a driver's license. The *Tarasoff* logic that a direct threat to others creates a duty on the part of clinicians to protect identifiable third par-

ties has also been extended by some to include medical conditions that could impair motor vehicle operation and result in either injury or death to third parties. A common scenario is that of a patient who suffers from uncontrolled seizures or syncope or dementia. Less obviously, the clinician may have to consider a patient who has a psychiatric condition (such as major depression or psychosis) or a medication regimen that could impair driving.

As discussed above, the courts in various jurisdictions have extended the initial *Tarasoff* decision into other areas and have established additional obligations for clinicians. There have been several cases where psychotherapists were found negligent because of motor vehicle accidents caused by their patients.[16] The case law is not as well established as the "standard" *Tarasoff* duty, but some scholars have noted that "the trend clearly suggests that courts regard the protection of the public as superior to confidentiality when the two are in conflict."[16]

Faced with a patient, who a clinician believes poses a potential threat, the clinician must decide whether the case warrants violating the patient's confidentiality. Certainly, the clinician should counsel the patient regarding the risks of driving and recommend voluntarily surrendering the motor vehicle license. If the patient insists on continuing to drive, a logical extension of the duty to protect with reasonable efforts would most likely include notification by the clinician of the state's motor vehicle authority. Indeed, some states require reporting of drivers with seizure disorders.[17]

Technology

The increasing use of electronic medical records and the creation of computerized databases, while clearly beneficial for many aspects of patient care, raise important questions regarding privacy and confidentiality. The easy retrieval and transmission of such records make them tempting targets for those interested in unauthorized access. A recent example includes a young woman who obtained access to a list of hospital admissions and, as a prank, left messages on answering machines informing the former patients that they were either pregnant or HIV-positive. The economic value of such data was demonstrated by a case in which clerks sold individual patient data from a state's Medicaid database to various insurance companies and HMOs.[18]

The practicing primary care clinician obviously is not personally responsible for the security of large databases or the creation of secure encryption systems for data transmission across the World Wide Web. However, clinicians are responsible for computerized records within their offices. The Council on Scientific Affairs of the AMA issued a report on the security of computer-based medical records in 1993.[19] Their recommendations include many routine steps that can minimize unauthorized access to the records. For example, individual passwords and/or key cards should be issued only to authorized users within the office. A strictly enforced office policy should prohibit disclosing or sharing of passwords or access codes. The access of individual users should be restricted to only those areas of the database necessary for the users to perform their jobs. Finally, the system should track record access by individual users to discourage unauthorized record viewing.[19]

Closing Comments

The notion of absolute confidentiality, as envisioned in the Hippocratic oath forbidding physicians from ever disclosing what they learn about patients, is no longer operative. While confidentiality remains central to the clinician-patient relationship, it must be understood that the right of an individual to privacy and confidentiality must be balanced with the rights of society and of innocent third parties. Clinicians have a duty, both ethical and legal, to maintain patient confidentiality in most situations. Clinicians also have a duty, both ethical and legal, to breach confidentiality in certain situations where third parties are at risk. The challenge for the practicing clinician is striking an appropriate balance between these competing duties.

References

1. Bindman AB, Osmond D, Hecht FM, et al: Multi-state evaluation of anonymous HIV testing and access to medical care. *JAMA* 280:1416–1420, 1998.

2. Gillon R: Medical oaths, declarations, and codes. *BMJ* 290:1194–1195, 1985.

3. Council on Ethical and Judicial Affairs of the American Medical Association: *Code of Medical Ethics.* Chicago, American Medical Association, 1998.

4. American College of Physicians: Ethics manual. *Ann Intern Med* 128:576–594, 1998.

5. American College of Occupational and Environmental Medicine: code of ethical conduct. *Occup Med* 36:27–30, 1994.

6. *Smith* v. *Driscoll*, 162 P. 572 (Wash. 1917).

7. Lawson CM: Tort claims against health care providers for breach of confidentiality. *Neb Med J* 150–157, June 1989.

8. Dickens BM: Legal limits of AIDS confidentiality. *JAMA* 259:3449–3451, 1988.

9. *Tarasoff* v. *Regents of University of California*, 529 P.2d 553 (Cal. 1974).

10. *Tarasoff* v. *Regents of University of California*, 551 P.2d 334 (Cal. 1976).

11. Almason AL: Personal liability implications of the duty to warn are hard pills to swallow: from Tarasoff to Hutchinson v. Patel and beyond. *J Contemp Health Law Policy* 13:471–496, 1997.

12. Ford CA, Millstein SG, Halpern-Felsher BL, et al: Influence of physician confidentiality assurances on adolescents' willingness to disclose information and seek future health care. *JAMA* 278:1029–1034, 1997.

13. Ubel PA, Zell MM, Miller DJ, et al: Elevator talk: observational study of inappropriate comments in a public space. *Am J Med* 99:190–194, 1995.

14. Tilton SH: Right to privacy and confidentiality of medical records. *Occup Med* 11:17–29, 1996.

15. American Psychiatric Association: AIDS policy: confidentiality and disclosure. *Am J Psychiatry* 145:541, 1988.

16. Pettis RW: Tarasoff and the dangerous driver: a look at the driving cases. *Bull Am Acad Psychiatry Law* 20:427–437, 1992.

17. Felthous AR: Substance abuse and the duty to protect. *Bull Am Acad Psychiatry Law* 21:419–426, 1993.

18. Council on Scientific Affairs of the American Medical Association: Feasibility of ensuring confidentiality and security of computer-based patient records. *Arch Fam Med* 2:556–560, 1993.

19. Woodard B: The computer-based patient record and confidentiality. *N Engl J Med* 333:1419–1422, 1995.

Gregory Luke Larkin

Suspected Abuse and Neglect

Dr. Smith sees Mr. Eberhard on morning rounds at the Golden Acres nursing home. Mr. Eberhard, an 83-year-old widower and a veteran of World War II, has a dense left hemiparesis and mild multi-infarct dementia. He gets little stimulation, since he has no family remaining and few friends. Dr. Smith notes that his bed linens are soiled and wet. His heels and sacrum have yellow-green decubiti. He is restrained to the bed and complains that the nurses never answer his call bell. Dr. Smith finds no record of any physician's order for restraints. Golden Acres is located in a state that has mandatory reporting of elder abuse and neglect. Dr. Smith explains to Mr. Eberhard that she is concerned about the care he is receiving and that she is obligated by law to report his case to the authorities. He reacts violently to this suggestion, and begs Dr. Smith, "Please don't report this; I'll only pay for it later! If they transfer me out of here, I will have no other place to go." Dr. Smith recognizes that Mr. Eberhard's concerns could indeed be genuine. Few other residences could take him on such short notice. As Dr. Smith turns to leave, he tells her "You are the only one I trust."

Dr. Jones is working in family practice clinic. A pregnant, 17-year-old single mother brings her 2-year-old daughter in for care because of a small forehead laceration from "bumping the coffee table." Dr. Jones notes that they have missed her last two vaccinations and 18-month checkup. The child appears somnolent but arousable. The red reflex appears to be absent in the right eye, suggesting a detached retina. Just above the right eye is a linear 2-cm laceration. There is a small postauricular ecchymosis in the right parietal-occipital area but no evidence of oto- or rhinorrhea, raccoon's eyes, or any other head trauma. The forehead laceration is superficial to the galea and Dr. Jones repairs it quickly with tissue glue.

The mother says she is grateful but must run to work. Dr. Jones explains that he really needs to examine her child further, but the mother refuses. For the first time Dr. Jones notices that the mother is wincing in apparent pain. He asks if she is in discomfort, and she says "it's just a stupid contraction." Dr. Jones asks the boyfriend to step outside, and, after some protestation, he agrees.

Alone with mother and child, Dr. Jones asks whether she has sustained any recent trauma; she says no. Concerned, Dr. Jones asks to check her abdomen. She agrees reluctantly, and Dr. Jones finds a 36-week-size fundus with focal tenderness 2 cm above the umbilicus with a brown, 8-cm periumbilical ecchymosis. When Dr. Jones inquires as to the mechanism of injury, the mother states that she bumped against the steering wheel. When Dr. Jones asks how the child sustained the bruises and cuts to the head, she sobs, stating that it happened when her boyfriend was baby-sitting last night.

She now admits that her boyfriend has slapped and kicked her in the abdomen recently, but she does not feel she can leave him. In fact, she says she loves him, relies on his income and baby-sitting, and does not want to report any of this. Dr. Jones tells her that he is very concerned for both her and her child and that she needs to go immediately to the obstetrician for an ultrasound and fetal monitoring. Dr. Jones also conveys the need to send her daughter to the local children's hospital, where they can get her retina and brain checked. She refuses, saying "Oh, she's fine, just a li'l tired. Thanks fer sewin up 'er head; but we really gotta go now."

Uncertain about how to stop her from leaving, Dr. Jones informs her that he will have to report his concerns to authorities, but she pleads with him not to report this. She says she is also fearful that child protective services might remove her daughter from the home. She promises to take her child to the children's trauma center if Dr. Jones promises not to report.

Scope of the Problem

Cases such as these representative vignettes offer obvious signs of abuse and neglect, yet family violence often creeps silently and insidiously into clinicians' offices. Examples would include a child in status asthmaticus who lives with chain smokers, an elderly parent in rapid atrial fibrillation who has not received his digoxin in weeks, or a pregnant woman who is denied prenatal care by her husband. If a family keeps a child unvaccinated or tries to send grandfather to a nursing home against his will, how should the primary care clinician intervene? These commonplace cases raise poignant questions about what really constitutes abuse and neglect and what clinicians are ethically bound to do about it.

This chapter describes some of the medical, legal, and ethical challenges that arise in treating patients and families who may be in the throes of interpersonal turmoil, violence, and neglect. The clinician's moral responsibilities in these situations are highlighted.

Prevalence

Calculating the true incidence of abuse and neglect is difficult, partly because these are often occult; for every reported case there are about 14 others going unrecognized and unreported.[1] Also, the definition of what constitutes reportable abuse or neglect varies across state lines. Estimates encompassing all forms of abuse vary from 1 to 4 million cases per year in the United States.[2]

Although acute trauma from abuse is present in approximately 2 percent of female emergency department (ED) patients, nearly 14 percent of women who present to an ED have experienced abuse in the past year and 37 percent have experienced abuse in their lifetimes.[3] Approximately 2 million women are battered by their intimate partners each year,[4] and partner abuse or battering results in an estimated $5 to $10 billion dollars per year in health care costs, lost productivity, and criminal justice interventions.[5] Injuries from partner assault result in more than a million ED visits annually.[6] Despite the widespread nature of this problem, only about 5 percent of victims of domestic violence (DV) are appropriately identified.[4,7,8]

Abuse and neglect are not limited to adult women. Over 500,000 adolescents give birth every year, and nearly one-third of the children of these teenage mothers end up abused. Male perpetrators of partner violence often batter their partner's children as well. In the United States, over one million children are victimized by an adult guardian and between 1200 to 5000 die from abuse each year.

Elder abuse is a similarly silent epidemic; since victims often cannot speak for themselves, the true prevalence is unknown. Improved public health and technology have led to unprecedented decreases in mortality at the extremes of the life cycle. Paradoxically, this increase in life span for both the neonate and the aged place them at increased risk of abuse and neglect, affecting between 3 and 10 percent of all newborns and elderly.[9,10] The House Select Committee on Aging has reported that between 1 and 2 million older Americans experience mistreatment each year.[11] Since well over half of the residents in nursing facilities have some form of cognitive impairment, they are at particularly high risk. Even in the wake of federal quality requirements for nursing homes,[12] up to 40 percent of nurse's aides from one state admitted to committing at least one act of physical violence and psychological abuse annually.[13] Other examples of elder abuse include the inappropriate use of chemical or physical restraints and isolation from other residents. Shared living arrangements, resentful adult children, substance abuse, social isolation, and prior exposure to violence all contribute to the more than 1.5 million cases of elder abuse reported each year.[14] Family disintegration, socioeconomic pressures, increased mobility, and an aging baby-boomer cohort will likely be associated with an increased prevalence of family violence in the twenty-first century.

Relevant Terminology

Any physical, psychological, or economic injury to an intimate or dependent adult or child resulting from willful or negligent acts or omissions by a partner or caretaker generally constitute *abuse*. Abuse itself may range from harsh verbal treatment to torture, but it is always destructive to the process of growth, development, and well-being of the victim. There are several types of abuse that include the following[11]:

PHYSICAL ABUSE

Physical abuse involves active violence (assault) or passive violence (negligence) that results in bodily harm or physical pain to the victim. The most common types of physical abuse include slapping, hitting, striking with objects, and inflicting burns resulting in injury to the skin, soft tissues, and bones.

SEXUAL ABUSE

Sexual abuse includes the nonconsensual sexual touching, infliction of humiliation, or using an unwilling or unlawful other for sexual stimulation or gratification. There does not always have to be sexual contact; for example, exposing a child or dependent adult to unwanted pornography or sexual activity is a form of sexual violation and abuse.

PSYCHOLOGICAL ABUSE

Psychological abuse typically accompanies most other types of abuse, but it may occur in relative isolation. Emotional pain may be inflicted by verbal humiliation, insults, and threats of abandonment or institutionalization. It also includes the infliction of harassment, duress, deception, intimidation, and other threats that cause mental anguish to the patient. It may manifest as recalcitrant anxiety, depression, poor sleep habits, weight loss, and anhedonia. Since behavioral norms are variably interpreted between different ethnic groups, psychological abuse is particularly challenging to define in a multicultural milieu.[15]

FINANCIAL EXPLOITATION

In general, *financial exploitation* implies taking unfair advantage of a person's money or property interests for one's own personal profit. This may include stealing money and the coerced transfer of property, wills, trusts, or other legal documents.

NEGLECT

Neglect includes acts or omissions with regard to the dependent adult or child including the deprivation of minimal food, shelter, clothing, supervision, physical and mental health care, and other care needed to maintain life or health. Neglect may be intentional or unintentional, active or passive, stemming from either malice, ignorance, or genuine inability. Cases of passive and active neglect often raise difficult questions of responsibility and are sometimes referred to as inadequate care or mistreatment, respectively. These more neutral terms avoid the label "abuse" and mollify the assignment of blame. Neglect constitutes the largest percentage of reported elder abuse cases (>40 percent)[9] and is also common among unwanted infants.

Background Theory and Context

The multitude of moral and social complexities surrounding family abuse and neglect can be daunting. One important remedy for the many ethical dilemmas encountered in cases of suspected abuse and neglect is to focus on patient safety and the ethics of duty. Once the moral obligation to protect the patient from immediate harm is secured, specific ethical and legal duties to report and refer such cases to authorities must be weighed against the competing duties to maintain patients' privacy and trust. These duties to families and individual patients ought not to be seen as mutually exclusive, however, as caring for the victim may give all family members an opportunity to heal. Depending on the circumstances, several specific duties must be considered. Each is discussed in turn (see Table 13-1).

Duty to Recognize Abuse and/or Neglect

The ethical duty of recognizing abuse and neglect befalls clinicians because of their unique opportunity for observation and detection. While elders and children may be unable to speak for themselves, 43 percent of battered women seek medical services as their primary and exclusive source of help,[16] and over 65 percent of women surveyed would disclose violence to a clinician before others, including clergy, family, and friends.[17] Thus, in 1991, the U.S. Department of Health and Human Services identified routine domestic violence screening as a national health objective for the year 2000.[18] In 1992, the Joint Commission on Accreditation of Healthcare Organizations (JCAHO) mandated hospital policies and proce-

Table 13-1

Duties in Cases of Suspected Abuse and Neglect

Duty to recognize abuse and/or neglect
Duty to protect the victim
Duty to honor patient autonomy
Duty to treat both victims and perpetrators
Duty to report to the appropriate authority or agency
Duty to maintain confidentiality
Duty to document important findings
Duty to testify in court when necessary
Duty to protect self and others

dures to enhance early identification and referral of abuse victims.[19] Today, many professional health provider associations—including the American Medical Association (AMA),[20] the American College of Emergency Physicians (ACEP),[21] the American College of Obstetrics and Gynecology,[22,23] the American Academy of Family Practice,[24] and others[25,26]—urge domestic violence screening of all patients who present to the office, ED, or clinic.[27–32] Although family violence is more commonly reported among poor minorities and heterosexual couples, more affluent and same-sex couples encounter similarly high rates of family and partner violence and should also receive routine screening. Hence, the ethical duty is to screen all patients, since abuse and neglect cross all ethnic, lifestyle, and socioeconomic strata.

History and physical exam data can also assist in meeting the ethical duty to uncover abuse. For example, a history of developmental delay, handicaps, prolonged neonatal hospitalization, or the presence of nonbiological parents place children at increased risk of victimization.

In cases of physical abuse, physical exam commonly reveals unexplained bruises, lacerations, abrasions, head injuries, and fractures. These lesions will frequently be in different stages of healing. The most common clinical manifestations of neglect are dehydration and malnutrition. More subtle examples of neglect may include poor hygiene, subtherapeutic levels of prescribed medications, or intoxication with narcotics that have not been prescribed. By displaying empathy, respect for privacy, and understanding, clinicians can greatly facilitate trust, thereby enhancing the likelihood of victim disclosure leading to earlier recognition.

Duty to Protect the Victim

The ethical duty to protect victims of abuse and neglect is difficult to fulfill.[33] When abuse is confirmed, the first ethical and medical priority is the patient's safety. This is particularly important when the victims are minors or elders who cannot protect themselves. In these cases it may be necessary for clinicians to act against the wishes of family; in some circumstances obtaining an emergency court order may empower the clinician to protect the victim from the poor judgment of family or guardians. It is critical that clinicians protect victims while honestly informing guardians of their suspicions in a way that will preserve the guardians' dignity and motivate them to help. Using a crisis as an opportunity to help families is an important perspective to maintain. A presumptive diagnosis of adult or child maltreatment also mandates removal from the threatening situation. Such cases may require court-appointed guardianship and the intervention of child or adult protective services and police. A patient in immediate lethal danger should be separated from the alleged abuser and, if necessary, emergently admitted or transferred to safety. Nevertheless, safety must be secured while respecting autonomous choice whenever possible.

Beyond ethical duties, clinicians have legal obligations to protect victims. Clinicians may be found negligent if they fail to identify, properly treat, and protect the welfare of victims of family violence. Courts have long held clinicians liable for failure to protect children from abuse,[34] and with the generation of professional guidelines in this area, it is only a matter of time before case law declares a professional responsibility to diagnose, treat, and protect adult victims as well.

Duty to Honor Patient Autonomy

Autonomy stems from the Greek *auto* and *nomos*—literally "self-law." A clinician's duty to respect the patient's right to "self-law" may conflict with the obligation to provide beneficent care when the victim refuses the clinician's help. This right to self-determination is relinquished only when the victim lacks decision-making capacity owing to age or cognitive impairment (see Chap. 18). For example, patients may lack capacity because of severe dementia, intoxication, coma, or psychiatric impairment, such that they pose a clear threat to themselves or others.

Many decisionally competent adults refuse help because of pride, denial, fear of retribution, loneliness, and abandonment. Other forces may affect the battered victim's ability to act independently, including ensnarement, low self-esteem, and dependency. *Ensnarement* into the cycle of violence is a type of traumatic bonding resulting from intermittent positive reinforcement; violent periods alternate with periods of atonement, contrition, gift giving, and offers of doing better in the future. Low self-esteem often stems from being abused as a child and feeds on perpetrator insults and emotional neediness. Dependence related to poverty, lack of family, child care, and other resources leads to a paralysis of decision making on the part of the victim. Having lost self, these victims are ill equipped to exercise autonomy in any meaningful way. But unless the situation is highly lethal, a competent adult's decisions for further care or protection, however misinformed, should generally be respected.

Children also need to have their right to self-determination respected. Although legal constraints may be in place, it is important medically and ethically that, as teenage children grow, they be treated increasingly in their own right, respecting their perspective and dignity whenever possible (see Chap. 14). The American Academy of Pediatrics recommends obtaining consent from both patient and parent when the child is between 13 and 18 years of age.

Duty to Treat Both Victims and Perpetrators

Caring for helpless victims comes naturally to many clinicians. A more ethically complex and morally challenging problem is caring for the perpetrator of violence. While it is difficult to generate good will toward the assailant of a defenseless child, elder, or partner, clinicians cannot ethically refuse care to those they dislike. Although principle VI of the American Medical Association's *Code of Ethics* suggests that "physicians may choose whom to serve," other codes of ethics and the Emergency Medical Transfer and Active Labor Act (EMTALA) suggest the opposite: patients deserve care based on their status as human beings in need, not based on merit, ability to pay, or moral culpability for their injury or illness. By acknowledging the problems of perpetrators, clinicians can create an opportunity to win trust, get them into treatment, and break the cycle of violence.

Duty to Report to the Appropriate Authority or Agency

Most studies reveal that clinicians are often derelict in their duty to identify and report mistreated patients.[35,36] Reporting remains a major ethical and legal obligation in cases of suspected abuse and neglect. All states and the District of Columbia have mandatory reporting laws for abused children and dependent adults. For these dependent populations, the very suspicion of abuse and neglect must be reported when clinicians, in the course of their employment, encounter a dependent who they reasonably believe has been abused. Typically, suspicion alone is grounds for reporting, even if the victim has not actually been seen by the clinician.[37] Under these statutes, health care providers are not generally expected to prove anything and are generally immune from civil or criminal liability for good-faith disclosure to appropriate authorities. Often the reporter remains anonymous. If clinicians discover potential abuse outside of their jobs, they are typically considered *permissive reporters*. A *mandatory reporter* who does not report is guilty of a simple misdemeanor and may also incur civil liability for any proximate damages. Some states require clinicians to meet state requirements for training on dependent abuse.

Although every state has mandatory reporting laws for suspected abuse and neglect of children, only five (California, Kentucky, Mississippi, New Hampshire, and New Mexico) currently have mandatory reporting for cases of partner abuse. However, only a minority of clinicians believe that mandatory reporting laws are effective in protecting victims.[38] Clinicians tend to fear that the implications of taking dependent elders and children out of homes, the potential for increasing perpetrator retaliation, and the lack of efficacy of overworked protection agencies militate against their duty to report.

Reporting the abuse of a nondependent adult is not mandatory in most states; thus no immunity from liability exists in those states for reporting against the wishes of a competent adult. Although many clinicians fear potential liability for unauthorized disclosure, others realize that reluctance to act protects the autonomy and privacy of the batterer as much as, if not more than, that of the adult victim.

It is certainly true that ending a relationship involving abuse and neglect may lead to increasingly lethal battering, but there are no data supporting fears that reporting per se increases lethality. On the other hand, there are data suggesting that incarceration is one of the only routes to successful perpetrator treatment. Many states also have mandatory arrest laws that require the police to make an arrest when called to investigate a domestic disturbance. When there is mutual combat, these laws sometimes mandate arrest of both parties if there is any physical sign of trauma on the perpetrator as well as the victim. Clinicians must also comply with laws in most states that mandate reporting any assault with a deadly weapon or injuries that appear to be result of criminal acts.[39]

Some state laws extend to the viable unborn child as well, but generally the best care for the fetus is to care for the pregnant woman first and foremost. Over 3 million child witnesses of domestic violence are often themselves considered victims in need of protection, but there are few statutes that speak to this concern.[40]

A final legal concern, based on tort law,[41] revolves around a duty to warn, either victims or even perpetrators, of the potential for lethality. The adult victim or foreseeable victim should routinely be informed of ways to assess the lethality of his or her situation and warned of the potential for abuse. The reverse would also be true, however, and if a victim threatened to retaliate lethally against a perpetrator (e.g., 12 percent of murdered men are killed by their female partners),[17] a clinician could be considered responsible for warning the alleged perpetrator, whether or not that individual was guilty of battering in the past.

Duty to Maintain Confidentiality

Although the duty to warn is an instance when confidentiality may be breached, such breaches ought to be rare. Confidentiality is derived from the Latin *confidere*, "to trust"; thus, patients confide in their clinicians trusting that what they reveal will not be disclosed further without explicit permission (see Chap. 12). Even when the police or third parties such as protective services are notified under mandated reporting, clinicians should make every effort to get permission for such disclosure from the patient or family member. Failing this, information should be shared in a minimalist fashion, guarding the dignity and privacy of patients as much as possible. Such discretion will make it easier for patients to rely on clinicians in disclosing deeply personal information again in the future. It is particularly challenging to maintain confidentiality when partner violence affects employees and VIPs. Even when cases involve celebrities, athletes, or other public figures, it is important that clinicians not discuss the case with the media or family members, as investigation and prosecution could be severely hampered.

Duty to Document Important Findings

Clinicians who encounter victims of abuse or neglect should document in as much detail as possible the patient's narrative of the event, the patient's affect and behavior, and, the extent and distribution of the patient's injuries. A body map silhouette is a useful way to document the distribution of injuries on the medical record. In the case of small children, a radiographic skeletal survey is a standard method of documenting the chronology and distribution of musculoskeletal injury.

Photographs are another effective means of collecting evidence. Instant photos that do not require processing at an outside lab further protect confidentiality. After the reason for photographs is explained, it is important to obtain patient or guardian consent whenever possible. Even if the victim is a competent adult who does not wish to report the abuse, this type of evidence collection and documentation will provide needed substantiation when he or she determines that the times is right for a legal intervention. (For additional information contact Physicians for a Violence-Free Society, PO Box 35528, Dallas, TX 75235, 214-638-4200).

Duty to Testify in Court When Necessary

Although careful documentation can save clinicians a trip to court at a later date, it is still necessary for them to testify in court when asked. This is a social duty of any citizen who is witness to a case of abuse and neglect, and since clinicians have special skills at evaluation and observation, they are especially well suited for this activity. Ethical dilemmas arise when clinicians perform this as paid service; opportunistically exploiting the misfortune of another is a violation of professional ethics. Providing expert testimony should never become a clinician's livelihood; however, obtaining reimbursement for reasonable expenses associated with testifying is acceptable. Testifying in court is certainly inconvenient, and clinicians are famous for avoiding the courtroom. Yet clinicians must promote beneficence toward their patients who may be victims of domestic violence. Moreover, assisting in prosecution promotes justice, helps perpetrators receive needed help, and decreases the heavy burden of family violence on society.

Duty to Protect Self and Others

A critically important consideration in caring for victims of family violence that is all too often overlooked is the care of the self. Fear of reprisal, litigation, failure to affect victims, and failure to grieve can build up a considerable psychological debt on the clinician. Perhaps touched by violence in their own personal lives, nurses, social workers, and others must not fail to recognize their own humanity when confronted with disturbing cases of abuse and neglect. It is not uncommon for health care providers to become traumatized emotionally by a child's untimely death, for example, or to have scars in their own past opened when they become embroiled in cases of family violence. It is vital, therefore, that clinicians talk and listen empathetically to their staffs, nurses, coworkers, and others involved in such cases to facilitate the expression of provider grief. Recurrent nightmares, intrusive thoughts, sleep disturbances, and other manifestations of post-traumatic stress disorder are common in health care providers.

Moreover, clinicians must address their own needs and should recognize that they too will require the support and understanding of their friends and loved ones when they are mourning the death of a patient. Critical incident stress debriefing (CISD) teams, group or individual counseling, clergy, and other opportunities exist for processing serious trauma. For clinicians, the grieving process is challenging, since they are not at liberty to talk openly about the details of their cases to others. Since many of these cases have legal implications, the need to discuss the case must be balanced with the strict duty to maintain confidentiality beyond those caring for the patient and family.

Toward Resolution

Resolving Elder Abuse and Neglect

Using the taxonomy of duty described above, the first priority in cases of abuse and neglect is the safety and well-being of the victimized patient. This overarching duty prefigures duties to recognize, treat, document, and maintain confidentiality. The crux of the ethical challenge here is to consider potentially countervailing duties to honor patient autonomy and the duty to report to an appropriate authority against the stated wishes of a victim/patient.

When the adult victim is incompetent or if the patient agrees to reporting, duties are less likely to conflict. However, if the dependent yet competent adult refuses such reporting, the clinician may either explain that he or she is obligated by law to report or may become conscientious objectors to an unjust law. If the former is chosen, the clinician should frame the report as an attempt to determine what services might benefit the patient. Although reporting would appear to violate patients' privacy interests, the AMA and ACEP both suggest that patient confidentiality is subservient to the duty to report.[42,43] This decision is better informed when the safety risks are weighed against the patient-centered benefits and burdens of reporting/not reporting as articulated by the competent victim. Otherwise, patient dignity is threatened when his or her ability to make reasoned decisions is ignored. For example, a victim's concerns that the investigation itself may disturb family relationships or provoke further abuse may be genuine. Inadvertent trampling of patient autonomy in this case may undermine trust in the medical profession and discourage the victim from seeking help in the future. Instead, clinicians would do well to remember that an inability to understand a patient's decisions does not necessarily render the patient "incompetent." One need only observe an endlessly bickering couple on their fiftieth wedding anniversary to understand what Blaise Pascal (1623–1662) observed long ago: "Sometimes the heart has its reasons, of which Reason knows nothing." Thus, unlike the wishes of children, adults' wishes, however peculiar, should generally be respected. The clinician should also emphasize an ongoing willingness to help in the event that a victimized adult or elder decides to get assistance at a later time. It is important to emphasize that victims need not remain in abusive situations, and clinicians should offer any interventions victims are willing to accept.

If a clinician suspects an elder adult to have impaired decision-making capacity, concrete examples of cognitive impairment should be elicited and documented before an appropriate surrogate decision maker is sought (see Chap. 18). When it is clear that the victimized patient lacks adequate decision-making capacity, the court may need to appoint a guardian or conservator to make decisions on the patient's behalf. A court appointed *parens patriae* conservator

may suggest day care, home health aides, visiting nurses, or other services. In cases of cognitive impairment, *benevolent parentalism*, wherein the provider unilaterally strives to protect the best interests of the patient, is an appropriate means of fulfilling the duty to patient safety. Similarly, if the patient's surrogate or durable power of attorney for health care is either an alleged perpetrator of abuse or appears to be making decisions that are not in the patient's best interest, patient safety must be secured first. Involving a new court-appointed guardian and/or use of Adult Protective Services can assist in this process.

In the hypothetical case of Mr. Eberhard, it would be important for Dr. Smith to thoroughly document the history and objective physical findings that suggest maltreatment, using photographs and x-rays when indicated. Photos of restraints and decubiti, for example, can help greatly, but should be obtained only with the patient's express permission. Further clarifying the threats to the patient, contacting nursing home administration to remove unwarranted restraints, and striving for improved skin care would give staff the opportunity to correct their errors and allow some time to elapse prior to reporting. A persistently refractory staff or institution should ultimately be reported (against the patient's wishes), as the long-term health and welfare of the individual patient (not to mention other resident patients) would likely be in jeopardy.

Resolving Mixed Child/Partner Violence

To facilitate the organization of information in cases of suspected abuse or neglect, grouping the known data into four areas may help: medical indications, patient preferences, quality-of-life issues, and contextual factors. *Medical indications* refers to information based on the medical needs of the patient, such as diagnostic and treatment needs. *Patient preferences* includes patient-centered values, preferences, or opinions as evidenced through patient behavior or statements regarding treatment choices. *Quality-of-life* information includes both subjective and objective evaluation of the patient's well-being and satisfaction with life. *Contextual factors* incorporates issues related to the situation at hand, including the needs of family, community, and society, as well as religious issues, legal constraints, and socioeconomic factors.

Organizing information about a case in this way constitutes a *case-based* approach to complex cases pioneered by Jonsen et al[44] that was later refined by Schmidt.[45] By focusing on cases in this systematic way, one can reach reasonable and defensible solutions. Below this model is used to analyze the hypothetical case above involving the battered adolescent and child.

MEDICAL INDICATIONS

The hypothetical case of the teenage mother and child involves two battered patients, both of whom need treatment. They exemplify several hallmarks of cases involving abuse and neglect. First, there has been a delay in seeking medical care; neither prenatal care nor routine immunizations have been procured in a timely fashion. Second, the mechanism of injury suggested by the caretaker does not account for the injuries incurred; for example, striking the coffee table is a possible mechanism for a laceration but not a retinal detachment. Abuse victims classically have bruises in various stages of healing, as evidenced by both new (red-purple, 0 to 4 days) and old (brown, more than 2 weeks) ecchymoses. Acute head trauma with possible vitreoretinal detachment (absent red reflex) represents a very serious threat, since head injury is the most common cause of death among abused children. This child is somnolent and in need of further evaluation, including computed tomography of the head, at an institution that can manage pediatric head trauma.

The paramount medical consideration is safety. For the teenage patient's safety, monitoring for preterm labor, fetal distress, and possible abruption are important. This suggests the need for a non-stress test (to ascertain that there is good beat-to-beat variability of the fetal heart) and an ultrasound. Further, social service referral may be indicated. If the abuse situation is highly lethal (escalating violence, perpetrator threats of suicide, firearms in the home, etc.), Dr. Jones should obtain a court order. If it is perceived that the patient is a threat to herself or others, involuntary psychiatric commitment must be considered. Medical concerns about suicidal or homicidal behavior take precedence over confidentiality and other patient preferences.

PATIENT PREFERENCES

The mother's expressed preference both for herself and her daughter is to go home. The child in this case does not have the ability to articulate preferences that can be construed as valid, but most children would prefer not to be separated from their mothers. Nonetheless, minors may certainly have other preferences that need to be considered. Although the mother may be considered emancipated, there is some question as to whether a minor is legally allowed to make all health care decisions for herself at the age of 17, let alone for her child. She would normally be allowed to get treatment for pregnancy, sexually transmitted diseases, HIV, and contraception without parental consent; however, in some states, if she is under age 18, she could not give consent for her own treatment unless it fit under at least one of the categories above. In addition, she may, like many victims of intimate partner violence, suffer from posttraumatic stress disorder, anxiety, depression, and other disorders affecting judgment; that is, her spoken preferences may not really be her own. Therefore her ability to exercise her own autonomous choice must be evaluated. Yet, she is not suicidal, homicidal, or psychotic. Respecting the liberty of such a patient often means respecting her opinion that things would only get worse if her case were reported.

QUALITY-OF-LIFE ISSUES

There is tension between the perspective of the patient and the clinician in assessing quality of life. The pregnant mother sees her quality of life diminished by the reporting of abuse, the removal of her child, and/or submitting herself and her child to treatment. As bad as the home situation may be, abuse victims often prefer known demons to unknown ones. The mother sees the perpetrator's removal as a loss to her quality of life, partly because he contributes financially through his job and through baby sitting while she is in school. The house or apartment may be in his name, the checks may be in his name, the utilities may be in his name, and—most importantly—there may be no support from her family of origin or friends. Since she is neither economically nor emotionally independent, she fears losing what little she has, so that there is the possibility that she may have to drop out of school or face losing her child. Without mobilizing the criminal justice system to provide emergency restraining orders, obtaining emergency shelter for herself and her child, and using available psychosocial services, the victim is probably correct to suggest that her quality of life will be worsened by reporting alone.

The victim's quality of life from the clinician's perspective may appear to be better if the patient is forced to leave her current situation, but threats of retaliation and retribution on the part of the perpetrator are genuine concerns. In the absence of a highly lethal situation, the woman's interpretation of quality of life would carry more weight than the clinician's assessment. However, there is also a young child involved. As long as the perpetrator remains in the home, there is a genuine threat to the toddler's safety. The paradox is that the family that threatens abuse is often the same family that

provides the only source of comfort and security for these children. The mother may risk emotional and financial ruin if she acts on the reality of the abuse. So it is up to the clinician to weigh carefully the various competing interests while trying to maintain integrity and trust in the therapeutic relationship.

CONTEXTUAL FACTORS

The contextual legal issues in this case revolve around the dual challenges of reporting the two victims involved (excluding the fetus). As mentioned above, the legal status of the emancipated minor would likely allow for reporting of the intimate partner violence when mandated by the law. Yet ethical considerations would probably lead one away from reporting, since the adult teen seems to be able to make reasoned decisions for herself. However, both ethics and law are more clear with respect to the child: reporting to child protective services would be mandatory. Even though the mother might be considered competent and could decline intervention for herself, she may not similarly decline protective services for her child. As reflected in mandatory reporting statutes, both children and dependent elderly are construed as highly vulnerable and therefore deserving of greater protection under the law. Using the criminal justice system to obtain an emergency court order to treat the child without parental consent would also be an important consideration here.

RESOLUTION

The clinician's first duty is to offer protection to the child and the mother if she will accept it. If not, providing her with referral information for temporary restraining orders, safe housing, support groups, and crisis hot lines would be essential. Although the mother may refuse care for herself and for her pregnancy, she may not, in most states, refuse care for her child. To ensure her safety, this child needs to be transported immediately to the nearest appropriate trauma center, either with or without her mother. The trauma center can conduct a skeletal survey to look for fractures in various stages of healing, do computed tomography of the head to look for intracerebral or subdural hemorrhage, and arrange for an ophthalmologic consultation, possibly including an ultrasound of the globe to ascertain the status of the retina. The clinician should empathize with and express compassionate concern for the teen mother and should try to maintain a therapeutic alliance with her, but under no circumstances would it be appropriate to allow the mother to take such a seriously injured child home. The clinician must not allow surrogates to refuse lifesaving care for dependent children and adults. An emergency court order can be obtained if necessary, but should be used as a last resort. After arranging for transport to a trauma center the clinician should get express permission to photograph the child and document on a body map carefully all injuries and bruises.

The care of a young mother is more problematic, since she is a pregnant minor and many jurisdictions have laws expressing a state interest in protecting the mother as well as the viable fetus.[46] It might be extremely valuable to contact this teen's own mother or a trusted friend or family member to help her get the needed obstetrical evaluation. However, it is important for the clinician to give this patient options, showing concern for her safety and the safety of her child, demolishing possible myths that it is her fault, and respectfully giving information, reassurance, and, most importantly, hope for a brighter future. Clinicians should remember that their role is primarily to help victims and their children escape the harmful effects of violence in their lives, not to serve as agents of the police. On the other hand, clinicians can greatly assist future prosecution by obtaining color photographs of the mother's injuries in the event that she should decide to pursue a legal course of action against the perpetrator at a later date.

In addition, mandatory arrest laws in some states enable the clinician to call police and facilitate perpetrator arrest.

Other Resources

The high acuity of some cases do not lend themselves to ethics consultations and or lengthy deliberation. In most localities there are 24-hour hotlines that link clinicians and patients to resources. Patients, families, and clinicians may avail themselves of these resources for questions about treatment and referral. Clinicians desiring more information or wishing to file a report should consult state government directories under the listings "Child Protective Services," "Women's Services," "Adult Protective Services," or "Department of Aging" in the local area. Otherwise, contact the National Center on Elder Abuse (c/o American Public Welfare Association, 810 First Street NE, Suite 500, Washington DC 20002) or call (202-682-2470) for referral to a local agency. Similarly, providers may contact the National Domestic Violence Hotline (1-800-799-SAFE) or the Children's Safety Network (617-969-7100) for additional resources and assistance for elders, children, and partners.

Closing Comments

The multitude of social, legal, and ethical dilemmas in the context of family abuse is bewildering. Yet in spite of this bewilderment, herein lies an opportunity for clinicians to make a real difference in the lives of families, couples, children, parents, and grandparents. Although the victimized patient often feels frightened, vulnerable, and helpless, the clinician can empower these victims with the hope, strength, and caring needed to effect positive change.

This chapter has covered some of the medical, ethical, and legal considerations involved when clinicians encounter a suspected victim of abuse or neglect. Clinicians must join in the war against violence as one of their many professional duties. It remains a challenge to strike a balance between tendencies to overlook this problem and zeal to overreport it. Treating patients and families scarred by suspected abuse and neglect is at once frustrating, disturbing, and painful; yet it remains among the most gratifying and important challenges of modern clinical practice.

References

1. Tatara T: Understanding the nature and scope of domestic elder abuse with the use of state aggregate data summaries of key findings of a national survey of state APS and aging agencies. *J Elder Abuse Neglect* 5:35–57, 1993.
2. Greenfield LA, Rand MR, Craven D: *Violence by Intimates: Analysis of Data on Crimes by Current or Former Spouses, Boyfriends, and Girlfriends.* Washington DC: U.S. Department of Justice, Bureau of Justice Statistics Factbook, March 1998.
3. Dearwater S, Coben J, Campbell JC, et al: Prevalence of intimate partner abuse in women treated at community hospital emergency departments. *JAMA* 280:433–488, 1998.
4. AMA Council of Scientific Affairs. Violence against women: relevance for medical practitioners. *JAMA* 267:3184–3189, 1992.
5. American Medical Association: 4 million American women abused annually (news). *Hosp Health Netw* 68:15, 1994.
6. Campbell JC, Pliska MJ, Taylor W, Sheridan D: Battered women's experiences in the emergency department. *J Emerg Nurs* 20:280–288, 1994.
7. Webersinn AL, Hollinger CL, DeLamatre JE: Breaking the cycle of violence: an examination of factors relevant to treatment follow-through. *Psychol Rep* 68:231–240, 1991.
8. Kurz D: Interventions with battered women in health care settings. *Violence Victims* 5:243–256, 1990.
9. Pillemer K, Finkelhor D. The prevalence of elder abuse: a random sample survey. *Gerontologist* 28:51–57, 1988.
10. Jones J, Dougherty J, Schelble D, Cunningham W: Emergency department protocol for the diagnosis and evaluation of geriatric abuse. *Ann Emerg Med* 17:1006–1015, 1988.
11. U.S. Congress, House Select Committee on Aging: *Elder Abuse: What Can Be Done?* Washington DC, U.S. Government Printing Office, 1991.
12. Elon R, Pawlson LG: The impact of OBRA on medical practice within nursing facilities. *J Am Geriatr Soc* 40:958–963, 1992.
13. Pillemer K, Moore DW: Abuse of patients in nursing homes: findings from a survey of staff. *Gerontologist* 29:314–320, 1989.
14. Fulmer TT: Mistreatment of elders: assessment, diagnosis, and intervention. *Nurs Clin North Am* 24:707–716, 1989.
15. Moon A, Williams O: Perceptions of elder abuse and help seeking patterns among African American, Caucasian American, and Korean-American elderly women. *Gerontologist* 33:386–395, 1993.
16. Bowker LH, Maurer L: The medical treatment of battered wives. *Women Health* 12:25–45, 1987.
17. Center for Disease Control and Prevention: *MMWR* 43:132–137, 1994.
18. Public Health Service: Healthy people 2000: *National Health Promotion and Disease Prevention Objectives* (full report, with commentary). Washington DC: U.S. Department of Health and Human Services, Public Health Service, 1991.
19. Joint Commission on Accreditation of Healthcare Organizations: *1996 Accreditation Manual for Hospitals.* Oakbrook Terrace, IL, Joint Commission on Accreditation of Healthcare Organizations, 1995, pp 39–50.
20. Council on Scientific Affairs AMA: Violence against women: relevance for medical practitioners. *JAMA* 267:3184–3195, 1992.
21. American College of Emergency Physicians: Emergency medicine and domestic violence. *Ann Emerg Med* 25:442–443, 1995.
22. American College of Obstetricians and Gynecologists: ACOG technical bulletin: domestic violence (no. 209–August 1995 replaces no. 124, January 1989). *Int J Gynaecol Obstet* 51:161–170, 1995.

23. American College of Obstetricians and Gynecologists: ACOG issues technical bulletin on domestic violence. *Am Fam Physician* 52:2387–2388, 2391, 1995.

24. American Academy of Family Practice. Family violence. *Am Fam Physician* 50:1636–1646, 1994.

25. Quillian JP: Screening for spousal or partner abuse in a community health setting. *Journal of the American Academy of Nurse Practitioners* 8:155–160, 1996.

26. ENA: *Emergency Nurses Association Position Statement: Domestic Violence* 1996. Wash D.C., Emergency Nurses Association.

27. Screening for family violence, in *U.S. Preventive Services Task Force Guide to Clinical Preventive Services*, 2d ed. Baltimore, *Williams & Wilkins* 1996:555–565, 1996.

28. Dutton MA, Mitchell B, Haywood Y: The emergency department as a violence prevention center. *J Am Med Women Assoc* 51:92–95, 1996.

29. Abbott J: Injuries and illnesses of domestic violence. *Ann Emerg Med* 29:781–785, 1997.

30. Feldhaus KM, Koziol-McLain J, Amsbury HL, et al: Accuracy of 3 brief screening questions for detecting partner violence in the emergency department (see comments). *JAMA* 277:1357–1361, 1997.

31. McFarlane J, Greenberg L, Weltge A, Watson M: Identification of abuse in emergency departments: effectiveness of a two-question screening tool. *J Emerg Nurs* 21:391–394, 1995.

32. Hoff LA, Rosenbaum L: A victimization assessment tool: instrument development and clinical implications. *J Adv Nurs* 20:627–634, 1994.

33. Wolf RS. Elder abuse: ten years later. *J Am Geriatr Soc* 36:758–762, 1988.

34. *Landeros* v *Flood*, 551 P.2d 389, 393, 131 Cal. Rptr. 69, 73 (1976).

35. Blakely BE, Dion R: The relative contributions of occupational groups in the discovery and treatment of elder abuse and neglect. *J Gerontol Soc Work* 17:183–199, 1991.

36. Clark-Daniels CL, Daniels RS, Baumhover LA: Abuse and neglect of the elderly: are emergency department personnel aware of mandatory reporting laws? *Ann Emerg Med* 19:970–977, 1990.

37. Berkowitz CD, Bross DC, Chadwick DL, et al: *Diagnostic and Treatment Guidelines on Child Sexual Abuse*. Chicago, American Medical Association, 1992.

38. Tilden VP, Schmidt TA, Limandri BJ, et al: Factors related to clinicians' assessment of family violence. *Am J Public Health* 84:628–633, 1994.

39. Flitcraft AH, Hadley SM, Hendricks-Matthews MK, et al: *Diagnostic and Treatment Guidelines on Domestic Violence*. Chicago, American Medical Association, 1992.

40. American Psychological Association: *Violence and the Family: Report of the American Psychological Association Presidential Task Force on Violence and the Family*. 1996, p 11. Wash. D.C. American Psychological Assn.

41. *Tarasoff* v *Regents of the University of California*, 551 P. 2d 334 (Cal. 1976).

42. American Medical Association: *Diagnostic and Treatment Guidelines on Elder Abuse and Neglect*. Chicago, American Medical Association, 1992.

43. Larkin GL, Moskop J, Sanders A, Derse A: The emergency physician and patient confidentiality: a review. *Ann Emerg Med* 24:1161–1167, 1994.

44. Jonsen AR, Siegler M, Winslade WJ: *Clinical Ethics*, 3rd ed. New York, McGraw-Hill, 1992.

45. Schmidt TA: Intoxicated airline pilots: a case-based ethics model. *Acad Emerg Med* 1:55–59, 1994.

46. Gazmararian J, Lazorick S, Spitz A, et al: Prevalence of violence against pregnant women. *JAMA* 275:1915–1920, 1996.

Lainie Friedman Ross
John Lantos

Treating Minors

Alan, 8 years old, presents with fever and sore throat. On physical exam, he has exudative pharyngitis with tender anterior cervical lymph nodes. A quick Strep test is positive. The clinician explains to Alan and his mother, Ms. Ackerman, that penicillin is the treatment of choice, but that penicillin comes in many forms. Alan can be treated with a strawberry-flavored liquid, with chewable tablets, with pills that must be swallowed, or with an intramuscular injection. Ms. Ackerman asks that Alan be given a shot, but Alan says he doesn't want a shot and will take the strawberry flavored liquid.

Betty, 15 years old, presents for a yearly physical examination, which is normal. She is getting B's and C's in school and participates in some extracurricular activities. She is popular with her friends and tells the clinician that she has recently fallen in love with a 16-year-old boy. Her father thinks she is too young to go out with boys and has prohibited her from dating. She says she is not sexually active yet, but she requests a prescription for birth control pills that she plans to take "just in case." She also asks that the clinician not tell her parents because she fears her father's rage. She seems to be mature and thoughtful.

Vicky, 15 years old, presents for a sports physical. Her mother, Ms. Vilardi, states that although she believes that Vicki is not sexually active at present, she has seen her kissing boys and she fears that her daughter might become pregnant. Ms. Vilardi is a single mother who became pregnant with Vicky when she was 14. To protect Vicki from the hardships she faced, she would like her to begin receiving a long-acting injectable form of contraception. Vicky acknowledges that she has a boyfriend but denies sexual activity and denies plans to be sexually active. She does not want the shots because they will "make her fat."

Jane, 15 years old, is brought to clinic by her mother, Ms. Jensen. The clinician has known Jane since she was 2 years old, when she was diagnosed with a seizure disorder. Her seizures have been well controlled with medications. However, Ms. Jensen reports that Jane has had two seizures in the past 2 months. She was taken to the emergency room after each seizure, at which time her medication level was found to be subtherapeutic. During the conversation with the clinician, Jane admits to noncompliance. She denies depression and says to the contrary, "What do you mean? Things are wonderful. I passed driver's education and my folks are planning to buy me a car for my sixteenth birthday." The clinician informs Jane and her mother that the seizures need to be reported to the Department of Motor Vehicles. They beg the clinician not to report the seizures, and Jane promises to comply religiously with her medications.

Scope of the Problem

In the medical care of children, ethical conflicts may develop in three different domains. First, family members may disagree among themselves about what is best for the child. If the child is a teenager, he or she may be a party in these disputes. Second, family members who are united in their opinions may disagree with health care professionals. Finally, health care providers and the family may all agree with each other but find themselves to be in conflict with the state. The preceding four hypothetical cases represent the types of ethical issues that commonly arise in the care of children. In this chapter, we discuss these issues and give our opinion about whether or not a societal moral consensus has been reached concerning them. If so, we explain the basis of the consensus. If not, we show where the disagreements arise.

Background Theory and Context

Competency and Authority

Clinical ethics in cases involving competent adult patients typically focus on the clinician-patient dyad. In contrast, pediatric clinical ethics involves a triad composed of the clinician, the child, and his or her parents. Until recently, all children were presumed to be incompetent and parents were legally empowered to make virtually all decisions for them. Currently there are movements around the world to increase the child's legal power and give the child, particularly the older child, his or her own voice. Some argue that mature children (specifically adolescents) should be allowed to make their own decisions without their parents' permission or, in some cases, even without their parents' awareness.[1,2]

Whether an individual has the cognitive or emotional capacity to consent to medical treatment cannot be determined simply by determining whether that individual has reached the age of majority. The age of majority is a legislative decision based on a particular social consensus. In the United States, the age of majority used to be 21. For some decisions, such as whether to purchase alcoholic beverages, it still is. For medical decision making, it is 18, although states have statutes that recognize mature minors and emancipated minors. For driving, it varies state-by state. All of these choices reflect political, economic, moral, and psychological factors.

No reliable or validated test presently exists to determine whether any individual of any age has the capacity to make decisions in any particular situation (see Chap. 18). This situation is glaringly apparent in treating children when a child's cognitive capacities and psychological maturity are evolving at different rates. Given the absence of a reliable test of decision-making capacity, clinicians must assess each child and each situation individually. This approach has the benefit of individualizing the decision to account for peculiar features of each case, each child, and each family. It involves the risk that competency could be biased, in either direction, by the personal values of the clinician.

Even if competency could be determined quickly, reliably, and precisely, we would still need to ask whether competency alone was the only factor that should determine the child's role in health care decision making. Some argue that parents have the moral right to play a significant or even exclusive role in making decisions about their child's health care.[3] Their arguments are based on the view that a strong family role in all decisions for a child is best for the child, the parents, and society. On this view, these parental rights would not necessarily end abruptly even when the child was competent. At the other extreme, some argue that even young children have a moral right to participate in decisions that affect them.[4,5] By this argument, children, like all human beings, are moral agents and deserve serious moral respect.

Most providers of pediatric health care negotiate a course between these two extremes. They try to include children whenever possible and in whatever ways seem feasible. The child's right to participate increases as the child matures and develops the capacity to understand and analyze complex information.[2] However, the weightier the consequences of the decision, the more likely the clinician would be to follow the parents' opinion when it differed from the child's.

Specialized Consent Statutes

Regardless of one's position about the moral authority of parents and the moral standing of children to make their own health care decisions, in the United States children have the legal right to make certain medical decisions under specialized consent statutes, which exist in all states. These statutes vary in their scope, but all give adolescents the legal autonomy to seek and consent independently to the diagnosis and treatment of drug and alcohol abuse, contraceptive counseling, and/or the procurement of contraceptives.[6] Some states allow minors to consent to abortions without disclosure or consent from the minor's parents. Such statutes were designed to encourage adolescents to seek health care for problems that they might deny or ignore or for which they might delay seeking treatment if they had to get parental permission. Although these statutes allow clinicians to provide this care, they do not compel them to do so. In addition, these statutes do not necessarily give adolescents the right to refuse medical care. This may be troubling to the provider of adolescent health care, even if it allows desired actions to be taken.

The issues addressed by specialized consent statutes are significant. By the age of 18, over half of all female adolescents in the United States have had sexual intercourse; even more are sexually active.[7] Over 1 million American adolescents become pregnant every year.[8] Many teens do not seek medical or gynecologic care or contraception for a year or more after they initiate sexual activity.[9] Most of the teens who become pregnant are unmarried and most of their pregnancies are unplanned.[8] Slightly more than half will decide to take their pregnancies to term, and virtually all of these teenagers will take on the responsibilities of parenthood.

The purported intent of the specialized consent statutes is laudable: to encourage early, responsible sexual health care for adolescents. The pragmatic justification is compelling: given the fact that adolescents can be and frequently are sexually active even when birth control and other sexual health services are relatively inaccessible, they should be given the opportunity to be responsible for their sexual activity. The pragmatist does not need to concede or refute whether the availability of such services increases the numbers of sexually active adolescents, because the number is sufficiently large, even when such services are unavailable, to portend a critical public health issue. The pragmatist's position depends on the empirical claim that the statutes will promote better health care for adolescents in the realm of sexual and reproductive services than if parental involvement were required. Unfortunately, empirical data in support of this position are lacking.

Even if such data were available, it is not clear whether such pragmatic arguments are sufficient to ground a moral decision about whether or not to empower adolescents to consent to sexual and reproductive health care. The pragmatic goal of minimizing adolescent pregnancy may lead us to empower Betty (who wants contraception) and to disempower Vicky (who does not want contraception) in the hypothetical cases described above.

The moral argument in support of the specialized consent statutes is based on the moral claim that if a child is competent to make such decisions, competency should entail autonomy. But this argument would imply that these children should have the right to make all health care decisions and not just decisions covered by the specialized consent statutes. Some clinicians lean in this direction. To do so, one must view health care as exceptional, since we do not allow these same "competent" children to drive, smoke, or make a binding financial contract.

Two moral arguments can be made against the special consent statutes. The first is that granting autonomy to adolescents regarding their sexual activity may be autonomy-restricting over a lifetime. As with many decisions that children make, we might justify restricting a child's autonomy now to give her greater lifetime autonomy.[10] The second moral argument against the statutes is that parents have a valid interest in their children's development and activities, even after the children become teenagers and have achieved a significant level of competency. In order to act on those interests and to participate in their child's moral development, they need to have the opportunity to try to inculcate their beliefs.[10,11] They can do this only if they are aware of what their teens are doing. That is, competency is necessary but may not be sufficient to grant an adolescent health care autonomy.

Whether or not one agrees with the special consent statutes, they clearly do not apply to Vicky's case. The statutes empower teens to get contraception but do not empower them to refuse contraception to which their parents consent on their behalf.[12] Legally, parents can request that clinicians provide long-acting injectable contraception to their daughters. However, they cannot *demand* that a clinician do so. Thus, providers of adolescent care must make a personal moral decision about how they will respond.

Concerns about Public Health

The focus of clinical ethics on the patient and family downplays concerns that the clinician may also have responsibilities and obligations to the wider community. Teen pregnancy is a serious problem for individual adolescents, but it is also a serious public health problem. In public health, it is acknowledged that the principles of maintaining patients' confidentiality and autonomy must be balanced against the duty to protect the community from threats to its well-being. This conflict may influence the decisions that a provider of pediatric health care might make in cases involving sexually active teenagers.

Societal considerations also include an obligation for clinicians to protect the community against potentially dangerous individual behaviors. In the hypothetical case involving Jane, a different type of public health threat exists. Jane is at risk for having a seizure while driving and thus for being involved in a serious car crash. Because this puts both Jane and others at risk, Jane's clinician has an obligation to make sure that she does not drive if she is at high risk of having a seizure. This "duty to protect" is similar to the duty of a clinician who diagnoses a communicable disease to report that disease to appropriate public health authorities (see Chap. 12).

Legal and moral duties are not always identical. In 1999, six states had mandatory reporting laws for clinicians whose patients had seizure disorders.[13] One of the main arguments against mandatory reporting laws is that patients like Jane will be less forthright about future seizures, and this may lead to suboptimal medical care. In general, however, drivers with seizure disorders are required to self-report their condition at the time of driver's license application or renewal.[13] Requirements at other times are less clear-cut.[13] In addition, some states require that the clinician inform patients with seizures of the risks that driving poses to themselves and others and to remind patients of their responsibility to report this condition to the proper authority.[13] States vary in how long individuals should be seizure-free to renew their driving privileges. A 1-year seizure-free interval is currently the most widely used criterion, although a consensus panel argued in favor of a 3-month interval.[14]

Driving is often viewed as a social and economic necessity in the United States, and the prohibition of driving may reduce an individual's self-esteem and potential for employment. However, driving is also a social activity, and unsafe driving places the driver and others at risk. The central question in the case above is how best to balance the benefits of Jane's driving against the risk to herself and to others on the road.

If Jane's physician does not believe that there is a duty to report in this particular situation, the issue is what moral obligations if any the clinician has to ensure that Jane or her parents report Jane's seizures. One compromise would be to encourage Jane to report herself to the Motor Vehicle Department or at least to agree to refrain from driving until she has been seizure-free for a negotiated period of time (ideally in compliance with state law). It may also be valuable to negotiate a contract of more frequent blood tests to ensure her adherence with her antiepileptic drug regimen. The contract should state that the clinician would report Jane if she failed to adhere to the drug regimen as established by blood test, regardless of whether clinician reporting was mandatory.

Toward Resolution

Children and Parents as Competing Moral Agents

With regard to the first case vignette described at the opening of this chapter, most would agree that Alan needs penicillin. However, there are a number of different forms of treatment, all with similar efficacy if used appropriately. Each may have different side effects. The child prefers one balance of the benefits and burdens, the parent another. Their different values, when brought to play on the array of therapeutic options, has created a conflict between the parent and child about which the physician, may feel indifferent.

The first step in any conflict such as this is further discussion. It is valuable to understand why Ms. Ackerman prefers the injection. Issues to be weighed include efficacy, cost, convenience, attendant risks, and compliance. Ms. Ackerman's choice is practical—she sees the shot as more convenient and thus more reliable. The advantage of the shot is that it is a one-time dose and Alan will be assured of appropriate treatment to prevent acute rheumatic fever and rheumatic heart disease, the most serious sequelae of untreated strep infections. Ms. Ackerman also fears, based on past experience, that her child will be poorly adherent once the symp-

toms are gone. She does not want to have a thrice-daily battle over taking the medicine. A shot is also less expensive. Alan hates shots. Just the sight of a needle petrifies him. He promises his mother that he will take the medicine.

In most discussions, parents and children will come to consensus. But sometimes their positions are intractable. Who, then, should have the final word? In February 1995, the Committee on Bioethics of the American Academy of Pediatrics published recommendations regarding informed consent in pediatric practice.[2] In their document, the committee stated that children should be included (empowered) to the extent of their capacity. The committee recommended that persistent conflicts might benefit from third-party conflict resolution, with the clinician or professional mediator as the third party.[2] Although this may be ideal, there may be some parents who are well meaning but intolerant of third-party scrutiny. These parents may see the clinician's attempt to forge consensus as threatening their legitimate parental authority.

What are the clinician's options if Alan and his mother cannot achieve consensus? If the clinician sides with the parent, the clinician will have to give the protesting child an injection. What if the child resists? And what does this tell the child about his right to participate in medical decision making? On the other hand, to side with the child on the grounds of developing maturity places the parent in an awkward position, as she must now buy the antibiotic and give it to her child three times a day. What if Ms. Ackerman resists and says, "Okay, doctor, at what time will you come by to give Alan the penicillin?" Her response demonstrates the dilemma that clinicians face in their relationships with their patients. "The professionals' challenge, as nonparents, is how to be caring without taking unnecessary control of the life of the child for whom they do not and cannot take full responsibility."[15]

In the case of a therapeutic decision between oral and intramuscular penicillin, we believe that the parents should have ultimate decision-making authority. The reasons behind our conclusion are as follows: The risks of either treatment are low, as are the burdens of therapy. The health care professional should be prepared to minimize the pain of injection with adequate topical anesthesia. Furthermore, the child is only 8 years old, and therefore probably less able to understand the need for medication and the future implications of nonadherence. It is also unlikely that he would be capable of taking responsibility for his own medication regimen. However, we also believe that clinicians have the right and perhaps the obligation to involve children in the decision-making process and to explain why the child's wishes and requests are overridden, even if parents complain that this threatens their autonomy. Parental autonomy is not absolute. Both clinicians and children are (or are becoming) moral agents.

Sexually Active Adolescents

In the second and third hypothetical cases presented at the opening of this chapter, both Betty and Ms. Vilardi are trying to act responsibly, and their requests should be interpreted as an opportunity for dialogue. With Betty, the clinician might try to obtain more family history to find out why she so fears her father's anger: Has he been violent in the past? What is her parents' marriage like? Can she talk with her mother or another adult figure? With the Vilardi family, the clinician might try to include Vicky and her mother in a more general discussion of contraception to see if an alternate might be acceptable to both of them. The clinician might also want to address the issue of whether Vicky finds a three-way conversation embarrassing. Perhaps the best way to protect Vicky from unwanted pregnancy would be to encourage her to seek medical advice and treatment confidentially. Ms. Vilardi and Vicky may be very receptive to this. This does not resolve, however, whether or not Vicky should receive treatment that her mother requests but which she rejects.

How should clinicians deal with sexually active adolescents? First, the role of confidentiality in treating minors needs to be established. In most cases, confidentiality applies between the clinician and the family against the state unless there is evidence of abuse or neglect (see Chap. 13). But do the clinician and the child have a right to confidentiality that excludes parents? One of us (J.L.) assumes that confidentiality applies, whereas the other (L.R.) believes that this ought to be negotiated. If parents refuse to permit confidential relationships, adolescents need to be made aware of this and discussions should be restricted to those issues that they would be willing to have shared with their parents. Of note, even when a confidential relationship is established, the clinician must explain to the adolescent that there are limits. For example, the clinician will break confidentiality if he or she suspects that the adolescent is suicidal or is the victim of familial abuse.

Second is a need to decide whether adolescents are competent to make health care decisions about reproductive and sexual matters and whether competency is sufficient for granting health care autonomy. Even when adolescents are not competent, one may still decide to provide contraceptive services on pragmatic grounds. Our responses to Betty and Vicky reflect the lack of consensus about the moral legitimacy of the specialized consent statutes and adolescent autonomy more generally. One (L.R.) would grant parents the moral authority to make these decisions and therefore would not prescribe oral contraceptives for Betty and would treat Vicky. The other (J.L.) would provide the contraceptives to Betty but would not treat Vicky without her agreement. Instead, he (J.L.) thinks, priority should be given to identifying the underlying issues that led to the disagreement between mother and daughter.

Balancing Obligations

The last case vignette raises the issue of the clinician's responsibility to the community. We believe that the clinician has a moral obligation to Jane and to the community, but we do not believe that these obligations are well served by mandatory clinician reporting laws. First, these laws single out one medical condition that may interfere with optimal driving while they ignore other conditions of equal danger (e.g., there are no similar laws requiring the reporting of strokes, transient ischemic attacks, or hypoglycemic syncope). Second, mandatory reporting does not allow for individualized assessments. Third and most important, these laws make the clinician a double agent, which may discourage patients' candidness about their seizure activity. This may lead to suboptimal care, as patients might not disclose seizure break-throughs even if other medical interventions may be available that could obviate the problem.

In general, we believe that clinicians should encourage their patients to self-report even if they believe that their patients are not posing serious and imminent driving risks. The only exception would be cases in which the clinician believes that the patients do pose a significant risk of harming themselves or others. In such cases, even if the patients do not meet the criteria of "serious and imminent" danger, we believe that the clinician must not only counsel patients to self-report but also explain that he or she will report the information if the patients do not.

We believe that the clinician should encourage Jane to self-report and to voluntarily refrain from driving for a negotiated period of time. One of us (L.R.) believes that the clinician has a moral obligation to report in Jane's case and that he or she should do so voluntarily, particularly because Jane is a minor who deserves greater protection from herself than might a similarly situated adult. The other (J.L.) would encourage Jane to self-report but would not report himself if he, Jane, and her mom could negotiate a contract whereby Jane voluntarily refrained from driving and showed herself able to comply with her antiseizure medication.

Clinicians should realize that they will probably not be required to report Jane's seizure and therefore will need to make a moral decision about whether or not to require that Jane self-report or whether they will report voluntarily. The question is how best to balance the benefits of Jane's driving against the risk to herself and others on the road. That is, the ethical principles in conflict are Jane's right to a confidential relationship with the clinician and the clinician's obligation to promote the common good.

Closing Comments

Much of the literature of pediatric ethics focuses on the extreme cases: the premature infant who weighs 600 g, the child with leukemia whose parents refuse chemotherapy, or the child whose sibling needs a kidney transplant. Nonetheless, in taking care of children and adolescents there is a plethora of complex ethical issues along with, parental struggles to do what is right for their children that occurs in a complex legal environment. In this chapter, we have examined some of the ethical issues that arise in treating children in daily practice.

Every case raises both procedural and substantive issues; that is, how clinicians should approach the case and what the final decision should be. In some cases, there are legal constraints on decision making. In others, there is wide consensus on the preferable ethical solution. We have tried to point out these areas of consensus and to highlight areas where there is less agreement. Through dialogue, we may be able to narrow these points of dissension and to promote policy changes that best reflect our moral understanding of the health care provider's obligations with respect to children, their families, and the wider community.

References

1. Alderson P, Montgomery J: *Health Care Choices: Making Decisions with Children.* London, Institute for Public Policy Research, 1996.

2. American Academy of Pediatrics, Committee on Bioethics: Informed consent, parental permission, and assent in pediatric practice. *Pediatrics* 95:314–317, 1995.

3. Ross LF: *Children, Families, and Health Care Decision-Making.* Oxford, UK, Oxford University Press, 1998.

4. Holt J: *Escape from Childhood.* New York, Dutton, 1974.

5. Cohen H: *Equal Rights for Children.* Totowa, NJ, Rowman and Littlefield, 1980.

6. Holder AR: *Legal Issues in Pediatrics and Adolescent Medicine*, 2d ed. New Haven, CT, Yale University Press, 1985.

7. American Academy of Pediatrics, Committee on Adolescence: *Adolescent Pregnancy—Current Trends and Issues: 1998. Pediatrics* 103:516–520, 1999.

8. Moore KA: Teen fertility in the United States: 1993 data—facts at a glance. *Child Trends,* January 1996.

9. Alan Guttmacher Institute: *Sex and America's Teenagers.* New York, Alan Guttmacher Institute, 1994.

10. Ross LF: Health care decision making by children: is it in their best interest? *Hastings Ctr Rep* 27:41–45, 1997.

11. Gaylin W: Competence: no longer all or none, in Gaylin W, Macklin R, (eds): *Who Speaks for the Child: The Problems of Proxy Consent.* New York, Plenum Press, 1982, pp 27–54.

12. Costello JC: If I can say yes, why can't I say no? Adolescents at risk and the right to give or withhold consent to health care, in Humm, SR, Ort, BA, Anbari MM, et al (eds): *Child, Parent and State.* Philadelphia, Temple University Press, 1994, pp 490–503.

13. Krumholz A. Fisher RS, Lesser RP, Hauser A: Driving and epilepsy: a review and reappraisal. *JAMA* 265:622–626, 1991.

14. American Academy of Neurology, American Epilepsy Society, and Epilepsy Foundation of America. Consensus statements, sample statutory provisions, and model regulations regarding driver licensing and epilepsy. *Epilepsia* 35:696–705, 1994.

15. Goldstein J, Freud A, Solnit AJ, et al: *In the Best Interests of the Child.* New York, Free Press, 1986.

Julia E. Connelly

Refusal of Treatment

Two 76-year-old women described the new onset of left anterior substernal chest pain that was tight, squeezing, and occurred with exertion. The pain increased in frequency for several weeks and, by the time they were each seen in the physician's office, it was occurring three or four times a day. Both patients stated that each episode of pain lasted less than 5 minutes and resolved with rest; shortness of breath sometimes accompanied the painful episodes. Both patients were concerned about having "heart problems," although neither had a history of heart disease. The physician's assessment indicated that indeed both patients had unstable angina pectoris, a condition that predictably leads to myocardial infarction and possibly death. The physician recommended immediate hospitalization. Both patients refused to be hospitalized and wanted to return home. The patients' personal stories provide a context for understanding the specific issues that led to the decision to refuse hospitalization.

Ms. Agee's husband died 6 months ago. Early in the morning of the day of his death, Ms. Agee called the physician requesting an urgent home visit. As she called, the rescue squad was performing cardiopulmonary resuscitation (CPR) on her husband, who had end-stage lung disease. Although she did not want them to continue the CPR, she could not convince them to stop without a physician's order.

Ms. Agee was a regular patient of the physician; she had had a checkup 3 months prior to her visit for chest pain. At that time she was adjusting to her husband's death, as she was becoming involved with her family and community in "new ways."

On the day of her office visit for evaluation of chest pain, she was informed that her pain suggested an impending heart attack and that she needed to be hospitalized. She refused. Her situation was explained to her again; she was informed about the probability of having a heart attack and was told that she could die. She listened carefully and asked "What will they do to me at the hospital?" It was explained that medicines to prevent a heart attack would be administered and that perhaps diagnostic tests would be needed to clarify her problem. Nonetheless, she talked about her husband's illness. She told the story about one hospitalization in which he refused to be intubated, yet he was intubated against his wishes. She said, "I don't want to go to the hospital, where they have all those machines. I don't want any tubes, tests, or surgery. I've had a good life and I'm ready to die if my time has come." She believed that she would be reunited with her husband in death, and she refused to be hospitalized.

Ms. Nelson lived with her 10 cats and, until the day of her office visit, had been actively attending to her daily needs. Six years ago she came to the office because of depression. With the physician, she discovered that she had not resolved the death of her husband 25 years previously. She missed him, yet she was angry that he left her with a "big mess." She had not known how to write checks, pay bills, or "survive" in the world. Through several months of counseling, she became aware of her conflict around grief and anger, and she gained confidence in expressing herself directly.

When Ms. Nelson was advised that she needed to be hospitalized, she said, "Oh! I have to take care of my cats." The physician reassured her that someone else could help, then reiterated that she had a problem that could result in a "heart attack" and that she could die if she were not hospitalized. She commented once again about her cats. There was little evidence that she understood the gravity of her situation. She was asked to state what she understood. "Oh yes, I might have a heart attack if I don't go. I understand; but I must take care of my cats." She continued to refuse hospitalization.

Scope of the Problem

Refusal of treatment occurs when a patient demonstrates an unwillingness to comply with medical interventions suggested or recommended by a clinician. This assumes that the clinician is making thoughtful, individualized recommendations commensurate with care offered by other members of the medical profession. Although primary care clinicians may also provide medical care in hospitals, this chapter focuses on refusals of treatment in the outpatient setting.

When a patient refuses a recommended intervention, whether a medication, a consultation, or a diagnostic test, the clinician faces a conflict between his or her assessment and the patient's wishes. As with the two elderly patients with unstable angina described in the vignette above, the clinician must decide on the appropriate course of action. Should the patient be allowed to return home, or should the rescue squad be called against the patient's wishes to transport the patient to the hospital? The most problematic refusals are those that have the greatest consequences to the patient. As the potential for harm to the patient increases because of the refusal, the conflict for the clinician—between paternalistic behavior and respect for the patient's autonomy—sharpens. The clinician wants no only to benefit the patient but also to prevent harm. However, the clinician's and patient's interpretation of "harm" and "benefit" may be in conflict with one another. For instance, Ms. Agee sees death as the natural end of her long life, but the clinician may see her death asa harm or a bad outcome that ought to be prevented.

Prevalence

Refusal of treatment occurs frequently in primary care. One study in an internal medicine practice demonstrated that refusals occurred during 4 percent of office visits.[1] Primary care clinicians have an average of 20 to 25 office visits per day, therefore they can expect to encounter about one patient each day who refuses some recommended intervention. Patients refuse a wide variety of interventions, including health maintenance recommendations (such as immunization, Pap smear, mammography, and rectal examination) to diagnostic testing, medications, and therapeutic interventions. In an adult patient population, the frequency of refusals increases as patients age.[2]

Cultural and Religious Issues

Cultural or religious beliefs held by patients may influence their understanding of their illnesses: Why am I ill? Why me? How does healing occur? What does God want me to do? Religious beliefs provide guidance and facilitate medical decisions for many patients. In hospital and emergency room settings, the case of a Jehovah's Witness who refuses blood transfusions represents the classic example of refusal of treatment on religious grounds. The primary care clinician is likely to care for such patients, who explain their religious beliefs in advance; but many other patients do not do so until the situation of the refusal arises. The courts have upheld the right of a Jehovah's Witness to refuse blood transfusion in emergencies, ruling that the principle of respect for autonomous persons prevails over the clinician's interest in beneficence and nonmaleficence.[3]

As startling as such cases may be, cultural beliefs are often subtle and may go unrecognized by clinicians, and communication barriers further the tendency toward misunderstanding. Conflicts arise between patients and clinicians when religious and cultural beliefs of patients are used to restrict the provision of health care, especially when treatment is important or life-saving.

Patients may express nondenominational religious beliefs that lead to refusals of treatment. They may hold beliefs about God and God's intention regarding life that influence their medical decisions. For instance, consider a patient who suffered from congestive heart failure caused by the new onset of atrial fibrillation. The arrhythmia was controlled, the congestive heart failure treated, and anticoagulation initiated. She was advised to have electrocardioversion in order to simplify her medications and improve her long-term condition. She refused, saying that now she felt well and that God did not want her to have such an intervention. The patient understood the medical recommendation and the potential problems if she remained in atrial fibrillation. Her refusal and reasons remained constant during conversations with two cardiologists and on several occasions with her primary care clinician. Her religious beliefs resulted in her refusal.

Repeatedly, court decisions have allowed adults to refuse medical treatment on religious grounds. Patient refusals due to religious beliefs are acceptable when they are based on the principle of respect for autonomy, even when consequences such as death are likely, as long as the elements of an informed refusal (discussed below) are present and the patient's underlying reasons for the refusal are not based on some misunderstanding or false information.

Pediatric patients whose families are members of religious traditions that refuse medical treatment for children, such as Christian Scientists, pose difficult issues for clinicians.[4] When families refuse treatment for children, the clinician's interest in providing benefit to the child comes into conflict with the parents views. This struggle, along with concern about child abuse, has led three states by 1993 to change their laws removing language that allowed refusal of medical intervention for children on the grounds of religious beliefs (see Chap. 13). However, with regard to adolescents who have refused medical interventions based on religious beliefs, the courts have ruled both for and against the application of interventions. An adolescent's refusal due to personal religious beliefs without parental coercion or fear of family abuse is likely to be accepted by the courts[4] (see Chap. 14).

Background Theory and Context

The central ethical issues that the patient and clinician face when a refusal of treatment occurs are (1) the patient's right to refuse a treatment or intervention if the refusal results in harm, particularly when a beneficial intervention is available, and (2) the clinician's right to override the patient's refusal in order to prevent harm. Responding to these issues is shaped by legal procedures, the context of primary care and permissability of specific interventions.

Patients' Rights to Refuse

As individuals, we have rights, one of which is to refuse treatment. Engelhardt argues for the fundamental right to be left alone, which leads to the principle that individuals have authority over their person and must give permission for others to intervene, e.g., to touch them.[5] Embedded in the notion of the right to be left alone is the right to refuse treatments or interventions proposed by others. In the clinical setting, this individual authority raises questions. What should the clinician do when a patient refuses the recommended course of action? Who is in control, the patient or the clinician? What is the basis for the clinician's acquiescence or rejection of the refusal? Other issues related to the right to refuse treatment include informed consent, the right to privacy and confidentiality, freedom from harm by others, and the clinician's struggle with balancing beneficence and respect for persons. If patients do not have the capacity to make decisions, their refusal is not valid. Other interventions, depending on the importance of the refusal, may be needed to determine the appropriate course of action. Patients' privacy and confidentiality must be respected. However, family members or friends should be involved in the decision making when patients request or agree to their involvement. They should not be involved in coercing the patient into making decisions that are deemed appropriate by the clinicians, but they should provide support and further information to patients.

Acceptance or Rejection of Refusals: Considerations of Patient Autonomy

The clinician must consider under what circumstances a patient's refusal can be accepted or rejected. Beauchamp and Childress describe three perspectives for considering patient autonomy: autonomous persons, autonomous choices, and respect for the person's autonomy.[6] An *autonomous person* is free of controlling interference from others and of personal limitations, such as inadequate understanding or other constraints imposed by illness that impair the process of making decisions. Such persons act in accordance with a freely chosen and informed plan. *Autonomous choices* are those choices that are intentional or made with understanding and without controlling influences, such as family pressure or coercion by the clinician. To *respect an autonomous person* is to recognize the "person's capacities and perspective, including his or her right to hold views, to make choices, and to take actions based on personal values and beliefs."[6] These autonomous actions or choices are not to be subjected to controlling constraints by others. However, if choices endanger public health, potentially harm others, or involve scarce resources for which the patient

cannot pay, it can be appropriate to restrict autonomy.

Legal Precedents

A 1914 opinion by Justice Cardozo in *Schloendorff* v *Society of N.Y. Hospital* favored the patient's right to consent to or refuse treatment:

> "Every human being of adult years and sound mind has a right to determine what shall be done with his own body; and a surgeon who performs an operation without this patient's consent commits an assault, for which he is liable in damages."[7]

This ruling emphasizes the centrality of the patient's authority in the process of consent or refusal but limits the right to adults of sound mind.

Discussions about the extent of patient's or individual's right to refuse treatment have continued since *Schloendorff*. For instance, when a competent patient makes a decision that seems odd or even ridiculous, does this decision need to be respected by clinicians or should it be overridden? The courts have upheld the individual's right to make "foolish, unreasonable, or absurd decisions," such as refusing medical intervention even when the risk is great.[8] Engelhardt adds

> ". . . if a decision is competent or authority-conveying only if it is well reasoned from well-established, firm premises, the range of patient wishes to be respected will be markedly restricted. If a decision is competent because it is the free choice of a competent individual . . . then the range of decision that must be expected will be much greater."[9]

For the clinician, this distinction is critical, otherwise the clinician will be allowed to judge from his or her personal beliefs and values what is "ridiculous or odd" whenever a patient refuses a treatment or intervention. The clinician should not be the judge of the quality of the patient's decision but rather should focus on assuring that a decision is informed. If the elements of an informed decision are not met, the refusal may be challenged or overridden.

The Context of Primary Care

Several features of primary care practice that may influence refusal of treatment also need comment. First, the relationship of the patient and the clinician is central to the care of the patient.[10] The importance of this relationship for diagnostic and therapeutic purposes can overshadow that of technological interventions. Patients need to be understood as individuals with unique stories that shape their reactions, preferences, and decisions regarding their health care. Knowing what to do and why is important in this relationship.[11,12] Second, as in other fields of medicine, the goals, decisions, and actual plans for ongoing care are all negotiated and developed with the patient.[13] Third, the patient treated in the office has an easier time expressing control than the hospitalized patient. The office-based patient can leave the office or change clinicians without much interference from anyone. The primary care clinician has less physical control over the patient who refuses treatment, emphasizing why the relationship is so important in facilitating ongoing communication in areas of disagreement.[12]

Paternalism

The term *paternalism* brings to mind treatment of one adult by another as a father with good intentions treats his children. Paternalism can be "weak" or "strong." In *weak paternalism*, one has the authority to intervene on the behalf of another person who is refusing treatment only when the choice that is being made is not autonomous.[14] An example from office practice is that of a severely depressed and thereby nonautonomous patient who refuses surgical evaluation for acute abdominal pain. Without intervention, the patient may die, but does this

depressed patient have the capacity to decide what is best for her? A psychiatric consultation, or, perhaps, involvement of the patient's family, with the aim of persuading the patient to allow the appropriate and potentially life-saving treatment, would be justified by the standards of weak paternalism. In contrast, *strong paternalism* limits the autonomy of the individual even if the patient's choices are autonomous.[14] Strong paternalism supports treatments intended to benefit the individual, even though the individual has the capacity to make his or her own decision and is refusing the intervention. In general, ethicists agree that weak paternalism is justified, while the use of strong paternalism is debated.[14] Regardless, as described above, strong paternalism, even if justifiable, would likely be difficult to enforce in office practice, since patients come and go as they choose.

Toward Resolution

Elements of Informed Refusal

When a patient refuses a suggested intervention, the clinician faces a difficult problem. What is the best course of action? Should the refusal be accepted or overridden? The refusal must be assessed for the presence of basic elements to ensure that the refusal is an *informed refusal*. These elements include (1) the clinician's obligation to disclose information that the patient needs for decision making, (2) an assurance that the patient understands the issues, including the consequences of the refusal, (3) consideration of the patient's capacity to decide, and (4) an assessment of the voluntary nature of the decision.[15] Each of these essential features is discussed in some detail below. The reader should also refer to Chap. 19, "Informed Consent," because much of the discussion regarding informed consent applies to informed refusal.

DISCLOSURE OF INFORMATION

Patients need information to make decisions. But how much information is necessary? What information is reasonable to provide to patients in order to ensure their understanding? As when patients receive bad news, the situation that results in a refusal of treatment may be overwhelming for the patient, particularly when the risks associated with the refusal are great. On a case-by-case basis, the clinician must decide how much information the patient needs and when it is appropriate to provide it.

PATIENT UNDERSTANDING

To be certain that a refusal is informed, patients should be able to demonstrate an understanding of the clinician's recommendations and the potential consequences of the refusal. What are the expected risks and benefits of the intervention? What is the diagnosis or explanation of the problem? What are the likely consequences of the refusal? Medical issues are often complex and difficult to understand. Sometimes clinicians must inquire into patients' comprehension by asking them to recount their understanding of the issues and choices involved. If a patient cannot demonstrate an adequate grasp of these issues, it would likely be inappropriate for the clinician to accept the patient's refusal. In this setting, the clinician will have to decide whether further explanation is necessary or other approaches, including strong paternalism, are needed.

CAPACITY TO DECIDE

The patient must be competent to decide to accept or refuse treatment. In health care, *competence* refers to the capacity of an individual to make an autonomous decision about the health-related issue being considered[16] (see Chap. 18). In clinical settings, competence is specific to the decision-making tasks at hand. This focus is important, as there is sometimes competence in one area of decision making but not in another. Competence may also come and go, because of the influence of medications or owing to the impact of illness, such as pain or depression. Questions of incompetence arise when a patient is assumed to have the legal right to act or choose but no longer demonstrates the ability to do so. For instance, an elderly diabetic person may be able to live alone with the help of others but may not comprehend the need for aggressive treatment of a foot ulcer. Or a depressed person who feels hopeless may not agree to take medications to treat the depression or other medical illnesses, such as hypertension. In primary care, issues of competence regarding a refusal of treatment are common among adolescents, the elderly, and those with acute and chronic mental health disorders.

VOLUNTARINESS

Finally, a voluntary decision is essential, whether acceptance or refusal of treatment occurs. Many factors may influence a patient's decisions. For instance, a patient's beliefs about illness, personal values regarding diagnostic tests, as well as previous experiences in the medical system influence the patient's decision to accept or refuse treatment. The clinician must recognize these factors and explore them with the patient. To coerce or seemingly threaten the patient with bad outcomes, as if to "scare the patient" into the preferred decision, is not acceptable. Caution must be exercised too when family or friends become involved. The patient's confidentiality and autonomy must be respected (see Chap. 12).

Are the Features of an Informed Refusal Present?

MS. AGEE

Ms. Agee, whose husband died recently, refused to be hospitalized. Is she depressed?

Does she feel hopeless about her life since she is now alone? Does she have the capacity to make such an important decision? She told the clinician that she was lonely at times and missed her husband. She had been sad and tearful on occasion, but those times have been limited to brief episodes. She remained interested in her usual activities: church, family, and needlework. Based on this constellation of findings, a diagnosis of major depressive disorder would not be correct.

The clinician did not want to accept her refusal, since it might result in her death. Yet the patient was able to restate the conversation: she repeated the diagnosis, the concern that she might have a heart attack and die. She restated that she did not want to go to the hospital, where aggressive interventions were likely. She reflected on her life and stated that she did not want to die, but if it were her time to die, she could accept it.

Ms. Nelson

Ms. Nelson refused to be hospitalized for treatment of unstable angina because she wanted to be home to care for her cats. When the clinician asked her to describe her situation in her own words, she did not mention the possibility of her death. The clinician was not convinced that Ms. Nelson understood the situation and again attempted to explain the issues. Still concerned that Ms. Nelson did not understand the seriousness of the situation, the clinician asked Ms. Nelson for permission to contact her daughter, which she granted. Her daughter responded, "Oh, of course, you must send her to the hospital." The clinician did not want to delegate the decision to her daughter, but the options were limited. The clinician spoke with the patient again but decided to use different language and said, "Some people want doctors to do everything that is possible to save their lives and others just want to die the natural

way." "Oh, Doctor," she exclaimed, "I don't want to die. I'll go to the hospital."

Why Did the Patient Refuse the Treatment?

A point of critical inquiry is to wonder: "Why is the patient refusing the suggested course of action?" The reasons that patients refuse treatments or interventions fall into broad categories.[1,17] Patients make refusals when they do not trust the medical system. Some patients have had bad experiences with clinicians, tests or medications. Some choose not to take such risks again. Others distrust the recommendations of clinicians regarding the suggestions offered. Problems in communication, such as misunderstanding the clinician, also arise and lead to refusals.[17] The presence of psychological reactions—such as anxiety, depression, fear, and denial—may interfere with the patient's decision-making ability. Still other factors, such as costs of treatments and personal beliefs and values, lead some patients to refuse interventions. Recognition of the patient's reason for the refusal is necessary for the decisions that follow and for the maintenance of an ongoing patient-clinician relationship.

True interest in the patient requires an open and curious approach leading the clinician to investigate many personal areas. Who is this person? What does she believe about illness onset and resolution? Where does she receive support in her life? What are her concerns or fears about illness and health? The patient's narrative description will reveal important and unique personal features: his or her beliefs, values, customs, ideas, wishes, desires, expectations, fears, and concerns.[11] The narrative achieved through such a patient-centered approach will lead the clinician to understand the patient's reasons for the refusal.

A patient-centered approach encourages and enables clinicians to enter into the patient's world, to see illnesses through the patient's eyes, and attempt to understand what the illness means to the patient.[18] Listening to the patient is a key feature of narrative, as both the teller and the listener need to clarify, discuss, and re-describe the story for the information to be accurate. This type of interviewing skill is essential to help the patient and for an informed decision-making process to proceed.

Language is an important component of communication, and interviewing. Note that when the clinician's language changed in the course of talking with Ms. Nelson—the patient who lived with her cats—she recognized that she might die.

What Is the Clinician's Response to the Patient's Refusal?

The patient who refuses to accept the clinician's recommendations may elicit a variety of responses from the clinician. Frustration, anger, and disengagement may result when the refusal seems irrational to the clinician. The clinician may not understand the patient's reasons for the refusal and may not be able to accept it. Also, when a patient refuses treatment, more of the clinician's time will be required. This may add stress to the clinician's already busy schedule. In a study of refusals among hospitalized patients, Applebaum and Roth demonstrated that many clinicians did not try to understand the refusal from the patient's point of view. They often accepted the patient's refusal, but never understood it.[17] Why does the clinician not inquire? Does the clinician really care about the patient? When patients refuse clinicians' recommendations, clinicians must assess their personal reaction openly and directly in order to avoid letting the refusal negatively influence the relationship. Zinn has described how clinicians' feelings influence medical care,[19] including the immediate situation and the long-term relationship.

Clinicians must move toward the Socratic moral imperative "Know thyself." Clinicians' awareness of the emotional responses to patients, families, and the health care team must be cultivated. Asking oneself, "How are my feelings affecting my interactions and decisions in this particular situation?" may be enlightening. Self-awareness is critical because of the pervasive role emotions play in the decision-making process and the process of communication. Unfortunately, medical education does not emphasize the art of cultivating self-awareness. Nonetheless, it is incumbent upon the current generation of medical educators to ensure that clinicians be aware of the need for this.[20,21]

Children

Parents and clinicians will determine most medical interventions for children.[22] Most pediatric patients who refuse treatment are considered incapable of deciding what is best for them or unable to understand the consequences of the refusal. The decisions are then referred to the parents. Conflicts regarding office-based refusals arise as children become adolescents. As an adolescent, the child is usually capable of understanding the issues, including the risks and benefits of the treatment and the consequences of refusing it (see Chap. 14). The question then arises: Do adolescents who adequately understand the issues related to their treatment have a right to refuse when their parents and clinicians judge the intervention to be necessary? Adolescent refusals must be evaluated using the elements described for adults. Reasons for their refusals, such as adolescent rebellion, may limit participation in the decision-making process and require assessment of the validity of the refusal. When the intervention is considered necessary but not lifesaving, most courts allow the adolescent to decide. Such a situation might arise when the young person does not want blood drawn or refuses intramuscular antibiotics. At times the patient's assent can be gained through simple solutions, such as giving an oral antibiotic or obtaining blood by finger-stick, if possible. Issues of individual preference as well as control are central in providing health care for adolescents.[22]

Mental Health

In primary care, patients with distressing emotional problems as well as mental health disorders are common. Many patients have emotional problems (such as anxiety, depression, denial, fear, and worry) that interfere with their ability to enter into a relationship and make sound health care decisions. Other patients have diagnosable mental health disorders (including major depressive disorder, generalized anxiety disorder, panic disorder). Still others are chronically mentally ill (due to bipolar disease, schizophrenia, or personality disorders).

Primary care clinicians will confront refusals among all of these patients.[23] The ability of the patient to understand the choices available and the consequences of these decisions varies.

Patients with psychological symptoms, such as anxiety and depression, that interfere with their ability to focus on issues, ask questions, and comprehend the consequences of the refusal are common in primary care. Repeated discussion over time is sometimes required to determine a course of action. If urgent decisions are needed, counseling or legal intervention may be required. At times, support from family or friends can help patients to ask questions, sort values, achieve a clearer understanding of the situation.

Chronically mentally ill individuals may not be competent to make health care decisions; many have legal guardians for making such decisions. On the other hand, competence may wax and wane depending on the phase of the illness or the presence or absence of pharmacologic interventions. The patient may be competent to make some but not all decisions. Does the patient have the ability to understand the issues, decisions, and consequences on his or her life? When the patient consents to or refuses an intervention, a careful assessment to ensure that he or she is informed as necessary (see Chap. 18).

To Accept or Override the Patient's Refusal?

Clinicians, too, must live with the decision to accept or override the patient's refusal, the interactions or the process leading to the decision, and the outcome of the situation.

Ms. Agee

Ms. Agee persisted in her refusal but agreed to call the clinician the next day. Medications were prescribed in an attempt to prevent a heart attack. She returned to her home. The next day she called; there had been no further pain. The following day she called again. The pain had recurred and had been present for an hour. The clinician encouraged her to go to the hospital immediately. Again she stated that she did not want surgery, tubes, or other tests but reluctantly agreed to go. She died that afternoon. Several weeks later a young woman stopped the clinician and said, "You were my grandmother's doctor. I wish you had made her go to the hospital earlier. Perhaps, she would still be alive."

Ms. Agee's discussion with the clinician met the elements of informed refusal, and her reasons for refusal were consistent and compatible with what the clinician understood of her life. Only strong paternalism could have overridden her decision. Perhaps her family should have been involved, but she would have had to allow the clinician to notify them and request their involvement.

Ms. Nelson

Ms. Nelson was admitted to the hospital, where she had a myocardial infarction. She recovered without complications; her grandson cared for her cats. Following her discharge from the hospital, she continued to come to the office for many years after the event. If she had continued to refuse hospitalization without demonstrating a clear understanding of the consequences, the clinician would have rejected her refusal and sought further means to clarify the situation.

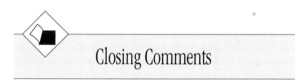

Closing Comments

Refusal of treatment, a common occurrence in primary care, presents the clinician with a challenging situation. No matter what the consequences of the refusal, before accepting or rejecting the patient's refusal, the clinician must review the interaction with the patient to ensure that the elements of informed refusal have been met. Does the patient have all of the information that is necessary? Does the patient understand the information, including the consequences of the refusal? Does the patient have the capacity to choose? Is the patient making a voluntary decision? In addition, recognition of the patient's reasons for the refusal will often help the clinician to put the situation into the context of the individual's life. Specific circumstances may influence the situation, such as the patient's religious beliefs, cultural background, or mental health status. The greater the risk or consequences of the refusal, the greater the challenge for the clinician in determining whether to accept the patient's refusal.

References

1. Connelly JE, Campbell C: Patients who refuse treatment in medical offices. *Arch Intern Med* 147:1829–1833, 1987.
2. Connelly, JE, DalleMura S: Ethical problems in the medical office. *JAMA* 260:6:812–815, 1988.
3. Latour, F: Ruling clarifies minors' rights: teen's court case points to age old confusion. *The Boston Globe*, Feb 19, 1999, p B01.
4. May L: Challenging medical authority: the refusal of treatment by Christian Scientists. *Hastings Ctr Rep* 25:15–21, 1995.
5. Engelhardt HT: Free and informed consent, refusal of treatment, and the health care team: the many faces of freedom, in *The Foundations of Bioethics*, 2d ed. New York, Oxford University Press, 1996, p 289.
6. Beauchamp TL, Childress JF: Respect for autonomy, in *Principles of Biomedical Ethics*, 4th ed. New York, Oxford University Press, 1994, pp. 68–72.
7. *Schloendorff v Society of N.Y. Hospital*, 211 N.Y. 125, 105 N.E. 92, 93 1914.
8. In re President and Directors of Georgetown College, Inc., 331F.2d 1000.1022 (D.C. Cir.) *cert denied*, 337 U. S. 978 (1964) (Burger, W. dissenting).
9. Engelhardt HT: Free and informed consent, refusal of treatment, and the health care team: the many faces of freedom, in *The Foundations of Bioethics*, 2d ed. New York, Oxford University Press, 1996, p 304.
10. Cassell E: *The Nature of Primary Care Medicine.* New York, Oxford University Press, 1977, pp 50–75.
11. Brody H: "My Story is broken; can you help me fix it?" *Lit Med* 13:79–92, 1992.
12. Smith H, Churchill L: Primary care: a moral notion, in *Professional Ethics and Primary Care Medicine.* Durham, NC, Duke University Press, 1986, pp 1–19.
13. Quill TE: Partnerships in patient care: a contractual approach. *Ann Intern Med* 98:228–234, 1983.
14. Beauchamp TL: Paternalism, in *The Encyclopedia of Bioethics.* New York, Simon & Schuster Macmillan, 1995, pp 1914–1920.
15. Beauchamp TL, Childress JF: Respect for Autonomy, in *Principles of Biomedical Ethics*, 4th ed. New York, Oxford University Press, 1994, pp 142–146.
16. Morriem EH: competence: at the intersection of law, medicine, and philosophy, in Cutter MAG, Shelp EE (eds): *Competency: A Study of Informal Competency Determinations in Primary Care.* The Hague, Netherlands: Kluwer, 1991, pp 93–125.

17. Applebaum P, Roth L: Patients who refuse treatment in medical hospitals. *JAMA* 250:1296–1301, 1983.

18. McWhinney I: The need for a transformed clinical method, in Stewart M, Roter D (eds): *Communicating with Medical Patients.* Newberry Park, CA, Sage Publications, 1989.

19. Zinn WM: Doctors have feelings too. *JAMA* 259:3296–3298, 1998.

20. Longhurst MF: Physician self-awareness: the neglected insight, in Stewart M, Roter D (eds): *Communicating with Medical Patients.* Newberry Park, CA, Sage Publications, 1989.

21. Connelly JE: Emotions, ethics and decisions in primary care. *J Clin Ethics* 9:225–234, 1998.

22. Holder AR: Parents, courts, and refusal of treatment. *J Pediatr* 103:515–521, 1983.

23. Curran WJ: The management of psychiatric patients: courts, patients' representatives, and the refusal of treatment. *N Engl J Med* 302:23:1297–1299, 1985.

Kathy Faber-Langendoen
Tania Chao

Pain Control

Mrs. Alou is a 72-year-old retired schoolteacher with metostatic breast cancer. Her disease progressed despite chemotherapy and several different hormonal treatments. Because he felt that "nothing more could be done," the oncologist returned Mrs. Alou to the care of her primary care physician. Mrs. Alou was given Tylox (a combination of oxycodone and acetaminophen) and took one every 6 hours as prescribed. She went to the emergency room because of worsened shoulder pain. Radiographs showed a stable lytic lesion in the left humerus but no fracture, and she was discharged with a refill for Tylox. In the primary care physician's office she is near tears. She reports that she has not slept for more than a few hours at a time because of pain.

Mr. McIntosh, a 31-year-old warehouse worker, comes to the physician's office as a new patient for routine care. Generally healthy except for mild obesity, he has been troubled by chronic low back pain since his discharge from the military 6 years earlier. Previous evaluations, including magnetic resonance imaging, have failed to elucidate any structural abnormality. Past medical history is notable for two hospitalizations for alcohol-induced pancreatitis. Nonsteroidal anti-inflammatory drugs (NSAIDs) have not lessened Mr. McIntosh's pain, and he is unwilling to engage in a weight-loss and exercise program. Instead, he asks for a codeine prescription.

Mr. Northrup, a 53-year-old telephone operator, has advanced rheumatoid arthritis. He has had multiple reconstructive surgeries of both feet, hands, and knees. His disease did not respond to nonsteroidal antiin-flammatory drugs (NSAIDs), oral gold, cyclophosphamide, or hydroxychloroquine sulfate. Methotrexate slowed the rate of progression of the disease but had to be stopped because of liver damage. He has been on daily prednisone for the last 4 years. Efforts to taper the steroids precipitate flares of his disease, requiring a boost in his steroids above his baseline. Because of the steroids, he has cushingoid features as well as decreased bone mineral density and now requires insulin for steroid-induced diabetes. He has no history of substance abuse.

Following his most recent reconstructive surgery, Mr. Northrup was discharged with a prescription for hydrocodone. For the 2 weeks he took this medication, his joint pain was markedly improved. Many days he was able to walk with canes instead of a walker, and he awoke in the mornings more refreshed than he had been in years. When he returns to his clinician's office for a scheduled follow-up visit, he asks if he could routinely be treated with hydrocodone, in the hope of maintaining his improved functional ability and of being able to decrease the prednisone.

Scope of the Problem

Primary care clinicians are frequently confronted with patients in pain desiring relief. While the use of nonopioid analgesics, psychosocial interventions, or other "conservative" measures gen-erally prompts no more ethical concern than does the pharmacologic treatment of hypertension, the use of opioids for pain has prompted substantial ethical reflection and regulatory oversight. The benefits of opioids as some of the most effective analgesics have been clearly established. Unfortunately, however, opioids have serious risks: addiction, respiratory depression, and social stigma for patients as well as medical board censure for physicians. The calculation in any particular clinical situation is complex as to whether the potential benefits are worth the risks both to patients and clinicians. In this chapter we address some of the ethical issues surrounding the use of opioids to control pain, delineating the extent of clinicians' duty to offer pain relief to patients in distress.

The Duty to Relieve Pain

The clinician's responsibility to alleviate pain and suffering is not a modern invention. Thomas Sydenham, the seventeenth-century British physician credited with bringing an empirical approach to clinical medicine, cited the following as one of his four precepts of doctoring: "The doctor, being himself a mortal man, should be diligent and tender in relieving his suffering patients, inasmuch as he himself must one day be a like sufferer."[1] Opioids have long been known to be effective in relieving pain, as noted by Sydenham in 1682: "Among the remedies which it has pleased Almighty God to give to man to relieve his sufferings, none is so universal and so efficacious as opium."[2] In the modern era, several prominent professional organizations (including the American Medical Association, the American College of Physicians, and the Institute of Medicine) have urged physicians to improve their treatment of pain with readily available measures, particularly the pain of those who are dying.[3–5] For example, a 1996 report of the American Medical Association decried the inadequate treatment of pain among patients at the end of life, saying:

> "The current patient care delivery system is deficient in regard to the care of the terminally ill. Expertise in pain management is often not available to patients, and comprehensive and enduring care is the exception."[4]

The 1998 U.S. Supreme Court decision upholding states' rights to outlaw assisted suicide also asserted a strong obligation to relieve the pain and distress of the dying, interpreted by some as establishing a right to pain relief and other palliative care.[6]

The Prevalence of Undertreated Pain

Undertreatment of pain persists despite these strong and unambiguous statements that the pain of dying patients can and ought to be relieved with therapies readily available. The Study to Understand Prognoses and Preferences for Outcomes and Risks of Treatment (SUPPORT), a multi-institutional study of the care given to patients hospitalized with serious illnesses, found that 50 percent of patients experienced unrelieved pain during their hospitalization and 15 percent reported extremely severe pain.[7] The exact incidence of pain among dying patients is not known; most reports in the literature are confined to patients with cancer, and estimates commonly range from incidences of 30 to 65 percent.[8] As such, Mrs. Alou, whose hypothetical case is described at the opening of this chapter, presents a classic and common example of the undertreatment of pain. A recent study of 54 cancer centers found that 67 percent of outpatients treated in these centers reported pain in the previous week, and 42 percent were not given adequate analgesia.[9] To some extent, clinicians recognize this undertreatment of pain. In a survey of clinicians about the care of patients near the end of life, 81 percent of nurses, attending physicians, and residents agreed with the following statement: "The most common form of narcotic abuse in the care of the dying is undertreatment of pain."[10]

Barriers to Optimal Pain Control

This persistent undertreatment of pain is due to several factors. Barriers to effective pain management include clinician barriers, patient barriers, and legislative and public policy barriers.

Clinicians may treat pain less than optimally because of lack of knowledge, inadequate pain assessment, and specific reluctance to prescribe opioids. Inadequate treatment of pain rests both with clinicians who do not prescribe adequate medication and nurses who give less than the maximally prescribed doses despite the patient's continued pain.[11–13] A knowledge assessment among nurses, physicians, pharmacists, and medical and nursing students showed significant ignorance about the use of opioids. For example, over one-third believed that patients should experience discomfort prior to receiving the next dose of pain medication.[14] The risk of respiratory depression is often cited as a reason to not escalate the dose of opioids in the face of unrelieved pain, even in dying patients. In reality, respiratory depression, particularly among patients who have chronically been receiving opioids yet continue to suffer pain, is rarely seen.[15] The major predictor of inadequate pain relief is inadequate assessment, and studies abound pointing to the failure of physicians and nurses to appreciate the severity of patients' pain.[13,16,17]

In addition, clinicians may undertreat patients with pain because of fears of addiction or tolerance (see Table 16-1 for definitions). Although the reported incidence of addiction among patients chronically receiving opioids is less than 1 percent,[18–20] only 28 percent of health care professionals surveyed disagreed with the statement "25 percent of patients receiving narcotics around the clock become addicted."[14] Similarly, the incidence of tolerance among cancer patients receiving chronic opioids is less than commonly believed, with requests for increased doses generally correlating with progression of disease.

The literature about opioid pharmacology and addiction is rapidly advancing, with reports of good outcomes after prolonged use of opioids in patients with cancer and other chronic diseases. Yet, opioids remain stigmatized because of concerns over dependence and addiction. The exact incidence of addiction has

Table 16-1

Key Terms in Assessing Risks of Opioids

Pharmacologic tolerance is the development of a need for escalating doses of a drug to maintain the drug's beneficial effects after repeated use.

Physical dependence is the capacity for developing a withdrawal syndrome if the drug is abruptly stopped.

Addiction (or psychological dependence) is manifest by compulsive drug use and aberrant drug-related behaviors, such as hoarding medications, losing prescriptions repeatedly, and seeking drugs from multiple sources.

SOURCE: From Portenoy,[18,21] with permission.

been variably reported, from zero out of over 10,000 burn patients with no prior history of substance abuse up to 10 percent in several smaller studies of patients with chronic headaches, back pain, neuropathic pain, and arthritis.[18] The incidence of addiction is highest among patients with prior histories of substance abuse. Opioid addiction is not simply an inherent property of a given drug but reflects an interaction between a drug and the patient's various psychological factors, neurochemical factors, and life situation.[21] Physical dependence ought not be confused with addiction. The human body becomes dependent upon several kinds of medications (e.g., corticosteroids, tricyclic antidepressants, some antihypertensives), which cannot be discontinued abruptly without significant adverse side effects.

Although some clinicians are reluctant to prescribe adequate analgesia, some patients are reluctant to report pain or take prescribed medication. In a survey of patients with cancer, leading barriers to adequate pain relief were fear of addiction, the belief that worsened pain means progression of the cancer, bothersome side effects, and fear of injections.[22] Patients who were older, had lower incomes, or had completed fewer years of formal education were less likely to report pain because of the belief that "good" patients do not complain of pain.

Finally, there are both regulatory and legislative barriers to the optimal treatment of cancer pain. Insurance policies may have "caps" on the number of opioid prescriptions or the number of tablets that can be dispensed in a month.[23,24] Such restrictions in Medicaid programs disproportionately affect women, the elderly, and minorities—groups already at risk for under-assessment and undertreatment of pain.[25] The federal government has categorized drugs into several "schedules"; most opioids are schedule II drugs, and prescriptions for them do not allow refills. Several states have further tightened access to opioids, passing laws requiring multiple copy prescriptions ("triplicate forms") for the dispensing of schedule II drugs. In states that have enacted such laws, prescriptions of opioids have decreased up to 60 percent.[26] The extent to which this 60 percent reduction reflects a reduction in inappropriate prescribing (as might be the hypothetical case of Mr. McIntosh, the warehouse worker with chronic back pain described at the beginning of the chapter), without adverse effects on other patients (like Mrs. Alou) is a matter of debate.

Although there is substantial consensus regarding the clinician's obligation to aggressively treat the pain of patients, such as Mrs. Alou, who have incurable cancers or who are dying, there is substantially less consensus regarding the appropriateness of using opioids for patients with chronic, noncancer pain, like Mr. Northrup or Mr. McIntosh, who do not have a predictably short life span. As was the case 20 years ago regarding the use of opioids for dying cancer patients, at the heart of this disagreement is the issue of the risk of tolerance or addiction to opioids in patients who may need these drugs for many years and whether this risk is justified in the care of patients who are not imminently dying.

Background Theory and Context

The Extent of the Duty to Relieve the Pain of Dying Patients

The obligation of clinicians to tend to patients' suffering is the essence of the medical profession. That is grounded in the principle of beneficence and the virtue of compassion. This obligation takes on added urgency in the care of dying patients where clinicians can assuage the suffering of the dying by careful management of pain and other symptoms as well as by acknowledging and addressing other aspects of suffering. By treating patients' pain, clinicians can facilitate dying patients' autonomy, freeing them to focus on achieving other goals such as spending time with loved ones, revisiting favorite places, and preparing emotionally and spiritually for death. Failure to treat patients' pain because of inattention or the hassle of complicated forms is no more acceptable than a failure to evaluate and treat other medical conditions, such as unstable angina.

This obligation extends to all patients. Studies demonstrate that certain groups of patients are at particularly high risk for not receiving adequate analgesia. The elderly, women, and ethnic minorities (particularly African Americans and Hispanics) are two to three times more likely to be undermedicated in a variety of clinical situations, including postoperatively,[11,27] for fractures,[28] and for cancer.[9,29,30] These differences persist even when patients are adequately assessed for pain,[29,31] suggesting that reports of pain from some groups of patients are systematically discounted. These differences may stem from biases about particular cultural expressions of pain or the limited ability of some clinicians to empathize with patients. Whatever the reason, the principle of justice and the virtue of compassion demand that all patients in pain be treated fairly, and systematic undertreatment of certain groups of patients is unacceptable.

Given the strong ethical basis for treating the pain of dying patients, are there any ethical concerns that might keep clinicians from prescribing appropriate analgesia, including opioids if needed? The risk of addiction in the setting of impending death seems inconsequential, given the patient's limited life expectancy. However, there are some immediate risks to opioid use that may lead clinicians to decide that their risks outweigh their benefits. Paramount among such concerns is the risk of respiratory depression from opioids. In a survey of almost 1500 nurses and physicians regarding care of patients near the end of life, 41 percent of respondents said that the fear of hastening death was the most common reason for giving inadequate pain medication. The actual risk of respiratory depression with opioids appears to be small but is not precisely known. Patients who have received opioids for several days often become tolerant to the respiratory effects of opioids, and some experts believe that accelerated doses of opioids rarely hasten death.[15]

THE RULE OF DOUBLE EFFECT

The primacy of the clinician's duty to relieve the pain of the dying, even if doing so hastens death by suppressing respirations, is generally justified under the ethical *rule of double effect*.[32] There are several formulations of the rule of double effect, but generally this argument claims that an action that has a bad outcome ("ill effect") is justified if:

- The act is not in itself morally impermissible (in the case of high doses of morphine for the pain of dying patients, administering morphine is not in itself morally problematic).
- The ill effect, while foreseen, is unintended (the respiratory suppression that hastens the patient's death is foreseen but not intended; the intent is to relieve the patient's pain).

- The ill effect is not disproportional to the good effect (the hastened death in a patient already imminently dying is not disproportional to the good of relieving the dying person's pain).
- The ill effect is not the means by which the good effect is achieved [in our example, the relief of pain results from the use of morphine, not by ending the patient's life. This is unlike the case of assisted suicide, where the relief of suffering (good effect) occurs by means of the ill effect (the patient's death)].

This line of reasoning is commonly invoked in clinical ethics. The American Medical Association relied on the rule of double effect when it argued that "the administration of a drug necessary to ease the pain of a patient who is terminally ill and suffering excruciating pain may be appropriate medical treatment even though the effect of the drug may shorten life."[33] Although this rule has its critics, it is widely cited as justification for aggressive pain treatment among patients with limited life spans, even at the risk of hastening death. One ought to remember, however, that in many cases the patient's death is not merely foreseen and may not be viewed as an "ill effect." For patients who have a sense of having completed their life's work, who suffer greatly despite maximal palliative efforts, or who have hope in an afterlife, death may be welcomed and not viewed as an unintended but unavoidable ill effect.

The Extent of the Duty to Relieve Chronic, Nonmalignant Pain

In the care of all patients, not just those categorized as "dying," patient comfort ought to be considered. Although the duty to relieve suffering is not absolute (for example, if meperidine is chosen to treat a vasoocclusive crisis in a patient with sickle cell disease, the dose may have to be limited in order to avoid the serious complication of seizures from toxic levels of drug metabolites). Nevertheless all patients have a right to have their pain taken seriously, not to be undertreated because of their demographic characteristics, and to be offered treatment with an accurate assessments of the associated risks and benefits.

If the essence of the medical profession is to tend to patients' suffering, this is no less the case with chronic, nonmalignant pain. Mr. Northrup suffers greatly from his rheumatoid arthritis and, given the nature of his disease, faces the prospect of continued unrelieved pain for many years. In comparison, Mrs. Alou, with liver metastases, faces a relatively short period of suffering even if her pain is not controlled. Yet despite Mr. Northrup's arguably greater burden of pain, clinicians are generally far more reluctant to treat the pain of patients like Mr. Northrup aggressively than that of patients like Mrs. Alou. Why?

Under the banner of "First, do no harm" (or "nonmaleficence"), many clinicians believe that the risk of addiction is too great or too serious to warrant the use of opioids in cases of chronic pain; they are consequently unwilling to let patients run that risk. Is the risk of addiction too great to allow Mr. Northrup to continue taking hydrocodone? In addition to carefully assessing the actual reported risk of addiction, one must consider the other risks this patient has taken previously in the treatment of his rheumatoid arthritis. Oral gold carries a 1 to 3 percent risk of serious hematologic effects. NSAIDs cause gastrointestinal bleeding and renal insufficiency. Methotrexate can (and did in this case) cause irreversible liver damage. Although each of these side effects is usually reversible or treatable, they are potentially fatal. Corticosteroids, the mainstay of Mr. Northrup's treatment, have been the most effective in controlling his disease. However, corticosteroids predictably carry several side effects, many of which he has already experienced. Steroids have caused diabetes and osteoporosis, both of which have increased Mr. Northrup's debility and shortened his expected survival. Steroids commonly cause proximal myopathy, cataracts, hypertension, lipid abnormalities, delayed wound healing, immunosuppression, and marked changes in body habitus, among a myriad of other ill effects. The body becomes physically tolerant to exogenous steroids, and abrupt cessation can precipitate an Addisonian crisis.

Despite these protean side effects and risks, few clinicians would invoke the principle to "First, do no harm" as justification not to prescribe steroids for this patient. His clinician likely believes that, despite the risks and foreseen toxicities of long-term prednisone use, Mr. Northrup ought to be allowed to take prednisone after being fully informed of the risks, even if some of its deleterious effects are virtually assured. The choice of whether to risk these protean side effects is one given to Mr. Northrup, recognizing his autonomy and right to decide what health outcomes he wishes to pursue and at what risk to himself.

The risks associated with chronic opioid administration arguably are no more devastating than the risks of chronic steroid administration, and the benefits of chronic opioids may be substantial. Enhanced functional status resulting from the use of opioids is a substantial health benefit to Mr. Northrup. A paternalistic clinician might argue that, for their own good, patients ought not be permitted to run the small but serious risk of addiction. However, an affirmation of the patient's autonomy and right to self-determination may embolden a clinician to offer Mr. Northrup chronic opioid therapy after fully informing him of its potential risks and benefits.

Risk to Clinicians in Prescribing Opioids

In addition to weighing the risks to patients of opioid use, clinicians may also take into account the professional risk to themselves if they prescribe opioids.[34] In an ideal world, the clinician's and patient's joint considered judgment about the merits of using opioids, with careful documentation of intent, would be sufficient to ensure appropriate use. In reality, however, abuse of these drugs has prompted regulatory oversight that at times may inappropriately limit clinicians' discretion. The exact prevalence of reprimands from medical boards to clinicians for legitimately prescribing opioids is unknown, and many reprimands are issued not for prescribing opioids but for prescribing them without first performing a suitable evaluation of the patient's medical problem and indications for pain medication. Nonetheless, even a rare case of overzealous censure has chilling effects on other clinicians. On the other hand, an Oregon physician was recently reprimanded by the state medical board for repeated undertreatment of pain.[35]

In the face of the specter of professional or public censure, clinicians might decide that the risk is not worth it and refuse to prescribe opioids except in the most unquestionable cases. Although this protects the clinician, it harms patients. Clinicians accept many other risks in the course of caring for patients. Exposure to potentially fatal transmissible diseases such as HIV and hepatitis C, long hours of separation from loved ones during training, and the high levels of stress intrinsic to the profession are routinely assumed by clinicians. A categorical decision to refuse to prescribe opioids when indicated because of risk to the clinician seems out of step with these other risks that are commonly taken.

Toward Resolution

Recommendations for Treating Individual Patients

Clinicians ought to recognize and address patients' reluctance to report pain or take opioids when indicated. Studies have shown that, in some patient populations, educational efforts addressing patients' concerns and misconceptions about analgesics can increase patient acceptance of strategies to relieve pain.[36] Too often, both clinicians and patients follow a "Don't ask, don't tell" policy when it comes to cancer pain, and clinicians must take the initiative in inquiring about patients' pain and allaying misplaced concerns.

Mrs. Alou ought to be able to expect competent, compassionate treatment of her medical condition, even if her breast cancer cannot be arrested. Although the oncologist's assessment when her disease progressed was that "nothing more can be done," in fact, much can be done for such patients, including addressing the psychosocial and religious issues that accompany the prospect of death, maintaining functional status as best as possible, and controlling pain. There are many options for better controlling Mrs. Alou's pain (e.g., increasing the Tylox dose, starting a long-acting opioid, administration of radiopharmaceuticals such as strontium 89, and using external beam radiation therapy).* These options—combined with a treatment plan that focused on relieving Mrs. Alou's symptoms and

---

*Discussion of the various strategies for managing pain is beyond the scope of this chapter. An excellent online source of information is the Agency for Health Care Policy and Research (AHCPR) website for clinical practice guidelines on pain, accessible at www.ahcpr.gov/clinic. Additional information can be found in Doyle D, Hanks GWC, MacDonald N: *Oxford Textbook of Palliative Medicine*, 2d ed. Oxford; UK: Oxford University Press, 1998.

helping her to achieve the best quality of life possible—would provide her with compassionate, competent, and ethically responsible care.

Pain management programs are increasingly likely to consider the use of opioids for patients like Mr. Northrup, the patient with refractory rheumatoid arthritis, under closely specified protocols. Common components of programs that use opioids for the treatment of chronic noncancer pain include those listed in Table 16-2.[21,37]

These same criteria suggest that Mr. McIntosh's back pain ought not be treated with chronic opioids. His unwillingness to try less risky therapies, his history of substance abuse, and the lack of a structural explanation for his symptoms suggest that treatment plans other than one involving opioids would be more appropriate.

If primary care clinicians believe that the use of chronic opioids for nonmalignant pain are out of their realm of expertise, referral to a pain clinic, if available, is appropriate. Some clinicians may feel that the risk of addiction is unacceptably high. Although such concerns limit the individual clinician's responsibility to prescribe opioids directly, compassion for the suffering patient—as well as the realization that the risks and benefits accrue to the patient and thereby fall under the patient's judgment—ought to encourage the reluctant clinician to refer the patient to a clinician willing to help.

Recommendations for Education

In a recent survey of over 900 oncologists, training in pain management during medical school and residency was rated as fair to poor by over 75 percent, and only 51 percent believed that their patients had good pain control.[38] However, the situation may be improving. Medical schools are increasingly including some formal instruction in pain control in their curricula; a recent study found that 62 percent of medical schools provided education on pain management for patients with chronic and terminal illnesses, although the quality and impact of these efforts remains largely a matter of speculation.[39] Since clinicians have an ethical obligation to treat patients in pain, medical schools and residency training

Table 16-2

Considerations in Using Opioids for Treating Chronic, Noncancer Pain

- Failure of all other reasonable strategies to control the patient's pain
- Pain attributable to an organic cause
- A single clinician designated to oversee the treatment program
- No history of substance abuse by the patient
- A reliable patient who is willing to comply with regular follow-up
- Patient's informed consent about the potential risks of addiction, cognitive impairment, and physical dependence
- Regular (often monthly) follow-up for monitoring, documentation of continued need, and writing of a new prescription
- Discontinuation of opioids for patients who show aberrant behaviors, including losing prescriptions, hoarding medications, obtaining opioids from other clinicians, etc.

programs have an obligation to promote competency in pain management among their graduates.

Recommendations for Regulatory Change

The inadequate treatment of pain is in part due to the chilling effect wrought by a perceived overzealous use of censure by medical boards of physicians who prescribe opioids appropriately for unremitting pain[34] as well as overly restrictive laws and regulations regarding opioid use. The American Medical Association, in its *Code of Medical Ethics*, states that physicians have "a responsibility to seek changes in those requirements which are contrary to the best interests of the patient."[40] Insofar as laws or regulations pose unreasonable barriers to patients who suffer, clinicians both individually and collectively ought to work to change them.

Clinicians and others concerned about good pain control have had success in shaping state laws regarding opioids (see Chap. 17). In the last decade, there has been an exponential growth in the number of laws and state medical board regulations addressing the use of opioids for chronic noncancer pain. *Intractable pain treatment acts* usually give clinicians immunity from disciplinary action for prescribing opioids for intractable pain, including pain from noncancer causes. By the end of 1997, a total of 14 states had intractable pain treatment acts, 8 had other relevant state regulations, and 23 state medical boards had issued pertinent guidelines. In total, 33 states have at least one these policies.[41*] Any public policy concerning medical practice has potential risks, particularly the overstipulation of medical practice in areas best left to the judgment of the individual clinician and joint decision making between the clinician and the patient. Yet it may be hoped that the enactment

of such legislation and guidelines will improve the care of patients with chronic intractable pain by giving official approval to the use of opioids in carefully selected and monitored patients.

Closing Comments

The use of opioids for pain raises difficult issues in patient care and its regulation. Clinicians and patients both have legitimate concerns about the level of risk it is reasonable to take in order to relieve pain—an essential aspect of the compassionate care of those who suffer. An accurate assessment of the risks—including their seriousness, prevalence, and proportionality to other risks taken by patients—should inform the decision as to whether opioids should be prescribed. Compassion for those who suffer, the clinician's obligation to relieve pain, and respect for a patient's autonomy in setting his or her own health goals and acceptable level of risk ought to embolden clinicians to treat pain with the same vigor, expertise, and commitment with which they treat other problems.

References

1. Sydenham T: The doctor, in Lammers S, Verhey A (eds:) *On Moral Medicine*, 2d ed. Grand Rapids, MI: Eerdmans, 1998, p 145.
2. As quoted in Andre J, Ogle K: Ethics, politics, and pain. *Med Hum Rep* 20:1–5, 1999.
3. Field MJ, Cassel CK (eds): *Approaching Death: Improving Care at the End of Life.* Washington, DC, National Academy Press, 1997.
4. American Medical Association: Good care of the dying patient. *JAMA* 275:474–478, 1996.

*States currently with intractable pain treatment acts: CA, CO, FL, MN, MO, NV, ND, OH, OR, RI, TX, VA, WA, WI; states currently with other regulations: AL, AR, IA, LA, NV, NJ, OR, TX; states currently with medical board guidelines: AK, AZ, CA, CO, FL, GA, ID, MA, MD, MN, MT, NM, NC, OH, OK, OR, RI, TN, TX, UT, VT, WA, WV.

5. American Board of Internal Medicine: Caring for the dying: identification and promotion of physician competency, educational resource document. 1996, pp 1–100.

6. Burt RA: The Supreme Court speaks: not assisted suicide but a constitutional right to palliative care. *N Engl J Med* 337:1234–1236, 1997.

7. Desbiens NA, Wu AW, Broste SK, et al: Pain and satisfaction with pain control in seriously ill hospitalized adults: findings from SUPPORT research investigations. *Crit Care Med* 24:1953–1961, 1996.

8. Ingham JM, Foley KM: *Hospice J* 13:89–100, 1998.

9. Cleeland CS, Gonin R, Hatfield AK, et al: Pain and its treatment in outpatients with metastatic cancer. *N Engl J Med* 330:592–596, 1994.

10. Solomon M, O'Donnell L, Jennings B, et al: Decisions near the end of life: professional views of life-sustaining treatments. *Am J Public Health* 83: 14–23, 1993.

11. Cohen FL: Postsurgical pain relief: patients' status and nurses' medication choices. *Pain* 9:265–274, 1980.

12. Paice JA, Mahon SM, Faut-Callahan M: Factors associated with adequate pain control in hospitalized postsurgical patients diagnosed with cancer. *Cancer Nurs* 14:298–305, 1991.

13. Whipple JK, Lewis KS, Quebbeman EJ, et al: Analysis of pain management in critically ill patients. *Pharmacotherapy* 15:592–599, 1995.

14. Lebovits AH, Florence I, Bathina R, et al: Pain knowledge and attitudes of healthcare providers: practice characteristics differences. *Clin J Pain* 13:237–243, 1997.

15. Buchan ML, Tolle SW: Pain relief for dying persons: dealing with physicians' fears and concerns. *J Clin Ethics* 6: 53–61, 1995.

16. Cherny NI, Cataine R: Professional negligence in the management of cancer pain: a case for urgent reforms. *Cancer* 76:2181–2185, 1995.

17. Choiniere M, Melzack R, Girard N, et al: Comparisons between patients' and nurses' assessment of pain and medication efficacy in severe burn injuries. *Pain* 40:143–152, 1990.

18. Portenoy RK: Chronic opioid therapy in nonmalignant pain. *J Pain Sympt Mgt* 5:S46–S62, 1990.

19. Porter J: Addiction rare in patients treated with narcotics. *N Engl J Med* 302:123, 1980.

20. Perry S, Heidrich G: Management of pain during debridement: a survey of U.S. burn units. *Pain* 13:267–280, 1982.

21. Portenoy RK: Chronic opioid therapy for persistent noncancer pain: can we get past the bias? *APS Bull* 1:3–5, 1991.

22. Ward SE, Goldberg N, Miller-McCauley V, et al: Patient-related barriers to management of cancer pain. *Pain* 52:319–324, 1993.

23. Foley K: The relationship of pain and symptom management to patient requests for physician-assisted suicide. *J Pain Sympt Mgt* 6:289–297, 1991.

24. Joranson DE: Are health-care reimbursement policies a barrier to acute and cancer pain management? *J Pain Sympt Mgt* 9:244–253, 1994.

25. Soumerai SB, Avorn J, Ross-Degnan D, Gortmaker S: Payment restrictions for prescription drugs under Medicaid: effects on therapy, cost and equity. *N Engl J Med* 317:550–556, 1987.

26. Angarola RT, Joranson DE. State controlled substances laws and pain control. *APS Bull* 2:10–11, 15, 1992.

27. McDonald DD: Gender and ethnic stereotyping and narcotic analgesic administration. *Res Nurs Health* 17:45–49, 1994.

28. Todd KH, Samaroo N, Hoffman JR: Ethnicity as a risk factor for inadequate emergency department analgesia. *JAMA* 269:1537–1539, 1993.

29. Cleeland CS, Gonin R, Baez L, et al: Pain and treatment of pain in minority patients with cancer: the Eastern Cooperative Oncology Group Minority Outpatient Pain Study. *Ann Intern Med* 127:813–816, 1997.

30. Bernabei R, Gambassi G, Lapane K, et al: Management of pain in elderly patients with cancer. *JAMA* 279:1877–1882, 1998.

31. Todd KH, Lee T, Hoffman JR: The effect of ethnicity on physician estimates of pain severity in patients with isolated extremity trauma. *JAMA* 271:925–928, 1994.

32. Garcia JLA: Double effect, in Reich WT (ed): *Encyclopedia of Bioethics*, rev ed. Vol 2. New York, MacMillan, 1995, pp 636–641.

33. Council on Ethical and Judicial Affairs of the American Medical Association: *Euthanasia Report C: Proceedings of the House of Delegates of the AMA*. Chicago, American Medical Association, 1988, pp 258–260.

34. Andre J, Ogle K: Ethics, politics, and pain. *Med Hum Rep* 20:1–5, 1999.

35. Barnett EH, Case marks big shift in pain policy. *The Oregonian* September 2, 1999 [www.oregonlive.com/news/99/09/st090201.html]

36. Wilder-Smith CH, Schuler L: Postoperative analgesia: pain by choice? The influence of patient attitudes and patient education. *Pain* 50:257–262, 1992.

37. Horning MR: Chronic opioids: a reassessment. *Alaska Med* 39:103–110, 1997.

38. VonRoenn JH, Cleeland CS, Gonin R, et al: Physician attitudes and practice in cancer pain management: a survey from the Eastern Cooperative Oncology Group. *Ann Intern Med* 119:121–126, 1993.

39. Association of American Medical Colleges: The increasing need for end of life and palliative care education. *Contemp Issues Med Educ* 2:1–2, 1999.

40. Council on ethical and judicial affairs of the American Medical Association: *1992 Code of Medial Ethics: Annotated Current Opinions.* Chicago: American Medical Association, 1992, p xiv.

41. Joranson DR, Gilson AM, Williams C, et al: State intractable pain policy: current status. *APS Bull* 7:7–9, 1997.

Paul Bascom
Susan W. Tolle

Chapter
17

Treatment at the End of Life

Zachary Coleman, 22 years old, lingers in a persistent vegetative state in a nursing home 6 months following a severe closed head injury. His grieving parents ask the doctor to discontinue artificial feeding. A week after the accident, the parents had agreed to the placement of a gastrostomy feeding tube and artificial feeding, on the assurance that the artificial feeding could be discontinued in the future if it became clear that their son's prognosis for recovery was inalterably poor. To their surprise, their son's physician now refuses to discontinue artificial feeding, claiming that such an act would be tantamount to murder.

Gretchen Sanders, 40 years old, has widely metastatic breast cancer; she is at home under hospice care, suffering from rapidly increasing pain despite the use of analgesic medications and increasingly higher doses of intravenous morphine. She has become sedated by the morphine but still moans frequently when moved or turned. The family pleads with the hospice nurse to call the physician to request a higher dose of morphine. The physician refuses to authorize the higher dose and asks that the patient be transferred to the hospital for evaluation and treatment. He believes that the patient's death is not imminent—that the patient could possibly live several more months. When the nurse persists in her request for higher doses of medication, the physician accuses her of attempting to euthanize the patient. He cites his fear that he might be investigated by the state licensing board for overuse of pain medication.

Tom Smith, 60 years old, has advanced lung cancer. He asks his physician to give him a lethal dose of medication to end his life. The request surprises the physician, as the patient's cancer, though already inoperable at the time of diagnosis, had progressed rather slowly. There had been minimal pain and no significant complications to manage. In recent months Mr. Smith had seemed more breathless and had been losing weight, but he seemed to be in good spirits. He was still able to care for himself alone at home. The physician had offered to refer Mr. Smith to the local hospice program, recognizing he likely would live less than 6 months, but the patient had refused, stating that he did not require any help.

Scope of the Problem

Ethical concerns arise frequently in end-of-life care. Through much discussion, debate, and landmark court cases, consensus has emerged regarding professional standards for ethical practice in many aspects of end-of-life care. Although cases arise that may challenge them, aspects of ethical and legal clarity include the ability of patients or their surrogates to refuse life-sustaining treatments, including artificial nutrition and hydration; the ethical acceptability of both withholding and withdrawing life-sustaining treatments; and the right of patients to receive high-dose pain medication even when such doses carry the risk of shortening life. On the other hand, debate rages about the ethics of physician-assisted suicide, which remains illegal in most jurisdictions.

In each of these aspects of medical practice—the refusal of life-sustaining treatments, the withholding and withdrawing of life support, the use of high-dose pain medication at the end of life, and requests for physician-assisted suicide—the decision-making process continues to be emotionally charged and challenging for clinicians, patients, and families. At times, despite legal clarity about ethical standards and patients' rights, a patient's values and choices may fundamentally conflict with those of the clinicians caring for them.

Definitions

Some of the conflicts that may arise in the context of decision making in end-of-life care originate from confusion over language. The terms used in discussions of end-of-life decision making carry strong emotional overtones. Similar actions may be labeled with differing terms, each carrying a distinct connotation. For example, "physician-assisted suicide" and "physician aid in dying" each describe a similar act, but, as described below, suggest particular points of view regarding the act. Therefore, a brief description of the terms used in this chapter follows.

CONSCIENTIOUS PRACTICE

Conscientious practice is defined as the "taking of professional actions that are consistent with one's ethical and moral beliefs, and avoiding actions that are contrary to one's beliefs."[1] The patient's right to refuse treatment or to pursue a given treatment does not oblige an individual clinician to participate in the provision of that treatment when the patient's choices conflict with the clinician's own moral beliefs. The clinician's right to conscientious practice allows the clinician to withdraw from the treatment of a patient once having assured that the patient can receive care from another clinician. Although when such a transfer of care is being formulated, the clinician should continue to ensure that appropriate measures are provided.

PHYSICIAN-ASSISTED SUICIDE/PHYSICIAN AID IN DYING

Physician-assisted suicide or *physician aid in dying* signifies the act of providing a lethal dose of medication for the patient to self-administer.

The term "physician-assisted suicide" seems to have achieved more common usage and is more specific. Accordingly, the former term, "physician-assisted suicide," is used in this chapter, rather than the more ambiguous "physician aid in dying."

EUTHANASIA

Euthanasia describes the act of ending the life of an individual suffering from a terminal illness or an incurable condition, usually by lethal injection. In contrast to physician-assisted suicide, euthanasia implies that direct action of the physician, with or without the consent of the patient. Ironically, the word euthanasia originates from the Latin roots *eu* ("good") and *thanatos* ("death"); thus it means "good death." Certainly those engaged in the tumultuous debate over euthanasia and physician-assisted suicide are motivated by the desire to provide a good death for patients, though reaching consensus regarding the attributes of a good death remains contentious.

THE PRINCIPLE OF DOUBLE EFFECT

The ethical *principle of double effect* may be invoked to justify the administration of high-dose pain medication when such administration carries the risk of hastening death.[2] This principle holds that any action may have two distinct effects, one desired and the other, while foreseen, undesired. If the primary goal of the action is to produce the desired effect, then the coincident occurrence of the undesired effect can be ethically permissible. (See Chap. 16)

TERMINAL SEDATION

Terminal sedation describes the use of high-dose medication to relieve pain at the end of life. However, its ambiguous connotations may lead some to equate the practice with euthanasia. The word "terminal" indicates that the expected and perhaps desired outcome is death.

The word "sedation" implies that medication will be administered not on the basis of pain relief but certainly until unconsciousness ensues.

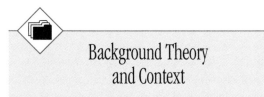

Background Theory and Context

Refusing Life-Sustaining Treatments

The right of patients or their surrogates to refuse life-sustaining medical treatments has been well established in courts of law. The *Quinlan* decision in 1975 established the right to discontinue mechanical ventilation and, by inference, other life-sustaining medical treatments.[3] The subsequent *Cruzan* decision by the U.S. Supreme Court in 1980 extended that right to include artificial nutrition and hydration.[4] When patients lack decision-making capacity, some states have established a higher standard for withdrawal of artificial nutrition and hydration. For example, Missouri requires "clear and convincing evidence" of the patient's preferences before surrogates have the authority to withdraw artificial feeding. Other states (e.g., New York) do not currently have surrogate laws, and the authority to withdraw life support is less clearly established for those patients who have not completed an advance directive (see Chap. 20).

THE ACCEPTABILITY OF BOTH WITHHOLDING AND WITHDRAWING TREATMENT

Ethical standards for clinicians hold that there is no difference between withholding treatment and withdrawing that same treatment once it has been initiated.[5] In both the Quinlan and Cruzan cases, the treatment in question—mechanical ventilation and enteral feeding, respectively—had already been initiated. Surrogates were petitioning for the right to withdraw those treatments. However, as the hypothetical case involving Zachary Coleman described above illustrates, in practice the act of withdrawing therapy may generate a deeper emotional response than choosing not to initiate a treatment in the first place. The act of discontinuing nutrition and hydration in a young, otherwise stable patient often engenders a greater emotional response than choosing not to perform cardiopulmonary resuscitation in an elderly patient with multiorgan failure. Nevertheless, the emotional reaction this case elicits does not alter the fundamental ethical principle that patients and their surrogates may choose to withdraw life-sustaining treatments, including artificial hydration and nutrition, once they have been initiated.[5]

The right to withdraw treatment protects patients and their surrogates from the pressure of urgent decision making. Such pressure may prompt choices to limit treatment in some who might otherwise choose a trial of treatment and might benefit from it. By initiating a treatment, two things may be gained. First, clinicians, patients, and surrogates may achieve greater certainty of prognosis, as occurred in this case. Second, time may allow greater clarity and consensus to develop about the patient's wishes.

CONSCIENTIOUS PRACTICE

The rights and values of the patient and his or her surrogates may at times conflict with deeply held beliefs of the patient's clinicians. In Zachary's case, the clinician believes that the withdrawal of nutrition and hydration from this young man would be "tantamount to murder." In fact, five percent of internists believe that withdrawal of artificial nutrition and hydration is morally wrong.[6] The right of conscientious practice allows the clinician to withdraw from the treatment of a patient without sanction while respecting the patient's right to refuse treatment.

Ethical standards of professional practice do not require that the clinician identify another clinician to assume care of the patient.[5] For those physicians with strong moral opposition to a patient's or surrogate's decision regarding treatment, providing assistance in this manner would also constitute a breach of their personal morality. Nonetheless, the clinician is obligated to provide all appropriate comfort measures until the time of transfer and to make all medical records available to the clinician assuming care of the patient.

High-Dose Pain Management at the End of Life

In the vast majority of patients near the end of life, pain treatments are administered without ethical conflict. In these patients, morphine and similar opioid pain-relieving drugs can be titrated to an effective dosage without intolerable side effects.[7] Patients on chronic opioid analgesics can often tolerate very high doses without significant side effects. If opioids are incompletely effective at controlling pain, then *coanalgesics* (such as corticosteroids, anticonvulsants, or antidepressants) may provide significant additional benefit. If sedation occurs, psychostimulants (such as methylphenidate) may be employed to offset the sedating effect of the opioid. More often, however, increasing sedation reflects the progression of the underlying disease, not the impact of opioid medications (see Chap. 16).

Nevertheless, there may arise rare cases in which pain is so severe and resistant to treatment that the dosages of opioids required to achieve analgesia may reach the level at which consciousness and even respiratory function are impaired. At times, the use of barbiturates to produce sedation may be the only effective recourse for control of overwhelming symptoms.[8] In these rare cases, decisions will be made that balance the expected benefit of pain relief with the undesired outcome of sedation and, perhaps, hastening of death. Under the principle of double effect, the goal of alleviating pain justifies and permits the hastening of death, which may occur as an unavoidable consequence of high-dose morphine administration to relieve pain.[2,5]

Although the administration of high-dose pain medication may appear to carry the same connotation of killing the patient as in euthanasia, in fact the two are fundamentally distinct. When high-dose pain medication is administered, the goal of treatment is relief of pain. Should pain relief occur without sedation and without hastening of death, the dose is not escalated. Only when pain relief is not achieved at nonsedating doses are doses increased until sedation occurs, with a possible though unavoidable hastening of death.[9] By contrast, in the case of euthanasia, the goal is to cause the death of the patient. The fundamentally different goal of treatment allows one to distinguish between the illegal act of euthanasia and the acceptable uses of pain medication at the end of life.

There are some commentators who find no distinction between euthanasia and the hastening of death from high-dose pain medication and who judge the use of the double-effect doctrine as unnecessary and artificial.[10] For those who approve of euthanasia and believe that the hastening of death can be an acceptable response to uncontrolled suffering, it follows that no additional ethical justification is needed to allow the use of aggressive attempts at symptom control. However, for patients, families, or clinicians who oppose euthanasia and the deliberate hastening of death, the principle of double effect provides justification for aggressive pain-relief measures to be employed free of the implication of euthanasia.[11]

Decisions to proceed with high-dose pain medication near the end-of-life must be made with the informed consent of patients or, when patients lack decision-making capacity, with their surrogates. Patients must be offered the opportunity to benefit from the wide array of treatments that may assist in managing their pain, though they may also choose not to avail themselves of those treatments. Patients and families choosing aggressive symptom control should be informed of the risks of sedation and hastening of death that may result from their decision. Clinicians must be careful, however, to remind patients and their families that, regardless of the outcome of the treatment, the proximate cause of death remains the underlying disease, not the pain treatment itself. Indeed, it may be reassuring to know that the relief of symptoms with high-dose pain medication rarely causes a hastening of death but that such an unavoidable outcome, if it does occur, is both ethical and legal.[12]

The hypothetical case of Gretchen Sanders, described at the opening of this chapter, involves a family and hospice nurse who ask a reluctant clinician to provide high-dose pain medication for the treatment of a dying patient with uncontrolled pain. There are clinicians who may remain uncomfortable with aggressive symptom control. In this case the clinician may truly believe that hospitalization and treatment would serve the best interest of the patient and may not agree with the choice to treat symptoms more aggressively at home. As in first case vignette involving Zachary Coleman, the clinician's right to conscientious practice would allow that clinician to withdraw from the care of that patient once another clinician had assumed responsibility for the patient's care.

Some of the physician's reluctance to pursue more aggressive pain management for Ms. Sanders may have arisen from a misguided fear of sanction by his state licensing board (see Chap. 16). In recent years, state medical boards, legislatures, and courts have been actively encouraging clinicians to increase their prescribing of pain-relieving medications near the end of life.[13] In the state of Oregon, the advance directive statute passed in 1993 mandates that "comfort measures," including appropriate doses of pain medications, be administered when life-sustaining treatments are withheld or withdrawn. The Oregon Board of Medical Examiners (BME), in 1998, publicly asserted their belief that the gross underprescribing of pain medica-

tions in a terminally ill patient with pain is equal grounds for investigation as is an inappropriate overprescribing for a patient with a chronic nonmalignant pain state. In a letter sent to all Oregon physicians, the BME stated their commitment to "investigate physicians for grossly under treating pain with the same interest and thoroughness as those who over prescribe controlled substances."[14] The U.S. Supreme Court, in its recent ruling on assisted suicide, affirmed the right of clinicians to provide very high dose pain relief at the end of life. While ruling that patients do not have a fundamental right to assisted suicide, the justices did signal their opposition to any restrictions on the ability of patients to receive adequate pain relief near the end of life.[12]

Physician-Assisted Suicide and Euthanasia

No other issues in end-of-life care create as much controversy as physician-assisted suicide and euthanasia. This controversy stems from the fundamental ethical questions raised by assisted suicide and euthanasia. Does a patient's right to autonomy encompass the right to have his or her physician hasten death? Does assisted suicide uphold the fundamental ethical principle of beneficence—of acting in a patient's best interest?[15] Or, conversely, does hastening a death violate the sanctity of life and the fundamental ethical principle of nonmaleficence—of doing no harm?[16,17] Deep divisions exist in many professional societies over the answers to these questions.

Nor is there unanimity of sentiment among those on either side of the debate. Some equate physician-assisted suicide and euthanasia, finding any hastening of death to violate the fundamental ethical code of physicians. Others find physician-assisted suicide to be ethically acceptable, since it represents ultimately a voluntary act by the patient, but continue to oppose euthanasia, citing a higher risk of abuse. Others approve of and equate both practices, believing that the mandate to relieve patients' symptoms justifies the use of either practice in certain situations.

It is not our purpose to discuss the merits of or objections to physician-assisted suicide.* Many others have written eloquently from both sides of the debate. Rather, our purpose in this chapter is to elaborate on the rights of the clinician to conscientious practice and on the compassionate and ethical response to a patient's request for assisted suicide. Clinicians who disagree on the ethics of assisted suicide find common ground, as described below, on the issue of how clinicians should evaluate a patient who requests assisted suicide.[1,16]

As mentioned previously, the debate over assisted suicide is clouded by confusion over terminology. This confusion may lead physicians and other health professionals to misclassify their actions. For example, some have employed the terms "physician-assisted suicide" and "euthanasia" to describe the act of escalating morphine doses to treat pain in the last days of life.[18] However, such an act represents an ethically and legally appropriate response to the patient's symptoms.[5] Conversely, when clinicians do deliberately hasten a patient's death by personally administering a lethal dose with the intent to shorten life, this is euthanasia and not assisted suicide. Physician-assisted suicide signifies specifically the act of providing a lethal dose of medication for the patient to self-administer.

Euthanasia is currently illegal throughout the United States. Although it remains officially illegal in The Netherlands, it is practiced under an agreement to not prosecute when certain protocols are followed. Assisted suicide is currently illegal in all jurisdictions in the United States except Oregon. Despite this, studies show that some physicians (4 to 7 percent) have written a prescription knowing that the patient intended

to use it to take his or her own life.[19–21] In Oregon, physicians are now legally permitted to write a prescription for a lethal dose of medication for competent, adult patients with terminal illnesses expected to cause death within 6 months.[1] Although this is legal, less than one dying person in a thousand utilized this law in 1998.[22]

Toward Resolution

Navigating the shoals of challenging cases concerning treatment at the end of life requires great sensitivity toward all involved and respect for each individual's own values and beliefs. Ethical and legal clarity about what individual patients may choose for themselves does not require that all those involved in the care of that patient agree with the choice. In a pluralistic society, there must be respect not only for individual autonomy but also for the ability of others to differ in their values and for those who differ to be respected in their refusal to participate in the care of such patients.

In responding to the cases described at the beginning of this chapter, creative responses were identified that reflect the background theory and context described above. Accordingly, we first provide the epilogues to these cases and then describe how clinicians might respond to requests for assisted suicide.

Epilogues

ZACHARY COLEMAN

The physician refusing to discontinue artificial feeding explained that such an act would

---

*Oregon Health Sciences University (OHSU) and the Center for Ethics in Health Care at OHSU stand officially neutral on the issue while working to improve the care of the dying in other ways.

violate his personal moral beliefs. The parents then asked for assistance in locating another physician who would honor their request. However, that second request was refused as well. Ultimately, the parents contacted the hospital where their son's feeding tube had been placed. The hospital ethics service helped locate a physician who would honor the parents' request. Their son was transferred to another facility, the artificial feeding was discontinued, and Zachary died 2 weeks later.

GRETCHEN SANDERS

The physician and family spoke directly. The physician informed the family that the transfer to the hospital and further testing might uncover some correctable source of Ms. Sanders' escalating pain and might extend her life by weeks or longer. However, the family replied that their mother's foremost desire was to be at home with her family when she died. She had consistently refused to be transferred to the hospital. The physician understood their wishes but still felt uncomfortable authorizing the increased dose of medication. He asked that the hospice medical director assume responsibility for prescribing the morphine. At the family's request, the hospice medical director increased the dose of morphine to the degree that the patient's moaning and grimacing ceased. He advised them that this was ethically permissible, though it might shorten the patient's life by days or weeks. The family regarded transfer to the hospital as unacceptable and chose to proceed with continued escalation of morphine dosage as needed to control her pain. Ms. Sanders died later that evening with her family at her bedside.

TOM SMITH

The physician asked to explore with Mr. Smith his reasons for seeking aid in dying. Mr. Smith explained that he wanted to continue to live alone in his small apartment. He had always lived a very solitary life, had very few friends,

and was estranged from his family. Even as death approached, he had no desire to reconnect with his family. His greatest fear was that he would be unable to care for himself and would be forced to leave his apartment. The thought of living in a nursing home horrified him. He sought the means to take his own life once his condition deteriorated to the point that he could not care for himself.

The physician inquired about the presence of depression. Mr. Smith admitted to some sadness over his approaching death and had some lingering regrets over abandoning his family many years before. On the whole, however, he felt that he had lived a good life, "had some wild times, some happy times," he said, smiling at these memories. The physician inquired about the patient's lack of social support. Mr. Smith replied that he had always been a loner and truly did not want anyone around.

The physician responded that her own personal beliefs and values would not permit her to honor the patient's request for a lethal prescription but that she would do her utmost to ensure that the patient could remain in his home until death. The patient agreed to accept the help of a home hospice team on the assurance that hospice would not require him to leave his home. In the ensuing weeks, the physician made several home visits and continued to acknowledge and honor the patient's desire to remain in his own home until the time of death. The patient was greatly relieved by the visits and by the knowledge that he could remain at home. In time he became weaker and less and less able to care for himself. Though nearly bed-bound, he still refused to be transferred from his home. One morning the hospice nurse arrived to find that he had died in the night.

Responding to a Request for Assisted Suicide

The compassionate and ethical response to a request for assisted suicide entails investigating with the patient the underlying concerns behind the request and endeavoring to address those concerns as much as possible.[1,16] Common wisdom presumes that uncontrolled pain or fear of unrelieved pain is the principal motivation behind requests for assisted suicide. Evidence indicates that terminally ill patients continue to experience uncontrolled pain, and improvement in pain management practices is an important priority.[23] Nevertheless, improvements in pain management are unlikely to eliminate all requests for assisted suicide. For many patients, hopelessness and concerns over loss of independence are more substantial factors in the request.[22,24]

REASONS BEHIND REQUESTS

The desire for assisted suicide often originates in patients' fears over loss of independence and loss of dignity.[22,24] Patients may seek assisted suicide as a means of regaining control over their lives as they confront the essentially uncontrollable, inexorable progression of terminal illness. Patients may seek to hasten their death as an antidote to their fears of protracted, lingering death. By addressing these underlying concerns, the desire for assisted suicide may often be alleviated. In the third case vignette presented at the opening of this chapter, the physician learns that Mr. Smith's request stems from a fear of having to leave his home. The physician acknowledges this as the patient's preeminent goal and pledges to help him remain at home, regardless of his desire to pursue assisted suicide.

Depression may be an important feature of those seeking assisted suicide. Diagnosing depression in those with terminal illness can be challenging. The physical signs of depression—such as fatigue; changes in sleep, energy, and libido; and weight loss—are often present as a result of the advancing illness. Most terminally ill patients will have periods of depressed mood or sadness. However, this is usually an appropriate emotional response to illness and impending death and is better described as grief

rather than depression. The diagnosis of depression in terminally ill patients is more reliably made on the basis of the cognitive signs of depression. Depressed patients commonly exhibit anhedonia, pervasive guilt and regret about the past, or loss of self-worth.

Social factors may also play a role in some patients' desire for assisted suicide. Many patients do not wish to burden their families or loved ones. Others have very limited social support.[22] When appropriate, patients should be reassured that their families are shouldering the burdens of care with love and affection. Resources such as hospice care should be made available.

CONSIDERATIONS IN RESPONDING

Ultimately, despite all efforts at improving care and providing comfort, some patients will persist in their desire for assisted suicide.[22] Each clinician will then decide on the basis of his or her own personal beliefs and values how to respond. The personal, ethical, and legal ramifications of participating must be carefully considered. This complex topic is explored in the book *The Oregon Death with Dignity Act: a Guidebook for Health Care Providers.*[2] This document was produced by a 25-member, multidisciplinary task force in response to the approval of Oregon's assisted suicide law.

Clinicians must decide to what degree they will be willing to assist a patient in hastening death. This intensely personal decision will challenge every clinician to examine carefully his or her own ethical beliefs. Those who are willing to assist a patient in principle may change their views depending on the patient and the circumstances.[19,22] The right to conscientious practice upholds the rights of the clinician to withdraw from the care of a patient who chooses a treatment to which the clinician is morally opposed. The right to conscientious practice also encompasses the right of physicians in Oregon, where assisted suicide is now legal, to assist patients in exercising their legally available options without fear of sanction. However, even in Oregon, where assisted suicide is legal, physicians in the employ of some health care systems are constrained by the policies of their institutions. Institutions also have the right of conscientious practice and thus the right to refuse to have their employees participate in practices at odds with the institution's fundamental values.[1]

Closing Comments

Up to this point, ethical standards in end-of-life care have originated largely from a foundation of respect for patient autonomy—primarily the right of patients to refuse unwanted treatments. As yet, there has been no universal right to receive treatment, as is evidenced by the ongoing epidemic of uninsured patients in the United States. In the future, we hope to witness an emerging right of patients to receive comfort at the end of life. The Supreme Court hinted at such a right in its rulings over assisted suicide, specifying that impediments may not be placed in the way of dying patients' access to pain relief.[12] In Oregon, legislation is being considered that would guarantee universal access to hospice care for all uninsured dying patients, regardless of income status. At the end of life patients have the legal and ethical right to refuse life-sustaining treatments. Will we as a society support a right to comfort in life's final months?

References

1. Haley K, Lee MA (eds): *The Oregon Death With Dignity Act—A Guidebook for Health Care Providers*. Portland, OR, The Center for Ethics in Health Care, 1998.
2. Pellegrino ED: Doctors must not kill. *J Clin Ethics* 3:95–102, 1992.
3. *Matter of Quinlan*, 348 A2d 81, 816 (NJ 1975).
4. *Cruzan* v *Director, Missouri Dept of Health*, 497 US 261 110 S Ct 2841, 111 L Ed2d 224 (1990).
5. Kitchens, LW Jr, Brennan TA, Carroll RJ, et al: American College of Physicians Ethics Manual, 4th ed. *Ann Intern Med* 128;576–595, 1998.
6. Hodges MO, Tolle SW, Stocking C, Cassel C: Tube feeding: internists' attitudes regarding ethical obligations. *Arch Intern Med* 154:1013–1020, 1994.
7. Fohr SA: The double effect of pain medication: separating myth from reality. *J Palliat Med* 1:315–328, 1998.
8. Troug RD, Berde CD, Mitchell C, et al: Barbiturates in the care of the terminally ill. *N Engl J Med* 327:1678–1682, 1992.
9. Buchan ML, Tolle SW: Pain relief for dying persons: dealing with physicians' fears and concerns. *J Clin Ethics* 6:53–61, 1995.
10. Billing JA, Block SD: Slow euthanasia. *J Palliat Care* 12:21–30, 1997.
11. Quill TE: Principle of double effect and end-of-life pain management: additional myths and a limited role. *J Palliat Med* 1:333–336, 1997.
12. Burt RA: The Supreme Court speaks: not assisted suicide but a constitutional right of Palliative Care. *N Engl J Med* 337:1234–1236, 1997.
13. Federation of State Medical Boards of the United States: *Model Guidelines for the Use of Controlled Substances for the Treatment of Pain*. Euless, TX, FSMBUS, May 1998.
14. Tolle SW, Haley K: *Pain Management in the Dying: Successes and Concerns: BME Report*. Portland, OR, Oregon Board of Medical Examiners, Fall 1998.
15. Angell M: The Supreme Court and physician-assisted suicide—the ultimate right. *N Engl J Med* 336:50–53, 1997.
16. Council on Ethical and Judicial Affairs. American Medical Association: *Code of Medical Ethics*. Report 59. Chicago, American Medical Association, 1994.

17. Foley KM: Competent care for the dying instead of physician-assisted suicide. *N Engl J Med* 336: 54–58, 1997.
18. Asch DA: The role of critical care nurses in euthanasia and assisted suicide. *N Engl J Med* 334:1374–1379, 1996.
19. Lee MA, Nelson HD, Tilden VP, et al: Legalizing assisted suicide—views of physicians in Oregon. *N Engl J Med* 334:310–315, 1996.
20. Meier DE, Emmons CA, Wallenstein S, et al: A national survey of physician-assisted suicide and euthanasia in the United States. *N Engl J Med* 338: 1193–1201, 1998.
21. Emanuel EJ, Daniels E, Fairclough D, et al: The Practice of euthanasia and physician-assisted suicide in the United States. *JAMA* 280:507–513, 1998.
22. Chin AE, Hedberg K, Higginson GK, Fleming DW: Legalized physician-assisted suicide in Oregon: the first year's experience. *N Engl J Med* 340: 577–583, 1999.
23. Field MJ, Cassell CK: Approaching death: improving care at the end of life. Institute of Medicine Committee on Care at the End of Life. Washington, DC, National Academy Press, 1997.
24. Ganzini L, Johnston WS, McFarland BH, et al: Attitudes of patients with amyotrophic lateral sclerosis and their care givers toward assisted suicide. *N Engl J Med* 339:967–973, 1998.

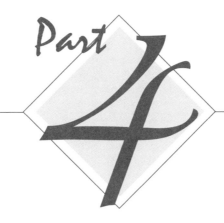

Part 4

Preventive
Ethics

Jason H. T. Karlawish
David Casarett

Competency and Decision-Making Capacity

Tom Zorn, 70 years old, discusses his diagnosis of mild Alzheimer disease with his primary care clinician. He says: "This is like cancer. I'll take whatever I can to slow this down. What can you give me?" The clinician describes treatment with vitamin E and nonsteroidal anti-inflammatory drugs (NSAIDs). Mr. Zorn has difficulty appreciating that the benefits of NSAIDs are relatively unproven and he has trouble reasoning about the risk of gastrointestinal bleeding associated with taking them. However, he experiences considerably less difficulty in considering the relevant features of vitamin E therapy.

Jane Tang, 17 years old, has insulin-dependent diabetes and a complicated reinfection of the bones of her right foot. Her options are partial amputation of her foot versus a 6-week course of antibiotics that can only be given in hospital. Jane is an honor student who plans to attend college to study ancient history. After several meetings with her parents, pediatrician, infectious disease specialist, and surgeon, Jane says she wants to have the amputation. She explains that surgical treatment will allow her to complete her studies with the best possible grades and go on to a competitive college.

Tim Nuthatch, 50 years old, has locally confined high-grade prostate cancer. He returns to his general internist after discussing treatment options with a urologist and an oncologist. Tim tells his physician, "There is nothing more powerful than my weapon of prayer. I'm going to let the Lord heal this plague upon my body."

Scope of the Problem

In most situations, clinicians will have little difficulty determining a patient's competency to participate in clinical decision making. Occasionally, however, a clinician will encounter cases such as these that are not so straightforward. Throughout this chapter, the term *competent* describes a patient who possesses *decision-making capacity* (*DMC*). DMC is a functional term.[1] It describes a patient's ability to make a specific health care decision such as whether to take an NSAID in effort to slow the progression of Alzheimer disease. A patient who is relatively or absolutely incapable of making this sort of decision is said to lack DMC. A clinician must judge whether that degree of decisional impairment—together with the risks, benefits, and complexity of the decision—means that the patient is incapable of making that decision.[2]

In this chapter we describe the standards for determining DMC, explain how to assess it, and suggests ways that clinicians can address common ethical challenges they will encounter in making such determinations.

Key Principles

A clinician who assesses a patient's DMC takes on a task with important medical, legal, and ethical elements. These elements are unified in the doctrine of informed consent, which allows patients with adequate DMC to make choices about their own health and health care (see Chap. 19).[3] The key is that this doctrine applies only to those patients who have adequate DMC. In informed consent, the determination of DMC is intended to assure that clinicians strike a proper balance between protecting patients' autonomy and promoting their welfare. In clinical terms, this avoids two potential harms: either incorrectly determining that patients lacks DMC, and thereby preventing them from exercising their choice, or permitting patients who lack DMC to make inappropriate or dangerous choices.

Although the concept of DMC has its roots in ethics and the law, the task of assessing DMC is akin to a diagnostic medical procedure. To accurately assess DMC, clinicians must understand how medical conditions can impair a patient's cognitive and affective abilities and must have robust diagnostic and interviewing skills. Therefore, as with any other basic diagnostic problem, clinicians should know how to assess DMC, just as they should know how to diagnose depression or pneumonia. Primary care providers should also be aware of the limits of their knowledge and expertise in making these assessments, just as they would know when to refer a patient with major depression or empyema to a specialist.

DMC is the clinical manifestation of a patient's cognitive and affective functions.[4] These functions, in turn, require a series of abilities including memory, judgment, attention, insight, language, calculation, and communication. These abilities may be impaired to varying degrees. For instance, a child's intellectual and emotional development may limit his or her insight and ability to communicate. In adults, a variety of conditions can impair these abilities, resulting in a lack of DMC. These conditions include dementia, delirium, substance abuse, and psychiatric disorders such as depression, anxiety, and schizophrenia. Of note, primary care providers may first become aware of one of these conditions because it has impaired a patient's DMC. That is, lack of DMC may be a presenting feature of one of these conditions and may be the only clue to its existence. This underscores the importance of assessing DMC as a basic medical skill.

Common Causes of Impaired Decision-Making Capacity

The prevalence of capacity-impairing conditions guarantees that clinicians practicing primary care will encounter these patients. In industrialized nations, where the elderly population is rising rapidly, dementia will become an increasingly common cause of cognitive impairment. In North America, for instance, the prevalence of persons over age 65 with moderate or severe dementia ranges from 4.5 to 10.2 percent.[5] In the United States, 4 million persons are estimated to have dementia, and this could reach 12 million by the year 2050.[6] These figures do not reflect the fact that the prevalence of dementia is substantially higher in certain primary care settings, such as the nursing home. Clinically significant decisional impairment is common among patients with Alzheimer disease, the most common cause of dementia.[7] Because *dementia* is defined as an impairment in two or more cognitive functions (such as memory and language), it has an evident causal link to decisional impairments.[8]

In contrast, psychiatric disorders indirectly impair DMC. For instance, a patient with major depression may not care about the outcome of a decision, and a patient with an anxiety disorder may be unable to pay attention to information required to make a decision. Depression, schizophrenia, and anxiety are extremely common psychiatric disorders.[9–12]

The association between serious and life-threatening or chronic illnesses and depression suggests that these patients may have decisional impairments. For example, depression has been reported in up to 25 percent of patients with cancer.[13,14] Clinical experience and research demonstrate that these diseases, like dementia, can cause significant impairment in DMC.[15]

To summarize, issues related to DMC are important in the practice of primary care. In primary care, clinicians will likely encounter patients with impaired DMC, and this may be among the initial diagnostic clues that a patient has a disease such as depression or dementia. Further, impairment may occur in patients with many diagnoses.

Nevertheless, although diseases such as dementia or schizophrenia may increase the odds of impairment, many of the patients with these conditions may have adequate DMC. Therefore, clinicians should not assume that patients lack DMC simply because they have a risk factor for impairment. For instance, depression does not always impair capacity, just as peripheral vascular disease is not always associated with coronary artery disease. However, in both cases, the effective primary care clinician must be alert to factors that increase the probability of an impairment in DMC.

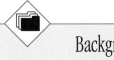

Background Theory and Context

Ethical Principles

Clinicians should respect the choices of competent patients and should promote their patients' well being. These duties are derived, respectively, from the principles of respect for autonomy and beneficence.[16,17] The clinicians' duty to *respect autonomy* follows from the recognition of the right of persons to be allowed to freely determine their lives. In health care, the principle of respect for autonomy is articulated clearly in the doctrine of informed consent.[3] *Beneficence* is the ethical principle stipulating that persons should be protected from harm and that their welfare should be promoted. A clinician who follows these principles may be faced with a dilemma—whether to respect a patient's choice or to protect the patient from harmful choices. However, the assessment of DMC may resolve such dilemmas. Patients with DMC should be allowed to choose, even if the choice

is harmful. In contrast, patients without DMC who express harmful choices need not have these expressions honored. This is not because the clinician objects to the patient's choice but because the patient cannot make an authentic choice. Thus, patients who have DMC are protected from unwanted influence by others, and patients who do not have DMC are protected from unwanted harm.

Sliding-Scale Concept of Competency

A clinician should select a level of adequate DMC according to the potential risks and benefits of the decision to be made.[1,4,18] Under this *sliding scale of competency* clinicians should use more stringent assessments when a patient chooses a risky course of action or refuses a beneficial, low-risk option.[19] It is analogous to the way in which clinicians set the cutoff for a diagnostic test. For example, if the disease is serious and the treatment is safe and effective, clinicians would be willing to accept occasional false-positive results and unnecessary treatments. Therefore, in order to maximize the test's sensitivity, a very low threshold for a positive test might be set. The same approach holds when clinicians assess DMC. If a patient makes a choice that has potentially fatal results, clinicians would occasionally be willing to risk overriding an authentic refusal of treatment. In these cases, clinicians would require considerable evidence of the patient's DMC, with the knowledge that this requirement might rarely result in incorrectly determining lack of DMC.

Clinicians must require more evidence of DMC before they allow patients to make choices that appear to be irrational or risky. This is illustrated by the hypothetical case of Mr. Zorn, the man with Alzheimer disease described above, who must choose among several disease-slowing therapies. The low risk and proven benefits of vitamin E warrant a less stringent assessment of the patient's DMC than do the higher risk and uncertain benefits of NSAID therapy. Therefore, the standards for defining DMC will be different in these two choices. Because DMC is task-specific, the patient may well be able to choose whether to take vitamin E but not an NSAID.

Standards for Assessing Decision-Making Capacity

The preceding discussion has raised two interrelated points. First, the choice of standards for DMC has a significant effect on its determination. Second, the rigor of the DMC assessment depends upon the risks and benefits of a decision. Therefore, clinicians need to know how to use a variety of standards.[7,20,21] Depending on the source, there are four or five accepted standards for determining DMC (see Table 18-1). What follows is a summary of the literature that defines and explains how to assess each standard. Table 18-2 provides a useful mnemonic that summarizes these standards.

ABILITY TO COMMUNICATE A CHOICE

This standard requires that the patient be able to make a choice and communicate it. To assess DMC according to this standard, clinicians need not assess the quality of a patient's decision.

Table 18-1

Standards of Decision-Making Capacity

1. Ability to communicate a choice
2. Ability to make a reasonable treatment choice
3. Ability to appreciate the decision and its consequences
4. Ability to rationally manipulate the information
5. Ability to understand the decision

Instead, they should only assess whether a decision is being made. This standard is so self-evident as to seem obvious, but it can be impaired by medical conditions, such as extreme anxiety, that lead to frequent changes in a decision. Patients may also be unable to express a choice if they suffer from impairments in communication caused by focal neurologic deficits such as aphasia.

ABILITY TO MAKE A REASONABLE TREATMENT CHOICE

This standard requires that patients be able to make a decision that a reasonable person would make in the same circumstances. It considers

Table 18-2

A "STANDARD" Approach to Assessing Decision-Making Capacity

Situation	The patient understands his or her situation
Treatment	The patient understands the proposed treatment
Alternative	The patient understands the alternatives to the treatment
No treatment	The patient understands the consequence of no treatment
Decision	The patient can communicate a decision
Appreciate	The patient can appreciate the decision and its consequences
Rational	The patient can rationally manipulate information
Durable	The patient's decision is durable over time

that a patient who refuses a reasonable choice, such as a low-risk, high-benefit procedure, may lack DMC. Deficits in judgment caused by dementia or affect (such as depression or anxiety) can impair a patient's ability to achieve this standard. This standard does not explore the patient's cognitive processing or rationale for a decision. The problem with this standard, of course, is that although patients who accept low-risk, high-benefit procedures are likely to be competent, they may not be. Conversely, patients who refuse beneficial procedures may actually have DMC. Because of unique values, such as extreme risk-intolerance or religious beliefs, patients may not adhere to the standards of "reasonable people."

ABILITY TO APPRECIATE THE DECISION AND ITS CONSEQUENCES

This standard requires that patients know that they are ill and that they are able to evaluate its effects upon themselves as well as the risks and benefits of treatment options. This goes beyond the second standard (the ability to make a reasonable treatment choice) by addressing the way in which patients justify their decisions. This focus requires patients to assign values to the information at hand. Deficits in the patient's ability to appreciate his or her illness or to focus upon a particular set of values can impair the ability to fulfill this standard. This can occur in illnesses that distort the perception of reality, such as delusional disorders, extreme anxiety, and dementia with frontal lobe dysfunction.

ABILITY TO RATIONALLY MANIPULATE THE INFORMATION

This standard requires that patients be able to weigh logically the risks and benefits of each option. Like the ability to appreciate a decision and its consequences, this standard focuses on the process and not the outcome of decision making. But, unlike that standard, the ability to rationally manipulate information focuses on patients' cognitive processes and not on the values patients assign to the information. Patients who are unable to calculate or manipulate information may be unable to meet the requirements of this standard. This can occur in illnesses that cause impairments in attention, calculation, and memory—for example, dementia, delirium, extreme emotional states such as mania, and thought disorders such as schizophrenia.

ABILITY TO UNDERSTAND THE DECISION

This standard requires that patients comprehend the fundamental meaning of a decision. It is the most common standard used by the law and it is featured as the measure of an autonomous person in the theory of informed consent.[3] It is also the most complex of the standards because "comprehending the fundamental meaning" is a condition that incorporates cognitive and normative elements. The term *meaning* has a number of legitimate definitions.[22] These range from the logical structure of facts (such as a statement of mathematical equivalence: 3 plus 2 equals 5), to an interconnected relationship of symbols and values (the Star of David means Jewishness). In the context of the moral aspects of medical decision making, *understanding* refers to a patient's ability to justify his or her choice using values. The task of the clinician is not to judge that these values are "right" or "wrong" but to decide that patients have examined their reasons and that the reasons are consistent and coherent. For example, in the hypothetical case described above of Mr. Nuthatch—who refuses surgical treatment of his prostate cancer because he intends to pursue prayer—the clinician assessing this patient's competency would focus on the consistency and coherence of his explanation. This concept of understanding has also been described as "effective communication."[18] Deficits in a patient's ability to process, manipulate, and assess information can impair his or her ability to fulfill this standard.

Applying the Standards

A clinician can assess DMC according to these standards by one of two methods: a structured assessment or a clinical interview.

Structured Assessment

In a structured assessment, the clinician uses an instrument to determine a patient's DMC. Available instruments include the 24-item Specific Instrument to assess a patient's capacity to complete an advance directive,[23] the "competency questionnaire" to assess a psychiatric patient's capacity to consent to hospitalization,[24,25] and vignettes to measure a long-term-care resident's DMC.[26]

Instruments are appealing because they can standardize judgments about DMC. Because these assessments have significant ethical and medical implications, it is important that clinicians make these determinations accurately and fairly. Instruments have the advantage of being "objective," in contrast to a "subjective" clinical interview. But the claim that an instrument is objective is only as good as the criteria against which it has been validated, and most studies validate instruments using a clinician's judgment of the patient's competency.[23,26–30] This criterion has poor validity, as shown by its poor interrater reliability[31] and by disparities in how clinicians understand competency assessments.[32] Moreover, most instruments are validated to assess a particular decision made by a particular kind of patient, such as an elderly person who executes an advance directive. They cannot be used appropriately for other decisions involving other kinds of patients.

Recognizing the limits of instruments and the subjectivity of a clinical assessment, a clinician should generally use an instrument to guide but not determine the assessment of a patient's DMC. In addition, an instrument should be used only for the kind of decision its developers intended. A good generic instrument is the MacArthur-Competence Assessment Tool (Mac-CAT),[33] which is normed to define decisional impairment as a score of 2.5 standard deviations or more below the mean score of healthy, non-hospitalized adults. A subject's MacCAT scores are intended to guide, not determine the clinician's judgment as to whether patients have DMC. Nonetheless, the instrument is lengthy and should be used only by those who have completed training in its use.

Clinical Interview

Whether clinicians use an instrument or not, they must also conduct an interview. Which standards should the clinician use in these interviews? This is a particularly important question, given the time constraints under which most primary care clinicians work, yet it is difficult to answer. If each standard builds on the others, then a busy clinician could simply assess the most difficult (e.g., the ability to understand the meaning of a decision). Several authors argue that each ability follows from the next and that a clinician can assume that the patient possesses the antecedent abilities.[7,34,35] Marson supports this with data that the number of patients with mild or moderate Alzheimer disease who are competent progressively decreases as they are assessed from standards 1 through 5.[7] Hence a patient who is competent according to standard 4—the ability to manipulate information rationally—is competent according to standards 1 through 3.

In contrast, Appelbaum and Grisso have shown that the competency of hospitalized patients with schizophrenia, depression, or angina varies according to the standard used.[15] When only one standard was applied at a time, the numbers of competent patients were 23 to 28 percent (patients with schizophrenia), 5 to 12 percent (patients with depression) and 0 to 7 percent (patients with angina). When three standards were combined, the prevalence of competent patients increased: 52 percent of patients with schizophrenia, 24 percent of patients with depression, and 12 percent of patients with angina. Depressed patients were more likely to be competent according to the standard of appreciation than the standards of understanding or rationally manipulating information.

These results suggest that it may often be incorrect to assume, for all kinds of patients, that an impairment in what may be the "highest standard," understanding, implies impairment in all other standards. Data suggest that different diseases may present with different hierarchies. For instance, a patient with an affective disorder such as depression or anxiety may retain cognitive abilities, but the disorder may impair the patient's ability to care about or appreciate the decision.[36] In contrast, a dementia caused by Alzheimer disease leads to a progressive loss of global cortical function, beginning with short-term memory and language. This pattern is more likely to cause a hierarchical loss of DMC. These findings imply that clinicians should select the standard for assessing DMC to fit not only the risks and benefits of the decision but also the patient's disease.

Toward Resolution

How to Assess Decision-Making Capacity

Just as clinicians follow steps when they are performing physical examinations, so too should they follow steps in assessing DMC. When faced with patients who may lack DMC, clinicians must exercise diagnostic judgments. As in the case of other diagnostic skills, practice is important. To be proficient, a clinician should perform numerous exams of patients with varied pathology and be able to describe these findings to colleagues using a common language. This section describes recommendations and practical suggestions for clinicians to acquire these skills.

As described above, there are two general approaches to performing the assessment: a structured assessment and a clinical interview. The steps for a clinical interview are outlined in Table 18-3.

Table 18-3

Steps in Assessing Decision-Making Capacity

1. Have a clear reason for why an assessment of DMC is necessary.
2. Verify that the patient can communicate.
3. Correct any medical or situational issues (such as anxiety, metabolic abnormalities, or severe symptoms) that may impair the patient's ability to make a decision.
4. Inform the patient of the purpose of the interview.
5. Assess the patient's affect and cognition with attention to affect, attention, calculation, language, judgment and memory, since the results will suggest likely reasons for any impairments that are uncovered (see Table 18-4).
6. Structure the assessment as a dialogue with open-ended questions (see Table 18-5).
7. Ensure that the patient talks at least half of the time.
8. Analyze the patient's answers to questions according to the standards of competency, because a patient's answers will likely mix elements of several standards (see Table 18-1).
9. Inform the patient of the results of the assessment.
10. Document the results.

After proceeding through this assessment, the clinician must make a judgment. Appelbaum and Grisso argue that this is most meaningfully expressed as "Does this patient have sufficient ability to make a meaningful decision, given the circumstances with which he or she is faced?"[37] The answer to this question decides whether the patient has adequate DMC.

When to Assess Decision-Making Capacity

A variety of diagnostic and clinical variables should prompt a clinician to consider assessing DMC. The diagnostic variables are those illnesses that impair a patient's affect and cognition, such as dementia, delirium, depression, schizophrenia, manic-depression, and substance abuse. A patient who has any one of these diagnoses should be assumed to have DMC, but these diagnoses should raise an index of suspicion about DMC. Other issues that might prompt the clinician to assess DMC include the refusal of a standard therapy, rapid changes in decisions, behavior that is difficult or disruptive, or changes in the patient's in cognitive or emo-

tional function (commonly called "changes in mental status").

What to Do When a Patient Makes an Irrational Choice

One of the most significant challenges in assessing DMC occurs when a patient makes an irrational choice. It can be very difficult to distinguish an irrational choice from a choice that reflects unique values or beliefs. The latter should generally not be the grounds for judging a patient to lack DMC, but it may or may not be evidence of impaired DMC. Whether an irrational choice is a sign of decisional impairment is controversial. Brock and Wartman cite several forms of irrational decision making, such as a bias toward the present rather than the future, fear of pain, and framing effects of probabilistic information. However, they argue that irrational choices are not sufficient to determine that a patient lacks DMC and do not justify overriding that patient's choice.[38]

A good rule of thumb is that decisions should be rational given the patient's values, even if a

Table 18-4

Standardized Tests of Affect and Cognition

Affect	Evaluate answers to simple open-ended questions (like "Are you depressed?" and "Are you anxious?"). Administer the Geriatric Depression Scale if appropriate.
Memory	Test patient's 5-min recall of three words; ask patient to give the day's full date, also his or her address and phone number.
Language	Ask the patient to name parts of objects, to generate a list of words in 1 min (e.g., "Tell me all the animals you can think of"), and to follow a multistep command.
Visuospatial	Ask the patient to draw the face of a clock showing that it is 2:30. (The instructions can be repeated if necessary; this is not a test of memory.)
Judgment	Ask the patient to interpret proverbs (e.g., "What does it mean that 'People who live in glass houses shouldn't throw stones?'").
Attention and calculation	Ask the patient to spell "world" backwards, to count down from 100 by threes.

decision appears irrational to others who hold different values. For example, in the hypothetical case described above of Mr. Nuthatch, who intends to rely solely on prayer to treat his cancer, the clinician must find out more about the basis for his belief in prayer, the duration of his beliefs, and whether his faith in prayer fits with other beliefs that he holds. This line of questioning may produce a picture of a man who has lived his life according to his faith. Alternatively, the clinician may find that his beliefs are newly acquired and relatively unexamined. The latter possibility would be grounds for further discussion and careful assessment of all of the standards of DMC. The outcomes of this assessment may be that both the clinician and patient better understand each other's values and goals.

What to Do When a Patient Refuses an Assessment of Decision-Making Capacity

Another challenge is how to manage the patient who refuses an assessment of DMC. In such a case, clinicians should not begin with the presumption that the patient lacks DMC but instead

maintain equal weights for the claims that the patient has DMC or does not. The clinician then gathers data from third parties, such as family and health care workers, to learn both the degree to which this refusal is typical for the patient and to obtain any evidence related to the patient's decisional abilities. The clinician weighs this information about the patient's decisional abilities together with the context of the decision (its risks and benefits) to arrive at a best judgment of the patient's capacity. The patient is then informed of this judgment and its consequences. The patient should be encouraged to discuss this finding with the clinician; the goal is to potentially open the patient up to a more thorough assessment.

The clinician of a patient who refuses an assessment of DMC faces some ethical and legal challenges as well. Although there is not space to examine this issue in adequate detail here, cases such as these may be one of the few exceptions to the general rule that a patient's medical information should kept strictly confidential (see Chap. 12). Even in the case of a patient who refuses an assessment of DMC, though, it is important that clinicians acquire

Table 18-5

Sample Questions to Guide a Clinical Interview to Assess Decision-Making Capacity

---

1. *The ability to communicate a choice*
   "What's your decision?"
2. *The ability to make a reasonable treatment choice*
   "What do you think a reasonable person in this same circumstance would do?" or
   "How might someone else argue that your choice isn't reasonable?"
3. *The ability to appreciate the decision and its consequences*
   "Tell me in your own words what's wrong with you and what are the options to take care of it."
4. *The ability to manipulate the information rationally*
   "Suppose I was in your situation and I asked you to help me think through the choice you face.
   Help me out by describing the choices I have and how to think through them."
5. *The ability to understand the decision*
   "Can you tell me why you chose that?" "In your own words, can you say back to me what we've been over?"

information from other health care providers and families without divulging more of the patient's medical information than is absolutely necessary. Second, as we have indicated, reliable assessments of DMC are difficult even with a patient's full cooperation. This task may be impossible without important data from the patient. Because decisions on DMC have important medical and legal ramifications, patients must be informed of these ramifications, since by refusing to participate in the process of determining DMC they may be forgoing an important opportunity to have their preferences honored. In any event, a determination of DMC made without any direct assessment of the patient should probably involve a psychiatrist and even legal counsel.

What to Do When a Family Member Disagrees with a Clinician's Assessment of Decision-Making Capacity

The judgment that a patient lacks DMC rests with the patient's clinician and other medical consultants. An instance may arise when a family member disagrees with this judgment. For example, a family may claim that their intimate knowledge of the patient grants them the authority to judge whether the patient has adequate DMC. This is a serious problem that can stall the patient's care. Its resolution relies upon two steps.[39]

The technical complexity of assessing DMC means that someone who is not familiar with this process will likely not articulate the reason for the disagreement as a matter of capacity. It is the clinician's responsibility to determine how much the disagreement turns upon conflicting assessments of the patient's abilities or the details of the decision itself. Once the cause of the disagreement has been identified, the next step is to mediate a resolution. Procedures that can achieve this include a joint assessment of the patient's decision making, so that both par-

ties can simultaneously witness it. Disagreements about the decision made by the patient can be addressed by learning the family member's perceptions of the risks and benefits of the various options. A third party, such as an ethics committee or another clinician, can help mediate a dispute, but both parties should agree on what the third party will do and how they will use that party's expertise.

When a Specialist Is Needed

The judgment that a patient lacks DMC can obviously have significant ethical and medical consequences for the patient. Given the importance of this determination a clinician may choose to consult a specialist for a number of reasons, as outlined in Table 18-6.

Table 18-6

Selected Reasons for Obtaining Consultation in Determining Decision-Making Capacity

- To obtain a second opinion on the judgment that a patient lacks DMC when making this determination is especially difficult.
- To assist is the diagnosis of a cognitive or emotional impairment that is hard to diagnose or to treat.
- To address particular aspects of the assessment (e.g., a speech therapist can address deficits that impair a patient's ability to communicate; a chaplain can help a patient discuss spiritual concerns; a palliative care specialist can guide the management of seemingly intractable symptoms that may impair the patient's ability to appreciate or understand).
- To address challenging situations (e.g., family members disagreeing on a patient's DMC).

Closing Comments

The knowledge and skills a clinician needs to assess a patient's DMC are essential to the practice of good medicine. Clinicians do not need to assess every patient's DMC. Just as a clinician must have knowledge and skills to identify and follow up diagnostic clues with a focused history and physical, clinicians should know when to assess a patient's DMC and the skills to assess the patient's abilities to achieve each of the standards for DMC. Instruments are useful aids, but they cannot substitute for professional judgment concerning whether patients have adequate DMC.

The assessment of DMC is not a quiz or a legal exercise but an opportunity to foster a dialogue between clinician and patient. Unlike the dialogues of the Socratics, whose goal was to arrive at truth as a universal form, the truth at stake in assessing DMC is personal, because the issue is what the information about a decision's risks and benefits means to the patient as well as to the clinician. Decisions about incompetence may be final in the eyes of the law, but in medicine they are situated within an ongoing negotiation upon what is the standard of care and the criteria for judging what is normal cognitive and emotional function.

References

1. Grisso T, Appelbaum PS: Thinking about competence, in *Assessing Competence to Consent to Treatment: A Guide for Physicians and Other Health Professionals.* New York, Oxford University Press, 1998, pp 17–30.
2. White BC: Current confusion surrounding the concept of competence, in *Competence to Consent.* Washington, DC, Georgetown University Press, 1994, pp 44–81.
3. Faden RR, Beauchamp TL: Part III: a theory of informed consent: in *A History and Theory of Informed Consent.* New York, Oxford University Press, 1986, pp 235–381.
4. White BC: The capacities that define competence to consent, in *Competence to Consent.* Washington, DC, Georgetown University Press, 1994, pp 154–184.
5. Rockwood K, Stadnyk K: The prevalence of dementia in the elderly: a review. *Can J Psychiatry* 39:253–257, 1994.
6. *Office of Technology Assessment: Losing a Million Minds: Confronting the Tragedy of Alzheimer's Disease and Other Dementias.* Washington, DC, U.S. Government Printing Office, 1987.
7. Marson DC, Ingram KK, Cody HA, et al: Assessing the competency of patients with Alzheimer's disease under different legal standards. *Arch Neurol* 52:949–954, 1995.
8. Geldmacher D, Whitehouse P: Evaluation of dementia. *N Engl J Med* 335:330–336, 1996.
9. Hafner H, Heiden Wad: Epidemiology of schizophrenia. *Can J Psychiatry* 42:139–151, 1997.
10. Flint AJ: Epidemiology and comorbidity of anxiety disorders in the elderly. *Am J Psychiatry* 151:640–649, 1994.
11. Kessler R, Walter E: Epidemiology of DSM-III-R major depression and minor depression among adolescents and young adults in the National Comorbidity Survey. *Depression Anxiety* 7:3–14, 1998.
12. Berry K, Fleming M, Manwell L, et al: Prevalence of and factors associated with current and life depression in older adult primary care patients. *Fam Med* 30:366–371, 1998.
13. Kathol R, Mutgi A, Williams J, et al: Diagnosis of depression in cancer patients according to four sets of criteria. *Am J Psychiatry* 147:1021–1024, 1990.
14. Derogatis L, Morrow G, Fetting J, et al: The prevalence of psychiatric disorders among cancer patients. *JAMA* 249: 1983.
15. Grisso T, Appelbaum PS: Comparison of standards for assessing patients' capacities to make treatment decisions. *Am J Psychiatry* 152:1033–1037, 1995.
16. White BC: Ethical foundations of competence to consent, in *Competence to Consent.* Washington,

DC, Georgetown University Press, 1994, pp 13–43.

17. Faden RR, Beauchamp TL: Foundations in moral theory, in *A History and Theory of Informed Consent*. New York, Oxford University Press, 1986, pp 3–22.

18. Faden RR, Beauchamp TL: The nature and degrees of competence, in *A History and Theory of Informed Consent*. New York, Oxford University Press, 1986, pp 288–293.

19. Beauchamp TL, Childress JF: The sliding-scale strategy, in *Principles of Biomedical Ethics*, 4th ed. New York, Oxford University Press, 1994, pp 138–141.

20. Meisel A, Roth L: What we do and do not know about informed consent. *JAMA* 246:2473–2477, 1981.

21. Grisso T, Appelbaum PS: Abilities related to competence, in *Assessing Competence to Consent to Treatment: A Guide for Physicians and Other Health Professionals*. New York, Oxford University Press, 1998, pp 31–60.

22. Peirce C: Logic as semiotic: the theory of signs, in Buchler J (ed): *Philosophical Writings of Peirce*. New York, Dover, 1955, pp 98–119.

23. Molloy DW, Silberfeld M, Darzins P, et al: Measuring capacity to complete an advance directive. *J Am Geriatr Soc* 44:660–664, 1996.

24. Appelbaum P, Mirkin S, Bateman A: Empirical assessment of competency to consent to psychiatric hospitalization. *Am J Psychiatry* 138:1170–1176, 1981.

25. Billick SB, Bella PD, Woodward Burgert III: Competency to consent to hospitalization in the medical patient. *J Am Acad Psychiatry Law* 25:191–196, 1997.

26. Pruchno RA, Smyer MA, Rose MS, et al: Competence of long-term care residents to participate in decisions about their medical care: a brief, objective assessment. *Gerontologist* 35:622–629, 1995.

27. Holzer JC, Gansler DA, Moczynski NP, et al: Cognitive functions in the informed consent evaluation process: a pilot study. *J Am Acad Psychiatry Law* 25:531–540, 1997.

28. Bean G, Nishisato S, Rector NA, et al: The psychometric properties of the competency interview schedule. *Can J Psychiatry* 39:368–376, 1994.

29. Kaufman DM, Zun L: A quantifiable, brief mental status examination for emergency patients. *J Emerg Med* 13:449–456, 1995.

30. Tomoda A, Yasumiya R, Sumiyama T, et al: Validity and reliability of structured interview for competency-incompetency assessment testing and ranking inventory. *J Clin Psychol* 53:443–450, 1997.

31. Marson DC, McInturff B, Hawkins L, et al: Consistency of physician judgments of capacity to consent in mild Alzheimer's disease. *J Am Geriatr Soc* 45:453–457, 1997.

32. Markson L, Kern D, Annas G, et al: Physician assessment of patient competence. *J Am Geriatr Soc* 42:1074–1080, 1994.

33. Grisso T, Appelbaum PS: Using the MacArthur Competence Assessment Tool—treatment, in *Assessing Competence to Consent to Treatment: A Guide for Physicians and Other Health Professionals*. New York, Oxford University Press, 1998, pp 101–126.

34. Drane J: Competency to give an informed consent: a model for making clinical assessments. *JAMA* 252:925–927, 1984.

35. Tancredi L: Competency for informed consent: conceptual limits of empirical data. *Int J Law Psychiatry* 5:51–63, 1982.

36. Elliott C: Caring about risks: are severely depressed patients competent to consent to research? *Arch Gen Psychiatry* 54:113–116, 1997.

37. Grisso T, Appelbaum PS: Making judgments about patients' competence, in *Assessing Competence to Consent to Treatment: A Guide for Physicians and Other Health Professionals*. New York, Oxford University Press, 1998, pp 127–148.

38. Brock D, Wartman SA: When competent patients make irrational choices. *N Engl J Med* 322:1595–1599, 1990.

39. Schneiderman LJ, Teetzel H, Kalmanson AG: Who decides who decides? When disagreement occurs between the physician and the patient's appointed proxy about the patient's decision-making capacity. *Arch Intern Med* 155:793–796, 1995.

Clarence H. Braddock III

Chapter

19

Informed Consent

Mr. Jackson, 53 years old, has hypertension and diabetes mellitus. He is of average intelligence and well involved in his own care. Nevertheless, he tends to defer to his primary care physician in almost all decisions, typically saying, "Whatever you think, doc." The physician is contemplating ordering a prostate-specific antigen (PSA) test to screen for prostate cancer. How much should the physician discuss this with Mr. Jackson?

Mrs. Thomas, 80 years old, has stable angina pectoris and mild multi-infarct dementia. She lives semi-independently but her son manages her financial affairs. She comes alone to regular office visits, and is able to communicate her concerns and voice understanding of routine issues. Today, her primary care clinician wants to discuss how to proceed in evaluating a newly discovered pulmonary nodule. The decision is whether to obtain a tissue biopsy now or follow the nodule with serial chest x-rays. How can the clinician be sure that Mrs. Thomas understands the implications of the decision and is able to give an informed opinion?

Scope of the Problem

For many clinicians, the mention of informed consent conjures images of having a patient sign an authorization form for surgery or an invasive procedure. Yet the overall purpose of informed consent is to foster the informed participation of patients in clinical decision making. There remains a gap between this idealized goal and the reality of practice, with clinicians having little guidance as to when and how to achieve meaningful patient involvement. This chapter summarizes some common ethical issues related to informed consent in primary care practice, reviews the ethical and legal foundations for the practice of informed consent, and provides some guidance for clinicians to help foster informed patient participation in clinical decision making.

Informed Consent in Primary Care

The task of obtaining informed consent in primary care practice is especially difficult. With ever-increasing pressures for time-efficiency,

clinicians have little time to devote to a thorough discussion of every clinical decision, particularly those that they believe are fairly routine. Furthermore, the types of decisions encountered in primary care practice are quite different from those of the inpatient, procedure-oriented world. However, even though many outpatient decisions may seem routine and unrelated to specific procedures, they may be as complex or more so than inpatient ones. For instance, decisions such as whether or not to order PSA testing as a screen for prostate cancer may be controversial or based on conflicting expert recommendations (see Chap. 5).

The primary care setting itself is quite varied, challenging the practice of informed consent. Some primary care clinicians may be caring for adolescents who, while considered minors without a legally recognized role in decision making, have strong and well-founded opinions about their health care (see Chap. 14). Primary care clinicians may encounter patients from a variety of cultural backgrounds, often creating conflict over assumptions implicit in Western medicine about mechanisms of disease or the relationship between self and others (see Chap. 11). Furthermore, in primary care, patients often come with explicit expectations for treatment, such as expecting antibiotic treatment for a common cold, that are at odds with what the primary care clinician understands are interventions know to be effective (see Chap. 1). These aspects of primary care increase the need for a clear understanding of the ethical foundations of informed consent and guidance in its effective application.

Empirical Data on Informed Consent

The growing empirical literature on informed consent gives insight into its epidemiology, such as the frequency and kinds of clinical decisions in primary care for which informed consent is relevant. Furthermore, it can shed light on prevailing attitudes toward informed consent, problems in its practice, and the influence of informed consent on important outcomes.

The occasion for informed consent happens commonly in primary care. In one study of routine office visits, there were an average of 3.2 clinical decisions per visit, typically involving medications or diagnostic laboratory tests.[1]

Numerous studies have shown that patients want to know their medical condition and be involved in treatment decisions.[2–4] In one study of patients' preferences for a role in decision making, 80 percent stated that they preferred to either share the decision or make it themselves.[5]

However, there is evidence that clinicians do not routinely involve patients in clinical decisions. Louis Harris and Associates evaluated physicians' self-reports of informed consent practices and found that although 96 percent of physicians reported routinely obtaining informed consent for surgical procedures, less than half did so for routine blood tests, diagnostic radiographs, or minor office procedures.[2] Sulmasy and colleagues found that physicians' disclosure of information to patients undergoing routine medical procedures ranged from 90 percent for explaining the procedure to 53 percent for explaining the alternatives.[6] Braddock and colleagues evaluated audiotapes of routine primary care office visits for the extent of informed

consent associated with outpatient clinical decisions, finding that discussion of alternatives occurred for 14 percent of decisions, risks and benefits, 9 percent; and assessment of understanding, 2 percent.[1] Several other studies have identified important deficiencies in the adequacy of informed consent in clinical practice.[7–10]

This is unfortunate, since several studies have identified an association between more effective informed consent and beneficial clinical outcomes, including compliance with medical regimens and satisfaction.[11–14]

Some Useful Distinctions

SHARED DECISION MAKING AND INFORMED CONSENT

The phrases "shared decision making" and "informed consent" have been used extensively and somewhat interchangeably in the medical ethics literature for over 20 years, yet there are some important differences between these terms. The concept of *shared decision making* forms a framework for guiding clinicians to involve their patients in routine but important decisions in primary care practice. It rests on the ideal of informed patient participation in important clinical decisions. Yet this concept differs in subtle but important ways from informed consent. Some authors, for instance, argue that shared decision making is an incorrect model in some contexts, such as emergency medical care and research. We will explore this distinction more extensively under the "Background Theory and Context," section below.

ASSENT AND CONSENT

The distinction between assent and consent signals the recognition of the difference between passive authorization of a health care intervention and informed participation in a health care decision. *Assent* implies passive acceptance of a clinical action or participation. For example, the clinician says, "Take this

medicine twice a day for your blood pressure."
The patient may agree (and may or may not
comply) but has not had an opportunity to be
an informed participant in decision making.
Thus, it is important to realize that while assent
from patients is clearly needed, in many cases
merely having assent is not sufficient.

Adult patients should usually be afforded the
opportunity to give informed consent for clinical
interventions. In some limited circumstances,
such as emergencies, it may suffice to have the
patient give assent to an intervention without
the benefit of substantive information disclosure.
In addition, there is a continuum of situations
involving minors and their participation in clinical decisions. For the most part, children are not
recognized as having the capacity to give
informed consent. Yet in certain jurisdictions,
"mature minors" may give informed consent for
some medical interventions (see Chap. 14). In
other situations, while an adolescent patient's
parents may sign informed consent for an intervention, it is important to obtain the "informed
assent" of the adolescent so as to foster cooperation with the proposed treatment.

Background Theory and Context

In this section, we review and analyze the primary ethical and legal foundations for informed
consent. Specifically, we analyze shared decision making as an ethical model for informed
consent and examine differing models of informed consent.

Ethical Foundations

SHARED-DECISION-MAKING MODEL

Shared decision making represents an ideal
of mutual participation in decision making by
clinician and patient, with the clinician having
an obligation to foster patients' participation
through information exchange and dialogue.
This phrase was introduced in the early 1980s
by a presidential advisory panel, which wrote:
"Ethically valid consent is a process of shared
decision-making based upon mutual respect and
participation, not a ritual to be equated with
reciting the contents of a form that details the
risks of a particular treatment."[15] Key to the concept of shared decision making is the role the
patient plays in it. A corollary to this is a clear
understanding of the clinician's role. First, it is
the clinician's role to make health care recommendations based on the desire to promote
well-being. Second is the duty to help patients
obtain both information and an opportunity to
participate actively in decision making.

The full meaning of this second role reveals
the distinction between more unilateral disclosure of risks and benefits and promotion
of an active role for the patient in decision
making. The former obligation could be met
by mere recitation of information, while the
latter must include efforts to foster patient
understanding.

For some authors, shared decision making is
informed consent.[15,16] That is, the purpose of
informed consent is to foster informed patient
participation, with the intent of shared decision
making between clinician and patient.

Shared decision making rests on the ethical
principles of respect for persons, respect for
autonomy, and promotion of patient well-being.
The principle of *respect for persons* derives from
the view that people are valuable in their own
right; thus clinicians have an obligation to show
respect for the intrinsic value of each individual.
One way in which the clinician can show
respect for persons is by fostering the meaningful participation of patients in decision making.

The concept of *autonomy* is central to Western ethical traditions and to U.S. politicocultural
norms. One meaning of autonomy is "self-
governing," so that in medical ethics this term
refers to respect for the patient's right to guide

what happens to his or her own body. An expression of respect for autonomy in the clinical context involves acknowledging and supporting the patients' right to have a role in clinical decisions that affect them.

The principle of *promotion of patient well-being*, often called beneficence, is also a central tenet of clinical medicine. Clinicians are guided by a strong professional obligation to use their knowledge and skill to evaluate patients' concerns and make recommendations for health care interventions that can be of benefit. The nature of clinical benefit may sometimes be fairly clear. For example, there is a clearly recognized and substantial reduction in cardiovascular risk associated with adequate blood pressure control. In some situations, the definition of benefit may vary substantially between clinician and patient. Again, using the example of blood pressure control, medication side effects may affect quality of life so much that a patient no longer perceives any net benefit. The purpose of shared decision making is to allow patients to have a role in determining the meaning of "benefit" in health care decisions affecting them.

AUTONOMOUS AUTHORIZATION

Some authors distinguish between shared decision making and informed consent. Their contention is that shared decision making is a worthy ideal for informed consent in some contexts but is not applicable in other situations—notably emergency medicine and biomedical research involving human subjects. Furthermore, they argue that shared decision making may be desirable but not necessary. What is ethically necessary is autonomous authorization to a proposed medical intervention. Thus, the clinician may not necessarily share the decision as to which intervention is proposed but must give the patient information about it and provide an opportunity to give autonomous authorization. Finally, shared decision making does not place sufficient emphasis on the authorization aspect of informed consent. That is, a patient may be thoroughly involved in decision making—and hence satisfy the shared-decision-making model—yet not give true authorization. Hence the ethical foundation rests in defining what constitutes "autonomous action" rather than in defining a process of sharing decision making.[17,18]

Autonomous action is typically defined in terms of a set of necessary conditions. That is, for an action to be called autonomous, it must involve certain features. Among those features most often proposed as constituting autonomous actions are intention, degree of understanding, and freedom from undue influence. *Intention* refers to having a conscious plan to engage in the action, rather than an accidental or inadvertent action. Understanding contributes significantly to autonomous action. As the depth and breadth of understanding of the nature and implications of action increases, so does the degree to which it is autonomous. Finally, an action cannot be considered autonomous if it is the result of coercion or manipulation. Thus the degree to which the action is not the result of undue influence also greatly influences the extent to which it is autonomous.

In the clinical context, when obtaining informed consent, the concept of "autonomous action" is translated into *autonomous authorization*.

THE SIGNED CONSENT FORM

Autonomous authorization stands in contrast to the mere signing of a consent form. Certainly the act of signing a consent form can serve as a valuable prompt for the dialogue suggested by the shared-decision-making model or for the kind of interaction depicted in the autonomous authorization model. However, it is a mistake to view the consent form alone as informed consent.

Furthermore, many decisions in primary care do not require signed consent forms, nor should they. Undue emphasis on signed authorization as the working definition of informed consent deflects focus away from meaningful informed consent for important clinical decisions.

In many states and localities, statutes list health care interventions for which signed authorization is required. Furthermore, institutional administrative policies may also contain such lists. It is important for clinicians to be aware of and follow such guidelines in order to support these risk-management and other institutional efforts. In these cases and those not requiring signed authorization, however, dialogue that fosters informed patient participation remain crucial.

SUMMARY

The models of informed consent discussed above are not necessarily in conflict. On one view, the shared-decision-making model serves as an ideal for the process of communication and interaction that should characterize the clinician-patient relationship. The autonomous authorization model then serves as the working model for meaningful informed consent across a wide range of clinical decisions, including those in which shared decision making is not realistic or applicable. The consent form mainly serves a legal purpose and is never a sufficient substitute for meaningful informed consent. It should always be accompanied by autonomous authorization and by shared decision making wherever possible.

Legal Foundations

CASE LAW

EARLY CASES The origins of informed consent in the law trace back to common law traditions in the nineteenth and early twentieth centuries. Early legal cases dealt with patients who had undergone a treatment or intervention without their permission. For example, in *Mohr* v *Williams* (1905), a physician obtained consent for surgery on the patient's right ear, only to find in the operating room that it was the left ear that needed the procedure. After learning that the incorrect ear had been operated on, the patient sued the physician for performing the procedure without her permission.[19] In such cases, judges relied on the legal doctrine of battery, based on the notion that unwarranted bodily invasion in the clinical context constitutes a form of unwanted touching.

In the case of *Schloendorff* v *Society of New York Hospitals* (1914), Justice Benjamin Cardozo articulated an important expansion of this battery model of consent, arguing that patients have a right to control decision about what is done to their bodies.

> "Every human being of adult years and sound mind has a right to determine what shall be done with his own body; a surgeon who performs an operation without his patient's consent commits an assault, for which he is liable for damages."[20]

This case established an important link between the legal doctrine of consent, expressed as the right to self-determination, and the ethical principle of respect for autonomy.

The term *informed consent* can be traced to a case in the 1950s, *Salgo* v *Leland Stanford University* (1957). In this case, a man suffered spinal cord ischemia following an angiogram, a complication he had not been warned of. The court argued that the patient's right to autonomy and control of decisions involving his body implied a duty upon physicians to disclose relevant information to patients to inform their thinking.[21]

REFINING THE DOCTRINE Case law since the 1960s refined the doctrine of informed consent primarily by addressing the amount of information that the physician is obligated to give to patients during the informed consent process. This evolved from the "professional practice" standard expressed in *Natanson* v *Kline* (1960) to the "reasonable person" standard outlined in *Canterbury* v *Spence* (1972).[22,23]

The *professional practice standard* requires that physicians share as much information as is customary for other physicians in practice to do in similar situations. For instance, in discussing a new medication, a clinician would be required to discuss only those side effects that other clinicians typically would discuss. The obvious shortcoming of this standard is that there is the potential for inadequate information sharing to become and remain the standard of care.

The *reasonable person standard* stipulates that the amount of information sharing needed is determined by asking what a hypothetical "reasonable person" would require. The advantage of this over the professional practice standard is that it creates an atmosphere of information sharing that is far more balanced in favor of the patient. As a practical matter however, it places physicians in an awkward position in determining the level of information exchange necessary. It is difficult to know what a hypothetical person might need to know, and no guidelines exist to guide the application of this standard. Furthermore, it does not recognize the diverse values, beliefs, and information priorities of individuals. In other words, the reasonable person standard does not respect the individual patient as a person.

One might argue that the most important gauge of how much information is needed to be an informed decision maker is the needs and values of the particular patient. This view is known as the *subjective standard.* That is, each person has his or her own set of unique information needs. Some patients, for instance, fearful of side effects, will need to have a more thorough discussion of these prior to feeling adequately informed. Another patient, concerned about long-term efficacy, may feel that this information about side effects is less important. Of note, the subjective standard is consistent with a strict interpretation of the shared-decision-making model of informed consent, suggesting that information sharing be guided by the individual's informational needs, not by the informational needs of a hypothetical "reasonable person."

Howard Brody proposed an alternative to the legal standards for information disclosure, which he called the *transparency standard.* This standard holds that disclosure is adequate if the clinician's thinking is made "transparent" to the patient, such that the patient understands by following along with the logic of the clinician's decision making. Operationally, clinicians talk through their decision making process with patients, revealing the relevant decision alternatives as well as their advantages, disadvantages, and uncertainties; then clinicians offer professional recommendations. For Brody, this standard has the advantage over legal disclosure standards in that it is an easier fit into the flow of communication among clinicians and patients as well as being more appropriate for the typical kinds of decisions that need to be made in primary care. By making the logic and considerations entering into the decision "transparent" to the patient, the clinician has met the ethical obligations of consent.[24]

STATUTORY LAW AND ADMINISTRATIVE POLICIES

In addition to case law, many states have statutes that describe procedures for ensuring adequate informed consent. Additionally, virtually all health care institutions have policies that define requirements for signed consent for certain interventions, such as surgery or invasive procedures, HIV testing, and other treatments with high risk-management implications. Health care accreditation bodies such as the Joint Commission for the Accreditation of Health Care Organizations evaluate the extent to which there is documented evidence of informed consent for certain interventions in the medical record. Finally, many professional societies provide guidelines on obtaining adequate informed consent.[24,25]

CONTRASTING LEGAL AND ETHICAL FOUNDATIONS

One major limitation to the legal foundation of informed consent is its focus on disclosure.

Case law created an obligation for physicians to share information but not to assure that patients understand that information or their role in decision making. Some authors see this as a critical flaw.[16]

Another major limitation of the case law origins of informed consent is its emphasis on surgery and invasive procedures. Most likely this arose because these kinds of cases are most common in medical litigation. Nevertheless, such a perspective might create the inaccurate impression that informed consent is a mere legal exercise to be done only prior to surgery or invasive procedures. In one case, *Malloy* v *Shanahan* (1980), the court was asked to consider whether a physician should have obtained informed consent from a woman before treating her for a prolonged period of time with a potentially toxic drug. The court asserted that the informed consent doctrine need not apply to routine health care decisions.[26] This is in clear conflict with the ethical foundations of informed consent discussed earlier. It also fails to recognize the realities of clinical practice, particularly in primary care. Here, most decisions are not related to procedures, yet many have complexities and risks that rival or exceed those of surgical procedures.

Although the legal foundation of informed consent has been enormously influential in developing a justification for the patient's participation in decision making, it is important to recognize the law's limitations. The ethical foundation provides a more robust version of informed consent, applying to a broader range of clinical decisions than does case law. The ethical foundation also places emphasis on the process of informed consent, not to the exclusion of the authorizing event but in a manner more consonant with the principles of respect for persons and promotion of well-being.

Toward Resolution

Translating Theory into Practice

Despite the wide acceptance of the need for informed consent in certain situations, such as those involving risky invasive procedures, clinicians have little guidance as to which clinical decisions need informed consent. Some authors have suggested that the ethical basis of informed consent requires patients' involvement in a much wider range of clinical decisions, including those involving medication prescriptions and laboratory tests.[15,16,27] Furthermore, many advocate greater involvement of patients in decision making than mere signing of consent forms. Lidz and colleagues called this focus on signing consent forms the "event model" of informed consent.[28] They suggest that this should be replaced by a "process model" focusing instead on promotion of the patient's active participation in decision making. As stated earlier, the most important ethical goal of informed consent is that the patient have an opportunity to be an informed participant in health care decisions. The discussion that follows outlines an approach to informed consent in primary care that has this ethical foundation but resonates with clinical reality.

The Spectrum of Informed Consent in Primary Care

Informed consent is relevant not only to invasive medical procedures but also to other decisions, such as prescription of potentially toxic medications or initiation of a diagnostic evaluation that might eventuate in expensive or invasive procedures. Clearly the extent of dialogue necessary to foster informed participation will vary. Among the factors influencing the needed dialogue are the duration of the clinician-patient relationship; the patient's experience with similar, prior decisions; and the patient's cognitive ability. Importantly, the nature and complexity of the decision will strongly affect the extent of discussion.

For some decisions of low complexity, only an abbreviated discussion is needed. *Basic consent* entails letting the patient know what the clinician would like to do and asking if that is acceptable. Basic consent is appropriate, for example, in drawing blood for simple tests. The level of discussion desirable for making such decisions can be derived from the shared decision making model of informed consent. Some discussion about the decision is always necessary, such as, "I'd like to order a blood count to make sure you're not anemic." For many basic decisions, there will be minimal if any "risk," and the alternatives are rather limited, such as not ordering a blood count. Thus it is not crucial to routinely discuss these elements. The conversation should, however, leave open the door for patients' questions or concerns, so that when the discussion is complete, patients have had their informational needs met. For basic decisions, this can be accomplished by clinicians merely asking, for instance, "Does that sound all right?"

Other decisions may be very *complex.* The typical example is a major surgical procedure, which involves substantial risk as well as clear alternatives. Here the need for discussion is greater. For such complex decisions, explicit discussion of alternatives, risks, and benefits and a full exploration of the patient's level of understanding and his or her opinion is essential.

Many decisions, such as prescribing a new medication, may need a level of discussion *intermediate* to these two extremes. The recommended extent of discussion of clinical decisions in primary care is shown in Table 19-1.

Characteristics of Meaningful Informed Consent

The ethical foundations of informed consent can be expressed in terms of domains that, if met, maximize the opportunity for a patient to participate meaningfully in his or her health care decisions. The domains critical to maximize patient participation are decision-making capacity, absence of coercion, adequate information, adequate understanding, and opportunity to express an opinion.

DECISION-MAKING CAPACITY

For patients to have an opportunity to play a role in treatment decisions, they must possess a minimum level of decision-making capacity, or competency (see Chap. 18). That capacity should include the ability to receive information, process and understand information, deliberate, and make and articulate their choices. In general, patients are presumed to have these capacities unless shown otherwise. Nevertheless, sometimes illness, medications, or mental dysfunction can limit the patient's ability to reason about and make decisions. Hence, in the informed consent process, the clinician should be vigilant to look for signs of impaired decision-making capacity.

When decision making is impaired, the clinician must resort to other mechanisms to have the patient's views represented. This is most often done through advance care planning or surrogate decision making, both of which are discussed further in Chap. 20.

Table 19-1

Elements of Informed Consent Needed According to Level of Decision Complexity*

Elements of Informed Consent	Basic	Intermediate	Complex
1. Discussion of the patient's role in decision making. Rationale: Many patients are not aware that they can and should participate in decision making. Examples: "I'd like us to make this decision together." "It helps me to know how you feel about this."	R†	R†	R
2. Discussion of the clinical issue and nature of the decision to be made. Rationale: A clear statement of what is at issue helps clarify what is being decided upon and allows the clinician to share some of his or her thinking about it. Examples: "This is what we need to decide." "The issue for us today is . . ."	R	R	R
3. Discussion of the alternatives. Rationale: A decision always involves among certain options, including doing nothing at all. This is not always clear to the patient without an explicit discussion. Example: "You could try the new medication or continue the one you are on now."		R	R
4. Discussion of the pros and cons (potential benefits and risks) of the alternatives. Rationale: Clinicians frequently discuss the pros of one option and the cons of another without fully exploring the pros and cons of each. This more balanced presentation allows the patient's decision to be more informed. Examples: "The new medication is more expensive, but you only need to take it once a day." "Screening for colon cancer using the stool cards is easier for you, but the flexible sigmoidoscopy is more precise."		R	R

	Basic	Intermediate	Complex
5. Discussion of uncertainties.			R
6. Assessment of the patient's understanding.		R	R
7. Exploration of the patient's preference.	R†	R†	R

5. Discussion of uncertainties.

Rationale: While often difficult, a discussion of uncertainties is crucial for patients' comprehensive understanding of the options. Thoughtful discussion can promote trust and encourage compliance.

Examples: "The chance that this will help is excellent."
"Most patients with this condition respond well to this medication, but not all."

6. Assessment of the patient's understanding.

Rationale: Once the core disclosures are made, the clinician must check with the patient to make sure what he or she has said so far makes sense. Fostering understanding is the central goal of informed decision making.

Examples: "Does that make sense to you?"
"Are you with me so far?"

7. Exploration of the patient's preference.

Rationale: Clinicians may assume that patients will speak up if they disagree with a decision, but patients often need to be asked for their opinion. It should be clear to the patient that it is appropriate to disagree or ask for more time.

Examples: "Does that sound reasonable?"
"What do you think?"

---

*This table demonstrates how the amount of information sharing in informed consent should vary with the complexity of the clinical decision. By convention, *basic* decisions are those with minimal risk, complexity, and controversy. Examples would include routine laboratory tests. *Complex* decisions are those involving invasive procedures or other interventions that are of high risk, high complexity, or controversial. *Intermediate* decisions lie between these extremes and might include such interventions as medication prescriptions, for which more than minimal disclosure is needed but less than formal, written informed consent. The letter **R** indicates which elements of informed consent ought to be required for these different levels of decisions. Also shown is sample dialogue illustrating how these elements might be met in the clinical encounter.

R: Required.

R†: Either element 1 or element 7.

ABSENCE OF MANIPULATION OR COERCION

Patients may feel pressure to "go along" with clinicians' recommendations. Having clinicians make recommendations and in some cases persuading patients to follow them are a core part of clinical care. However, the vulnerability of illness or the disparity in power that is ever-present in the clinician-patient relationship can, on occasion, create a coercive atmosphere. For example, clinicians may be tempted to present positively one treatment alternative while presenting negatively another. If the clinician says, "Medication A is very effective and safe while medication B is a lot of trouble," almost any patient will opt for medication A. Presenting information in this fashion should be avoided, since it undermines the patient's ability to weigh health care alternatives (see Chap. 11). Clinicians must be aware of this potential and make an effort to present information and alternatives in a balanced fashion so as not to mislead or manipulate. It is then appropriate for the clinician to offer an opinion that reflects his or her own judgment. Finally, frank coercion, as when the clinician expresses anger with treatment refusal or threatens to disengage from the relationship unless the patient agrees to the recommended treatment, is never appropriate.

ADEQUATE INFORMATION

It is essential that the patient have adequate information on which to act as an informed participant in treatment decisions. The key question that emerges is what quantity and type of information is enough?

There are several standards for the appropriate amount of information sharing in informed consent. As discussed above, these approaches include what a typical clinician would say about this intervention; what the average patient needs to know in order to be an informed participant in the decision; what would this patient need to know and understand in order to make an informed decision; and the extent to which the clinician makes the clinical reasoning behind his or her recommendation transparent. Most states have legislation or legal cases that determine the required disclosure standard for informed consent. The best approach to the question of how much information is enough is one that meets the professional obligation to provide the best care and also respects the patient as a person with the right to a voice in health care decisions.

The next question is what kind of information should be shared? Although patients may have some unique informational needs, there are several generally accepted relevant categories of information: the nature of the decision, the relevant decision alternatives, the pros and cons (or risks and benefits), the alternatives, and any uncertainties inherent in the proposed intervention and its alternatives.

ADEQUATE UNDERSTANDING

Understanding is the key element for informed participation in decision making. The patient cannot be an informed participant unless he or she understands the nature of the decision and other relevant information. Furthermore, it is clear from the shared-decision-making model of informed consent that fostering understanding is an integral part of the collaborative decision making process. Despite its conceptual centrality to the informed consent process, the assessment of understanding is not a common part of clinical practice. In one recent study of the adequacy of informed decision making in routine office practice, "assessment of understanding" was infrequently observed.[1]

The emphasis on understanding fundamentally changes the nature of decision making. If the sole goal of informed consent is merely adequate disclosure, then a one-way conversation in which the clinician recites risks, benefits, and alternatives might suffice. On the other hand, if understanding is the focus, the norm becomes a conversation in which the clinician evaluates the patient's understanding, asks questions, and allows for clarifying remarks.

It is also important to distinguish two kinds of understanding. The first is the need for the patient to understand the information relevant to the decision. This can often by examined by clinicians asking simple questions, such as, "Does that make sense to you?" If such questions do not elicit clear evidence that the patient understands what is being discussed, more in-depth questioning is needed, such as, "Tell me in your own words what you understood me to say."

The second level of understanding is the need for patients to understand their role in decision making. Without some effort to explicitly discuss their role, many patients will assume that they are to play a passive role in decision making. In primary care, the clinician can discuss his or her view of the patient's role in decision making early in the relationship and thus set a pattern for subsequent decision making.

OPPORTUNITY TO EXPRESS A PREFERENCE

Many patients may be reluctant to ask questions or voice uncertainty about a planned intervention. In some cases, this doubt may translate instead into nonadherence with a medical regimen (see Chap. 4) or dissatisfaction with the patient-clinician relationship. It is therefore critical for patients to have an explicit opportunity to express their preferences regarding clinical decisions.

Some patients may decline or even refuse to participate in informed consent. When this occurs, it should prompt some explicit discussion of the rationale for patient's involvement. This will enable the clinician to distinguish the patient's informed refusal to give informed consent from other factors, such as embarrassment or disinterest, that may masquerade as refusal to participate in the informed consent process. In the rare event that a patient clearly waives the right to participate in informed consent, the clinician may proceed with the proposed interven-

tion. When one is in doubt in these unusual situations, consultation with an ethics committee or an attorney can be beneficial.

Guidelines for Practice: Common Clinical Challenges in Informed Consent

In this final section, the prior discussion is summarized by addressing some common practical questions about informed consent. The answers to these questions represent suggested approaches to obtaining informed consent in primary care practice.

HOW MUCH INFORMATION SHOULD BE PROVIDED TO ENABLE "INFORMED" CONSENT?

The best approach depends in part on regional legal and administrative requirements and in part on the clinician's preferred ethical model of informed consent. In Mr. Jackson's hypothetical case, described at the opening of this chapter, obtaining a PSA to screen for prostate cancer is being considered. At a minimum, the clinician should review the main advantages and disadvantages of PSA screening, the potential implications of an elevated value, and other approaches to screening, including not screening at all. A clinician might also compare and contrast alternative views of PSA testing from different professional organizations. Mr. Jackson may still choose to follow the clinician's recommendation for testing, but by engaging him in the decision-making process, the clinician will be affording Mr. Jackson the opportunity to give input based on his own values and beliefs.

HOW CAN INFORMED CONSENT BE OBTAINED FROM PATIENTS WITH IMPAIRED CAPACITY TO PARTICIPATE IN DECISION MAKING?

Informed consent requires that patients possess the cognitive capacity to participate in decision making. Part of the process of informed consent, then, is to assess whether there are conditions that might impair decision-making capacity. In the second case vignette described above, involving Mrs. Thomas, the patient has mild multi-infarct dementia, raising the question of whether she will understand the implications of the decision regarding her lung nodule and be able to make an informed choice.

In most cases, it is clear whether or not patients are competent to make their own decisions. Medical conditions that impair cognitive capacity or impose significant stress associated with illness should not necessarily preclude patients from participating in their own care (see Chap. 18). However, precautions should be taken to ensure that patients have the capacity to make good decisions. This includes the ability to understand their situation, understand the risks associated with the choices at hand, and communicate a decision based on that understanding. When this is unclear, a psychiatric consultation can be helpful.

On occasion, a patient's refusal of treatment raises the question of decision-making capacity. It is important to recognize that a treatment refusal does not necessarily imply a lack of decision-making capacity. Competent patients have the right to refuse treatment, even those treatments that may be lifesaving. Treatment refusal may, however, be a signal to pursue further the patient's beliefs and understanding about the decision (see Chap. 15).

Conversely, treatment acceptance may obfuscate impaired decision-making capacity. The patient who is content to do "whatever you say" may have some cognitive impairment that interferes with the possibility of obtaining meaningful informed consent. This highlights the importance of some exploration of patients' understanding as part of any informed consent dialogue.

With Mrs. Thomas, a reasonable approach would be to discuss the possible implications of a lung nodule and the pros and cons of potential interventions to evaluate it more fully. Using care to avoid technical jargon, the clinician should then carefully explore Mrs. Thomas's understanding. It might be helpful for the clinician to explain the rationale for the recommended course of action. If Mrs. Thomas seems confused or unable to offer any informed preference, it would be useful to seek discussion with a surrogate, as discussed further in Chap. 20.

HOW CAN PATIENTS BE MEANINGFULLY INVOLVED IN IMPORTANT DECISIONS WHEN TIME IN THE TYPICAL PRIMARY CARE ENCOUNTER IS LIMITED?

This is a particularly difficult challenge in contemporary primary care practice as the pace increases and the time spent with each patient comes under more pressure. Between the extremes of no informed consent for any decisions and full informed consent for all decisions, clinicians might adopt a graduated approach. As shown in Table 19-1, discussion can be abbreviated for most simple, basic interventions, saving more lengthy dialogue for complex or risky interventions. Another strategy that can be effective is to discuss particularly significant decisions over several visits, to allow adequate time for discussion to meet the criteria for meaningful informed consent.

WHAT SORTS OF INTERVENTIONS REQUIRE WRITTEN INFORMED CONSENT?

Most health care institutions have policies that state which health interventions require written informed consent. For example, surgery, anesthesia, and other invasive procedures are usually in this category. Signed consent forms should be viewed as the culmination of a dialogue designed to foster the patient's informed participation in the clinical decision.

For a wider range of decisions, signed authorization is neither required nor needed, but some meaningful discussion is essential. For instance, a man contemplating having a PSA screen should know the relevant arguments for and against it. The degree of discussion should be guided first by the level of complexity of the decision and second by the patient's individual informational needs.

IS THERE SUCH A THING AS PRESUMED/IMPLIED CONSENT?

The patient's consent should only be "presumed," rather than obtained, in emergency situations when the patient is unconscious or incompetent and no surrogate decision maker is available. In general, the patient's presence in the hospital ward, intensive care unit, or clinic does not represent implied consent to all treatment and procedures. The patient's wishes and values may be quite different from those of the clinician. Although the principle of respect for the person obligates clinicians to try to include patients in the health care decisions that affect their lives and bodies, the principle of promoting well-being may require clinicians to act on the behalf of patients, without obtaining formal consent, when life is at stake.

HOW DOES ONE OBTAIN MEANINGFUL INFORMED CONSENT IN EMERGENCY SITUATIONS?

In truly emergent situation, such as acute trauma, the ethical principle of beneficence takes precedence over respect for autonomy, permitting treatment to proceed without informed consent. This is primarily because the gravity of the situation makes time of the essence. For example, the time taken to explain procedures to a patient in hypovolemic shock may come at the expense of organ damage or death. Nevertheless, conscious patients should be afforded a sense of what is being done. In some cases, this will more closely resemble "assent" rather than "consent." In less emergent conditions, there may be time to more closely approximate the ethical models of informed consent described earlier in the chapter.

WHAT ABOUT OBTAINING INFORMED CONSENT FOR PARTICIPATION IN CLINICAL RESEARCH?

Informed consent for clinical research is typically more extensive and formalized than informed consent in clinical practice. Although a full description of informed consent for research is beyond the scope of this chapter, it is important to recognize some major distinctions between informed consent for clinical care and informed consent for research. First, the clinician acts primarily to seek benefit for the patient, while the researcher seeks first to benefit society through scientific investigation, often with only hypothesized benefit for the research subject who may be a patient. A second important difference between clinical care and research involves the vulnerability of the patient to harm. In many types of clinical research, the subject may be exposed to harms of unknown likelihood or magnitude. Consequently there is a strong obligation to make this clear to the potential subject and to emphasize that participation is voluntary.

Closing Comments

Informed consent is a process of discussion of health care decisions with patients. The primary reason for these discussions is not the law but rather the ethical principles of respect for persons and promotion of well-being. As such, informed consent discussions are relevant for all clinical decisions. This is particularly critical in primary care practice, where the application of this approach may positively influence the provider-patient relationship and enhance clinical outcomes. The reality of practice makes thorough discussion of all decisions impractical, but some discussion of more basic decisions is feasible, using guidelines such as those provided in this chapter.

References

1. Braddock CH, Fihn SD, Levinson W, et al: How doctors and patients discuss routine clinical

decisions: informed decision making in the outpatient setting. *J Gen Intern Med* 12:339–345, 1997.

2. Louis Harris and Associates: Views of informed consent and decision making: parallel surveys of physicians and the public, in *Making Health Care Decisions, President's Commission for the Study of Ethical Problems in Medicine and Biomedical and Behavioral Research*. Washington, DC, U.S. Government Printing Office, 1982.

3. Deber R, Kraetschmer N, Irvine J: What role do patients wish to play in treatment decision making? *Arch Intern Med* 156:1414–1420, 1996.

4. Strull W, Lo B, Charles G: Do patients want to participate in medical decision making? *JAMA* 252:2990–2994, 1984.

5. Mazur D, Hickham D: Patients' preferences for risk disclosure and role in decision making for invasive medical procedures. *J Gen Intern Med* 12:114–117, 1997.

6. Sulmasy DP, Lehmann LS, Levine DM, et al: Patient's perception of the quality of informed consent for common medical procedures. *J Clin Ethics* 5:189–194, 1994.

7. Lidz C, Meisel A, Holden JL, et al: Informed consent and the structure of medical care, in *Making Health Care Decisions: President's Commission for the Study of Ethical Problems in Medicine and Biomedical and Behavioral Research*. Washington, DC, U.S. Government Printing Office, 1982, pp 317–410.

8. Katz J: Informed consent and the prescription of nonsteroidal antiinflammatory drugs. *Arthritis Rheum* 35:1257–1263, 1992.

9. Boreham P, Gibson D: The information process in private medical consultations: a preliminary investigation. *Soc Sci Med* 12:409, 1978.

10. Wu W, Pearlman R: Consent in medical decision making: the role of communication. *J Gen Intern Med* 3:9–14, 1988.

11. Donovan J: Patient decision making: the missing ingredient in compliance research. *Int J Technol Assess Health Care* 11:443–455, 1995.

12. Greenfield S, Kaplan S, Ware J: Expanding patient involvement in care: effect on patient outcomes. *Ann Intern Med* 102:520–528, 1985.

13. Kaplan SH, Greenfield S, Ware J: Assessing the effects of physician-patient interactions on the outcomes of chronic disease. *Med Care* 27:S110–S127, 1989.

14. Hulka B: Patient-clinician interactions and compliance., in Haynes R, Taylor D, Sackett D (eds): *Compliance in Health Care*. Baltimore, Johns Hopkins University Press, 1979, pp 63–77.

15. A report on the ethical and legal implications of informed consent in the patient-practitioner relationship, in *Making Health Care Decisions: President's Commission for the Study of Ethical Problems in Medicine and Biomedical and Behavioral Research*. Washington, DC, U.S. Government Printing Office, 1982.

16. Katz J: *The Silent World of Doctor and Patient*. New York, Free Press, 1984.

17. Faden RR, Beauchamp TL: *A History and Theory of Informed Consent*, New York, Oxford University Press, 1986.

18. Beauchamp TL, Childress JF: *Principles of Biomedical Ethics*, 4th ed. New York, Oxford University Press, 1994.

19. *Mohr* v *Williams* 98 Minn. 261, 104 N.W. 12 (1905).

20. *Schloendorff* v *Society of New York Hospitals* 211 N.Y. 125, 105 N.E. 92 (1914).

21. *Salgo* v *Leland Stanford Jr University Board of Trustees* 317 P. 2d 170, 181 (1957).

22. *Canterbury* v *Spence* 464 F.2d 772 (D.C. Cir. 1972).

23. *Natanson* v *Kline* 186 Kan. 393, P.d. 1093 (1960).

24. American Medical Association Council on Ethical and Judicial Affairs: *Code of Medical Ethics, Current Opinions with Annotations: Including the Principles of Medical Ethics, Fundamental Elements of the Patient-Physician Relationship and Rules of the Council on Ethical and Judicial Affairs*. Chicago, American Medical Association, 1998.

25. American College of Physicians Ad Hoc Committee on Medical Ethics: *American College of Physicians Ethics Manual*, 3d ed. Philadelphia, American College of Physicians, 1993, p 68.

26. *Malloy* v *Shanahan* 421 A.2d 803 (Pa. Sup. Ct. 1980).

27. Ubel P: Informed consent: from bodily invasion to the seemingly mundane. *Arch Intern Med* 156:1262–1263, 1996.

28. Lidz C, Appelbaum P, Meisel A: Two models of implementing informed consent. *Arch Intern Med* 148:1385–1389, 1988.

29. Brody H: Transparency: informed consent in primary care. *Hastings Cent Rep* 19(5):5–9, 1989.

James A. Tulsky

Advance Care Planning

Isabel Goldstein, age 83, has Alzheimer disease. Initially, she lived at the home of her daughter Debra, who cared for her conscientiously with the help of her brother, Scott. However, as the disease progressed, they reluctantly admitted her to a local nursing home. They continued to visit her several times a week and closely supervised her care. After a year in the nursing home, Mrs. Goldstein stopped eating. Debra and Scott held long talks with her clinician, Dr. Williams, about whether their mother would want to receive tube feeding. After considerable reflection on their mother's past statements and general values, they concluded that she would not have wanted to be kept alive in this way. Sadly, they decided to withhold tube feeding and provide palliative care until her expected death. They contacted their sister, Julie, who lived across the country, and notified her of the situation. Julie, who had seen her mother only twice in the previous 3 years and had been marginally involved in her care, immediately flew to her mother's hometown and angrily confronted her siblings about the decision. She accused them of killing their mother and "giving up." She called the clinician and threatened legal action if enteral feeding was not started. After believing that a plan of care had been determined, Dr. Williams now felt confused and caught in a situation from which she was not sure how to extricate herself.

Bruce Adams, age 73, has inoperable coronary artery disease, NYHA class III congestive heart failure, diabetes, and gout. He was followed closely by his general internist, Dr. Kelly. During one visit, Mr. Adams brought in a copy of the advance directive that he had completed with his lawyer when he was updating his estate will. Several months later, Mr. Adams was admitted unexpectedly to the hospital with pneumonia. After 2 days on antibiotics and oxygen, he decompensated further and required intubation and transfer to the intensive care unit. During the following week he suffered a myocardial infarction with cardiogenic shock, acute renal failure, and worsening oxygenation. In addition, he remained febrile and lapsed into obtundation. His clinician became skeptical that he would ever leave the intensive care unit alive and decided to discuss the possibility of withdrawal of support with Mr. Adams's family. Dr. Kelly recalled the advance directive and brought it with him to the family meeting. It stated: "I wish that my life not be prolonged by extraordinary means if my condition is determined to be terminal and incurable or if I am diagnosed as being in a persistent vegetative state." No one could determine whether this advance directive applied to the present situation, and they decided to continue treatment. He died 2 weeks later.

Mary McIntyre, age 78, has a long history of severe chronic obstructive pulmonary disease. She was short-of-breath even at rest and unable to walk across the room or go up a flight of stairs without stopping to rest. She had chronic lower extremity edema and signs of right heart failure. She had recently been admitted with a severe exacerbation of her lung disease and spent 2 days in the intensive care unit, barely escaping intubation. Dr. Mancini decided that she ought to speak with Ms. McIntyre, about completing an advance directive.

Dr. Mancini asked the patient about her preferences for cardiopulmonary resuscitation, and Ms. McIntyre replied, "If my heart would stop right now, it would be a blessing. I would not want the doctors to try to restart it. I'm afraid of dying slowly and of suffering with shortness-of-breath." Dr. Mancini then asked about her preferences for mechanical ventilation. Ms. McIntyre told her, "If I couldn't breathe, I would want to be on a breathing machine." Dr. Mancini replied, "Even if you would be stuck on the ventilator and not be able to get off?" To this question, Ms. McIntyre responded, "I would still want it. I am so scared of suffocating to death." Dr. Mancini was not quite sure how to reconcile these preferences but wrote a note in the chart and sent the patient to a social worker to help her complete advance directive forms.

Scope of the Problem

Clinicians must frequently make difficult decisions about life-sustaining treatments for patients about whose preferences little is known. Informed consent is the guiding principle for respecting patients' values in medical decision making. Advance care planning is simply a means to allow for informed consent should the patient be unable to participate in medical decision making owing to illness. That is, through advance care planning, a patient's self-determination may be preserved even after the patient has lost decision-making capacity.

However, the primary care provider must negotiate a variety of obstacles standing in the way of a useful advance care planning process. The hypothetical cases above highlight several of the predicaments that clinicians face when advance directives do not exist or are prepared inadequately. These include potentially unwanted aggressive treatment in the face of uncertainty, advance directives that are not informed, difficulties in interpreting directives, communication problems with patients when treatment preferences are being discussed, family conflict, and advance directives that appear to conflict with patients' best interests.

This chapter covers the history and theory behind advance care planning, several legal and ethical issues associated with advance directives, approaches to use in communicating about them, and potential solutions to common problems encountered with advance care planning in clinical practice.

Defining Terms

A variety of terms have been used, sometimes interchangeably, to describe the components of advance care planning. The following defini-

tions reflect the most common understanding of their meaning.

ADVANCE CARE PLANNING

This refers to the entire process of planning for decision-making incapacity. Advance care planning centers on clarifying a patient's values and articulating those values in a statement of general goals for care as well as specific treatment preferences. It is not just about forms or documents. If advance care planning is done well, patients who complete it while they still possess decision-making capacity should find the process useful as they confront future decisions.

ADVANCE DIRECTIVE

This is a written or oral statement that describes a patient's preferences for care in the setting of decisional incapacity. An advance directive may include specific treatment preferences, a statement of general values, or a designation of surrogate decision makers.

DECISION-MAKING CAPACITY

Patients are considered to have decision-making capacity if they are able to understand the nature of the proposed test or treatment, with its attendant risks, benefits, and likely outcomes; appreciate the alternatives to treatment; and express a preference. Patients may have adequate decision-making capacity even in the setting of dementia or mental illness (see Chap. 18).

DURABLE POWER OF ATTORNEY FOR HEALTH CARE

This legal document allows a person to designate a surrogate to make health care decisions if that person loses decision-making capacity.

LIVING WILL

A living will is a document that specifies a patient's treatment preferences when he or she is decisionally incapacitated. Frequently, living wills apply only to specific scenarios, such as terminal illness or persistent vegetative state.

SURROGATE

A surrogate is a person designated to make decisions on the patient's behalf in the setting of loss of decision-making capacity. When this individual is formally selected by the patient and appropriate procedures are followed, he or she may also be referred to as the *health care proxy* or the *attorney-in-fact for health care.*

Prevalence

The majority of patients would like to engage in advance care planning and believe that advance directives are important to their care. Surveys have demonstrated that between 66 percent and 93 percent of outpatients would like to discuss advance care planning with clinicians.[1–3] Despite patients' interest, a consensus among experts that advance care planning is necessary, and a variety of local and national policies that encourage its use, the number of patients who actually discuss and complete advance directives remains low. Between 6 percent and 33 percent percent of patients have actually discussed advance directives[1,2,4,5] One study found that in a population of men with AIDS, only 38 percent percent had discussed their preferences for resuscitation.[6] A number of other studies have demonstrated that completion rates for formal advance directives are even lower.[7–9]

In the case of patients who complete advance directives, a number of obstacles may prevent the directives from influencing patient care. In one study among patients who had completed advance directives, only 26 percent of the forms were noticed by health care providers when the

patients were hospitalized.[10] Furthermore, even when identified, in many cases the directives are ignored.[11]

Similarly, in the absence of directed interventions to increase completion of advance directives, fewer than 10 percent of patients are likely to appoint surrogate decision makers.[4] Perhaps more important, if patients do not explicitly discuss their preferences with their appointed surrogate, the likelihood that the surrogate will predict accurately the patient's preferences is no better than chance.[12]

Background Theory and Context

History

Although it is important to maintain the distinction between ethics and the law, the force of court cases has moved the use of advance care planning forward. Historically, clinicians faced with treatment decisions for incompetent patients made the decisions themselves or consulted family members, who did their best to make what they believed was the right decision. Until the 1960s and the introduction of technologies that could keep severely incapacitated patients alive indefinitely, problems of patients being kept alive against their will rarely arose. However, as the technology that was developed to reverse complications of acute illness began to be applied to chronically ill and severely debilitated patients, patients and their families began to raise questions.

First was the question of whether a competent patient could refuse the application of life-sustaining therapies. Two cases in particular established this right. William Bartling, 70 years old, had chronic obstructive pulmonary disease and lung cancer when he developed a pneu-mothorax after lung biopsy and became ventila-tor-dependent.[13] After 2 months, he requested that the ventilator be withdrawn, but his clini-cians and hospital refused. In 1994, a California court ruled that "if the right of the patient to self-determination as to his own medical treat-ment is to have any meaning at all, it must be paramount to the interests of the patient's hospi-tal and doctors."[14] Thus, the court established that Mr. Bartling's request should be respected.

At approximately the same time, Elizabeth Bouvia, a 26-year-old with severe cerebral palsy, requested that a hospital discontinue her enteral tube feedings and provide her with pain and symptom relief while she starved to death.[15] Although one court initially refused this request, equating it with assisted suicide, a subsequent court overruled this finding in 1986 and deter-mined that Ms. Bouvia had the right to refuse all treatments, including tube feedings. The court wrote, "We find nothing in the law to suggest that the right to refuse medical treatment may be exercised only if the patient's motives meet someone else's approval."[16] This ruling declared firmly that patients may have idiosyncratic rea-sons for their requests but that, in the face of decision-making capacity, clinicians must honor all such requests.

Both of these cases concerned competent patients. They were able to assess their current quality of life, discuss their options, and make choices. However, what could be done for patients in similar situations who could not express their wishes? Would they be con-demned to lives supported by medical technol-ogy? Perhaps the two best-known and most important cases to help answer this question involved the tragedies of two young women, Karen Ann Quinlan and Nancy Cruzan.

Karen Ann Quinlan was 22 years old when, for unclear reasons, she was found to be in a persistent vegetative state.[17] She was being maintained by mechanical ventilation, although all physicians agreed that she would never recover cognitive function. Ms. Quinlan's father requested that the ventilator be withdrawn, with the understanding that she would die. Her clini-cians refused to accommodate this request and the case ultimately went to the New Jersey Supreme Court. The court ruled that Karen Ann Quinlan's father, as guardian, could make the decision to withdraw the ventilator by rendering his best judgment as to what she would have wanted. This case affirmed the role of surrogates in decision making about life-sustaining treat-ments. However, the limitations of this ruling were unclear. What treatments would be included in such decision making, and how cer-tain did the family need to be about the patient's prior wishes?

Nancy Cruzan, age 33, had been in an auto-mobile accident in 1983 and was in a persistent vegetative state thereafter.[18] Unlike Karen Ann Quinlan, she was not on a mechanical ventila-tor. However, she was being kept alive by feed-ings via a gastrostomy tube. Three years after her accident, realizing that her condition would not improve, her family asked that her tube feedings be discontinued. A year before her accident, she had told her housemate that if she "couldn't do for herself things even halfway, let alone not at all, she wouldn't want to live that way and she hoped that her family would know that." Because the hospital refused to withhold feedings, the case went to court. The Missouri Supreme Court ruled that life-sustaining treat-ments could not be withdrawn without clear and convincing evidence of the patient's prior wishes. In 1990, the U.S. Supreme Court affirmed this ruling and declared that although competent patients have the right to refuse med-ical treatment, states may establish "procedural safeguards" to guide the exercise of that right in incompetent patients.[18] This ruling left to the state the right to determine the level of evidence that would be required to prove that an individ-ual would have wanted a treatment withdrawn.

The greatest implication of this ruling was the promotion of written advance directives that would meet the criteria that might be set by any state. To facilitate this process, in 1990 the U.S. Congress passed the Patient Self Determination Act (PSDA).[19] This law required all recipients of Medicare funding (nearly all hospitals, nursing homes, and home health agencies) to notify patients on admission of their right to create advance directives and to provide them with appropriate information about this process. This law was followed by the promulgation of guidelines from the Joint Commission on Accreditation of Healthcare Organizations (JCAHO) that further increase the likelihood that advance directives will be written and implemented.

Although these laws do not currently apply directly to the outpatient primary care setting, there is an increasing emphasis in most institutions of the need to begin advance care planning with outpatients rather than waiting until they are hospitalized. In the outpatient setting clinicians can have conversations about potential future scenarios without the pressure of decision making in a crisis. Also, in outpatient primary care the conversation is more likely to be conducted by a patient's primary care provider, who typically has a preexisting relationship with that patient.

Ethical Theory

Several ethical principles undergird the moral authority of clinical decision making. In particular, the principles of autonomy, nonmaleficence, and beneficence form the ethical backbone of advance care planning.

Autonomy demands that patients have the right to self-determination. Advance directives are an obvious expression of self-determination. Patients are able to control what happens to their bodies even after they lose decision-making capacity.

The principle of *nonmaleficence* requires clinicians to avoid causing harm. Many interventions that clinicians employ risk serious adverse effects, and these potential consequences must be balanced judiciously with the treatment's beneficial effects. When life-sustaining treatments such as cardiopulmonary resuscitation are being considered, the greatest risk is that the use of interventions with little likelihood of prolonging or improving life will result in a degrading death or a prolonged period of severe cognitive disability.

Beneficence is the principle that requires doing what is in the patient's best interests. Clinicians are to advance those interests. Best interests must be decided from the patient's perspective so as to allow for the tremendous variability in values and goals among individuals in a pluralistic society. However, in the absence of explicit expressed wishes, deciding what is in someone's best interests can be quite challenging. Useful advance directives contain statements that will make this assessment easier. Nevertheless, the obligation of beneficence motivates some providers to consider overriding directives when they appear to conflict with what they perceive as a patient's best interests.

Types of Advance Directives

The most important aspect of creating advance directives is the conversation between a patient, the patient's designated surrogate decision makers, and the clinician. In fact, such conversations, if sufficiently detailed, constitute oral directives that can be upheld legally.[18,20] Yet written documents offer greater assurance that a patient's wishes will be honored. This is the case because of some restrictive state laws; potential challenges to a patient's previously expresssed preferences by family members, friends, and caregivers; lack of continuity of clinicians from the outpatient to inpatient setting; and the potential unavailability of surrogates when decisions need to be made. These documents take different forms.

TREATMENT DIRECTIVES

Treatment directives are the most common type of advance directive. Frequently, treatment directives are also referred to as *living wills*. Such documents generally describe the conditions under which the directive is to be implemented (e.g., terminal illness, persistent vegetative state, or any condition resulting in decisional incapacity) and the patient's preferences for treatment under varying scenarios. Some of these forms are highly specific with regard to treatments and scenarios; others are rather vague or narrow, stating only a refusal of "extraordinary care" in case of terminal illness or a persistent vegetative state.[21] Still others are quite expansive, encouraging the patient to complete a "values history" that describes a broad set of patient values which may be applied in a variety of situations.[22] Although most states have created suggested documents to use, nearly all will accept other types of forms as long as they meet that state's criteria for notarization and are written within the scope of that state's advance care planning law. Most treatment directive forms meet these requirements, but clinicians should become familiar with local documents and statutes. Clinicians should also choose one or several legally valid forms and make them available to their patients (Table 20-1).

DURABLE POWER OF ATTORNEY FOR HEALTH CARE

The *durable power of attorney for health care* (also called a *health care proxy form*) is a document that allows patients to name a surrogate decision maker for themselves in the case of future decisional incapacity. The individual identified in such a document takes on complete decisional authority for the patient's health affairs only after the patient is no longer able to do so. When no such form is available, clinicians generally turn to next of kin and close friends to assist in decision making. The form is particularly useful when a potential conflict is suspected or patients wish to designate someone as proxy who may not otherwise have legal standing (e.g., a same-sex partner). However,

Table 20-1

Resources for Advance Care Planning

Choice in Dying
1035 30th Street NW
Washington, DC 20016
202-338-9790
800-989-WILL
Web site: http://www.choices.org
This organization is a good resource for advance directive documents and laws in all states.

American Association of Retired Persons (AARP)
601 E Street NW
Washington, DC 20049
202-434-2277
800-424-2277
Web site: http://www.aarp.org
Distributes (for free) a popular booklet for patients entitled *Shape Your Health Care Future with Health Care Advance Directives.*

Pearlman R, Starks H, Cain K, et al: *Your Life Your Choices: Planning for Future Medical Decisions: How to Prepare a Personalized Living Will.*
For information contact:
    Patient Decision Support
    4218 50th Avenue, Northeast
    Seattle, WA 98105
    (206) 527-4786
Website: www.patientdecisions.com
This workbook guides the patient through a series of exercises to help him or her complete comprehensive advance care planning.

studies show that designated surrogates are frequently unaware of patients' preferences for treatment.[12] Therefore, patients who complete such documents must be encouraged to discuss their values and preferences for life-sustaining treatments with their designated surrogates.

Changing Advance Directives

Although patients' preferences for life-sustaining treatments are fairly stable over time, some patients may wish to change or modify their treatment directives after completing the forms. This is perfectly acceptable and simply requires revising the existing forms. It is good practice for clinicians to revisit advance directives annually with patients and to allow them the opportunity to update forms and replace deceased or unwilling surrogate decision makers.

Toward Resolution

It is one thing to know the background, theory, and procedures related to advance care planning but another to discuss the issue with a patient in a manner that will result in good decision making and that will leave the patient feeling supported and understood. Audiotape studies of actual discussions about advance care planning demonstrate that information is frequently presented in ways that may not be understood by patients and that leave uncertainty insufficiently addressed—further, that the scenarios and treatments discussed often do not reflect the most challenging situations confronted in real medical settings.[23,24] These data are not surprising. Patients struggle to understand the issues underlying hypothetical future treatment decisions while confronting the emotional impact of discussing their own mortality. Clinicians must respond to patients' cognitive and affective demands, yet few clinicians receive formal training in such communication.

Elements of Advance Care Planning

This section describes an approach to communicating with patients about advance care plan-

Table 20-2

Elements of Good Discussions about Advance Care Planning

Introducing the topic
  Private setting
  Significant others present
  Reassurance that such discussions are routine
  Purpose is to respect patient's wishes

Information giving
  Patient must understand course of illness and prognosis
  Treatments should be discussed in terms of patient's experience
  Treatment outcomes should be mentioned

Eliciting preferences
  Understanding of patient's goals regarding treatment
  Unacceptable life states—what risks are acceptable to avoid these states?
  Patient's approach to uncertainty
  Specific discussion of artificial nutrition and hydration
  Emphasis on what will be done for the patient

Proxies
  Identification of proxy decision maker
  Patient encouraged to communicate with proxy
  Determine and communicate how much leeway proxy should have

Documentation
  Patient given opportunity to complete written advance directive
  Clinician documents in chart

Communication
  Clinicians need to attend to patient affect
  Need to avoid and define vague terms
  Must ensure shared understanding of conversation
  Patient must have ample opportunity to ask questions

ning (Table 20-2). Although all of the elements below are essential for good discussions, as discussed below the primary care clinician need not and probably should not attempt to do all of this in one conversation. Advance care planning is completed as a process over time, allowing patients and clinicians an opportunity for thoughtful reflection and interaction with others.

INTRODUCING THE TOPIC

The setting for such a conversation should be private and conducive to open and relaxed communication. This may include placing the clinician's pager on silent mode or requesting from office staff that they withhold interruptions. The patient should be advised beforehand that important issues will be discussed and encouraged to bring one or two significant family members or friends to the next visit.

Introducing the subject can be awkward. The clinician wishes to explain to the patient that the purpose of advance care planning is to respect the patient's wishes; however, when the topic is brought up, many patients wonder whether their doctor believes that their death is imminent. Therefore patients ought to be reassured that such discussions are a standard part of the clinician's medical practice and that advance care planning is therefore raised with all patients. Of course, in some cases, the patient may be quite ill, and the clinician must confront this reality with the patient. Frequently, relating the discussion to a recent sentinel event, such as a hospitalization, can provide a seamless transition to this difficult topic. In today's climate of managed care, it may be important to allay patients' fears that advance directives are simply a means to achieve medical cost savings.

INFORMATION GIVING

Patients require accurate information to make decisions that reflect their values and goals. Clinicians must elicit patients' understanding of their medical condition and prognosis and correct any misperceptions. Although it is not always necessary to describe potential treatments in great detail, patients should understand the relationship between the treatment and potential outcomes. The primary reason for patients to consider withholding treatments is to avoid an outcome judged by them to be worse than death. The other reason is that the burden of the treatment, on themselves or their loved ones, outweighs the potential benefit. Therefore, patients should achieve an understanding of the impact of common life-sustaining interventions on their quality of life.

ELICITING PREFERENCES

Patients state their preferences after learning about potential options and evaluating these in light of their personal values. *Values* are deeply held beliefs, such as a desire for personal independence or the importance of a religious practice. By exploring patients' values and goals, clinicians can help them clarify their particular preferences. Sometimes clinicians can ask explicitly about such values (e.g., "what makes life worth living for you?"). Alternatively, values may be elicited in the process of asking about specific treatment preferences. For example, after a patient makes a statement about end-of-life care (e.g., "I'd never want to be on one of those machines"), the clinician may respond by simply asking why. The answer to this question (e.g., "Because I never want to be a burden on my family or society") may uncover a patient's core values that will greatly influence treatment decisions. In the third hypothetical case above, Ms. McIntyre repeatedly stated that she wished to receive mechanical ventilation even though she does not want CPR. Dr. Mancini, frustrated by trying to interpret this apparent contradiction, accepted this statement at face value. Had he addressed her fear of suffocation, by reassuring her that palliation of terminal dyspnea is possible without ventilation, the patient might have chosen this alternative and forgone the choice to use a respirator.

Identifying what conditions the patient would find unacceptable can also help clarify his or her preferences. A useful question is, "Can you imagine any situations in which life would not be worth living?" Typically, patients mention a persistent vegetative state or similar dire scenarios. This question can be followed by asking what the patient would be willing to undergo in order to avoid such states.

For many patients, dealing with uncertainty is the most difficult aspect of decision making. Everyone responds to uncertainty differently, and the patient's approach to this issue should be discussed explicitly as well. Some patients will state that any possibility of recovery is worth pursuing, while others will refuse curative treatment when the likelihood of recovery drops below a particular threshold. Some patients are comfortable using numbers in talking about probabilities, others are less quantitatively facile. The patient's preferences should dictate the extent to which numbers are used in this discussion. Although clinicians do not need to ask about all specific treatment preferences, they should inquire about artificial nutrition and hydration. This is particularly true if the patient states a desire for treatment in any situation, since a feeding tube is a highly controversial treatment option that is commonly considered for cognitively impaired patients.

Several things may be done to support the patient's emotional response to the discussion. Patients should be encouraged to take their time with these decisions. An immediate decision is rarely necessary, particularly in the outpatient setting, and patients should not feel rushed. Furthermore, they should be reminded that they may always change their minds and restate their preferences. Finally, the clinician must emphasize what will be done to meet the patient's goals. The patient needs to hear that the clinician will remain actively involved and not abandon the patient regardless of the stated goals and preferences.

PROXIES

Identifying who is to act as the patient's health care proxy may be the most important outcome of a conversation about advance care planning. Does the patient wish this to be a single individual or his or her entire family? Given the literature demonstrating poor concordance between patients' preferences and surrogates' perceptions of those preferences, the clinician would be wise to stress the need for the patient to communicate with the selected proxy decision maker.[12] Patients should also be asked how much leeway their proxies should have in decision making.[25] Should proxies adhere strictly to patients' stated preferences, or ought they have more flexibility in making actual decisions?

DOCUMENTATION

To help ensure that a patient's stated preferences will be respected, discussions about advance directives must be documented. Patients should be given the opportunity to complete a written advance directive. Nevertheless, whether or not such a document is completed, clinicians can promote a patient's interests and improve future decision making by writing a note in the medical record that describes the patient's values, goals for care, specific preferences, and choices for a health care proxy.

COMMUNICATION

The quality of the communication determines the success of the advance care planning discussions and greatly affect the patients' satisfaction. Discussions of end-of-life treatment goals and surrogate decision making raise complex and emotionally laden issues, including mortality, spirituality, and personal relationships. The clinician discussing advance care planning with a patient must attend carefully to the patient's affect and respond to expressions of emotion. Clinicians must take care not to dominate discussions and to provide an environment in which patients are able to express their concerns and share their most important values.

Patients and clinicians often use vague terms that ought to be avoided. For example, a statement that a treatment should be continued as long as "quality of life is good" begs for further clarification. How does the patient (or the surrogate, or the clinician) define a good quality of life? In fact, it is always important to ensure that the patient and clinician have a shared understanding of the conversation and its implications. Similarly, medical jargon should be avoided when possible, and clinicians should always define technical terms. Finally, patients must be encouraged to ask questions.

Practical Matters

EFFICIENCY

Some clinicians may be overwhelmed by the demands placed on them with regard to advance care planning. How can all of these issues be covered in a thorough and compassionate manner within the context of a busy office practice? Should advance care planning be initiated with every adult patient that enters a clinician's office?

Clinicians should remember that the entire process of advance care planning need not occur in one sitting and that many members of the health care team can share this responsibility. A clinician can raise the issue at a first visit while providing written information. This will result in a more educated and engaged patient at a future visit, when questions may be answered and deeper issues explored. The completion of specific treatment directives may even be put off to a later appointment. In addition, the clinician may be able to send the patient to a social worker or other member of the team to assist with the actual paperwork of an advance directive. With the use of such assistance, advance care planning can become a regular component of care for all chronically ill and elderly patients. In contrast, although all patients should be informed of their options (probably through written materials provided in medical offices), extensive advance care planning is not necessary for many young and healthy patients.

In considering questions of time efficiency, clinicians should recognize the potential for future time savings due to good advance care planning. Time spent up front discussing the patient's values and goals may decrease the difficulty and duration of decision making should serious illness arise.

RESOLVING DISPUTES

Advance care planning can help to prevent the types of dilemmas that challenged the clinicians and families in the first two representative vignettes described at the beginning of the chapter. In the first hypothetical case, an appropriate advance care planning process would have educated Julia, Mrs. Goldstein's estranged daughter, about her mother's true preferences and, if necessary, provided legal and moral support to Dr. Williams and Mrs. Goldstein's other two children in making the decision to withhold tube feeding. Although family conflict cannot always be avoided, the knowledge that actions being taken are in accordance with a patient's predetermined wishes certainly reduces the burden of decision making.

The dilemma in the second vignette, involving Mr. Adams, could have been avoided if the patient, in discussing his advance directive with his clinician prior to the illness, had been asked about scenarios besides persistent vegetative state and terminal illness. A discussion about "states worse than death" would likely have revealed that the patient would not want continued aggressive care in the scenario that ultimately confronted him.

Nevertheless, even with excellent advance care planning and communication, situations are bound to arise in which advance directives are unclear or when the choices of surrogates or health care providers as well as advance directives are in conflict. These cases may be complex and are often appropriate to refer for ethics consultation.

Closing Comments

Advance care planning provides patients with the opportunity to ensure that medical care throughout their lives, even after the loss of decision-making capacity, is consistent with their lifelong values and preferences. Conversations about advance directives demonstrate to patients that clinicians are interested in respecting these values and frequently serve to strengthen the clinician-patient relationship. However, empathic, explicit, and careful communication is necessary to ensure that advance care planning meets the goals of patients and clinicians.

References

1. Emanuel LL, Barry MJ, Stoeckle JD, et al: Advance directives for medical care—a case for greater use. *N Engl J Med* 324:889, 1991.
2. Lo B, McLeod GA, Saika G: Patient attitudes to discussing life-sustaining treatment. *Arch Intern Med* 146:1613, 1986.
3. Shmerling RH, Bedell SE, Lilienfeld A, et al: Discussing cardiopulmonary resuscitation: a study of elderly outpatients. *J Gen Intern Med* 3:317, 1988.
4. Meier DE, Fuss BR, O'Rourke D, et al: Marked improvement in recognition and completion of health care proxies: a randomized controlled trial of counseling by hospital patient representatives. *Arch Intern Med* 156:1227, 1996.
5. Steinbrook R, Lo B, Moulton J, et al: Preferences of homosexual men with AIDS for life-sustaining treatment. *N Engl J Med* 314:457, 1986.
6. Haas JS, Weissman JS, Cleary PD, et al: Discussion of preferences for life-sustaining care by persons with AIDS: predictors of failure in patient-clinician communication. *Arch Intern Med* 153:1241, 1993.
7. Reilly BM, Wagner M, Ash J: Promoting completion of health care proxies following hospitalization. *Arch Intern Med* 155:2202, 1995.
8. Richter KP, Fawcett SB, Paine-Andrews A, et al: Promoting the use of advance directives: an empirical study. *Arch Fam Med* 5:382, 1996.
9. Rubin SM, Strull WM, Fialkow MF, et al: Increasing the completion of the durable power of attorney for health care: a randomized, controlled trial. *JAMA* 271:209, 1994.
10. Morrison RS, Olson E, Mertz KR, et al: The inaccessibility of advance directives on transfer from ambulatory to acute care settings. *JAMA* 274:478, 1995.
11. Danis M, Southerland LI, Garrett JM, et al: A prospective study of advance directives for life-sustaining care. *N Engl J Med* 324:882, 1991.
12. Seckler AB, Meier DE, Mulvihill M, et al: Substituted judgment: how accurate are proxy predictions? *Ann Intern Med* 115:92, 1991.
13. Lo B: The Bartling case: protecting patients from harm while respecting their wishes. *J Am Geriatr Soc* 34:44, 1986.
14. *Bartling v Superior Court*: 209 Cal Rptr. 220 163 Cal. App. 3d 186 (1984).
15. Steinbrook R, Lo B: The case of Elizabeth Bouvia: starvation, suicide, or problem patient? *Arch Intern Med* 146:161, 1986.
16. *Bouvia v Superior Court*: 225 Cal. Rptr. 297, 179 Cal. App. 3d 1127 (1986).
17. *In the matter of Karen Quinlan*: 70 N.J. 10, 335 A. 2d 647 (1976).
18. *Cruzan v Missouri Department of Health*: 497 U.S., 111 L.Ed.2d 224,110 S.Ct. 2841 (1990).
19. U.S. Congress: Patient Self-Determination Act, 1990; Omnibus Budget Reconciliation Act (OBRA) (PL 101-508).
20. Lo B, Rouse F, Dornbrand L: Family decision making on trial: who decides for incompetent patients? *N Engl J Med* 322:1228, 1990.
21. Emanuel LL, Emanuel EJ: The medical directive: a new comprehensive advance care document. *JAMA* 261:3288, 1989.
22. Doukas DJ, McCullough LB: The values history: the evaluation of the patient's values and advance directives. *J Fam Pract* 32:145, 1991.
23. Tulsky JA, Chesney MA, Lo B: How do medical residents discuss resuscitation with patients? *J Gen Intern Med* 10:436, 1995.
24. Tulsky JA, Fischer GS, Rose MR, et al: Opening the black box: how do clinicians communicate about advance directives? *Ann Intern Med* 129: 441, 1998.
25. Sehgal A, Galbraith A, Chesney M, et al: How strictly do dialysis patients want their advance directives followed? *JAMA* 267:59, 1992.

Jeremy Sugarman

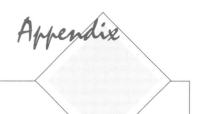

Resources in Medical Ethics

The contributors to this volume have provided rich reference sections to guide the reader to valuable resources in medical ethics. For interested readers some additional resources are identified in this Appendix in several categories: "Bibliographic Resources," Centers and Organizations, "Journals," and "Useful Works."

Bibliographic Resources

The National Reference Center for Bioethics Literature at Georgetown University maintains an electronic database, BIOETHICSLINE, which includes a wealth of materials related to medical ethics, including books, journal articles, news materials, and videotapes. The staff at the National Reference Center can provide valuable insight into available materials and currently will perform free searches in BIOETHICSLINE (1-800-MED-ETHX). BIOETHICSLINE can also be searched over the Internet [http://igm.nlm.nih.gov/].

The American Society for Bioethics and Humanities web site offers links to a variety of resources in medical ethics [http://www.asbh.org/links/], as do several of the centers and organizations listed below.

Finally, a good starting place for questions in medical ethics is the *Encyclopedia of Bioethics*, edited by Warren T. Reich (New York: Simon & Shuster Macmillan, 1995).

Centers and Organizations

There are many centers and organizations whose work is in some way related to medical ethics. No attempt is made here to identify all such entities. Rather, a few have been selected based on those whose web sites currently offer additional resources in medical ethics (along with links to other centers and organizations) or that provide regular conferences which may be of interest to readers.

267

Centers

Center for Bioethics, University of Minnesota
[http://www.med.umn.edu/bioethics/]

Center for Biomedical Ethics, University of Virginia
[http://www.med.virginia.edu/medicine/inter-dis/bio-ethics]

The Center for the Study of Bioethics, Medical College of Wisconsin
[http://www.mcw.edu/bioethics/]

The Hastings Center
[http://www.hastingscenter.org/]

The Joseph and Rose Kennedy Institute of Ethics, Georgetown University
[http://www.georgetown.edu/research/kie/]

The Midwest Bioethics Center
[http://www.midbio.com/]

University of Pennsylvania Center for Bioethics
[http://www.med.upenn.edu/bioethics/index.shtml]

University of Toronto Joint Centre in Bioethics
[http://www.utoronto.ca/jcb/]

Organizations

The American Society for Bioethics and Humanities
[http://www.asbh.org/]

The American Society for Law, Medicine and Ethics
[http://www.aslme.org/]

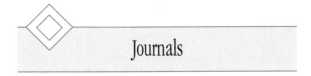

Journals

Medical journals now publish articles related to medical ethics on a regular basis. In addition, some journals specialize in publishing this work. The latter include the following:

Bioethics
Cambridge Quarterly of Healthcare Ethics
The Hastings Center Report
The Journal of Clinical Ethics
The Journal of Law, Medicine and Ethics
The Journal of Medical Ethics
The Journal of Medicine and Philosophy
The Kennedy Institute of Ethics Journal

Useful Works

The growth in the discipline of medical ethics has been associated with the publication of much work that would be virtually impossible to catalogue in any meaningful way in this Appendix. Therefore, provided here is a listing of works that may be useful to those looking for systematic ways of approaching ethical issues that arise in clinical practice as well as some texts dealing with major theoretical approaches to ethics in primary care.

Ethics in Practice

1. American College of Physicians: Ethics manual. *Ann Intern Med* 128:576–594, 1998.
2. English DC: *Bioethics: A Clinical Guide for Medical Students.* New York, Norton, 1994.
3. Garrett TM, Baillie HW, Garrett RM: *Health Care Ethics: Principles and Problems,* 3d ed. Upper Saddle River, NJ, Prentice-Hall, 1998.
4. Hebert PC: *Doing Right: A Practical Guide to Ethics for Physicians and Medical Trainees.* Toronto, Oxford University Press, 1996.
5. Jonsen AR, Siegler M, Winslade WJ: *Clinical Ethics: A Practical Approach to Ethical Decisions in Clinical Medicine,* 4th ed. New York, McGraw-Hill, 1998.

6. Lo B: *Resolving Ethical Dilemmas: A Guide for Clinicians.* Baltimore, Williams & Wilkins, 1995.

Theory

1. Brody H, Tomlinson T: Ethics in primary care: setting aside common misunderstandings. *Primary Care* 13:225–240, 1986.

2. Christie RJ, Hoffmaster CB: *Ethical Issues in Family Medicine.* New York, Oxford University Press, 1986.

3. Smith HL, Churchill LR: *Professional Ethics and Primary Care Medicine: Beyond Dilemmas and Decorum.* Durham, NC, Duke University Press, 1986.

Index

Page numbers followed by the letters *f* and *t* indicate figures and tables, respectively.

Notes